Hospital Neurology

Editors

VANJA C. DOUGLAS
MAULIK P. SHAH

NEUROLOGIC CLINICS

www.neurologic.theclinics.com

Consulting Editor
RANDOLPH W. EVANS

February 2022 • Volume 40 • Number 1

ELSEVIER

1600 John F. Kennedy Boulevard • Suite 1800 • Philadelphia, Pennsylvania, 19103-2899

http://www.theclinics.com

NEUROLOGIC CLINICS Volume 40, Number 1
February 2022 ISSN 0733-8619, ISBN-13: 978-0-323-81349-5

Editor: Stacy Eastman
Developmental Editor: Hannah Almira Lopez

Neurologic Clinics (ISSN 0733-8619) is published quarterly by Elsevier Inc., 360 Park Avenue South, New York, NY 10010–1710. Months of issue are February, May, August, and November. Periodicals postage paid at New York, NY, and additional mailing offices. Subscription prices are $343.00 per year for US individuals, $916.00 per year for US institutions, $100.00 per year for US students, $420.00 per year for Canadian individuals, $953.00 per year for Canadian institutions, $475.00 per year for international individuals, $953.00 per year for international institutions, $210.00 for foreign students/residents, and $100.00 for Canadian students/residents. To receive student/resident rate, orders must be accompanied by name of affiliated institution, date of term, and the *signature* of program/residency coordinator on institution letterhead. Orders will be billed at individual rate until proof of status is received. Foreign air speed delivery is included in all *Clinics* subscription prices. All prices are subject to change without notice. **POSTMASTER:** Send address changes to *Neurologic Clinics*, Elsevier Health Sciences Division, Subscription Customer Service, 3251 Riverport Lane, Maryland Heights, MO 63043. **Customer Service: Telephone: 1-800-654-2452 (U.S. and Canada); 314-447-8871 (outside U.S. and Canada). Fax: 314-447-8029. E-mail: journalscustomerservice-usa@elsevier.com (for print support); journalsonlinesupport-usa@elsevier.com (for online support).**

Reprints. For copies of 100 or more of articles in this publication, please contact the Commercial Reprints Department, Elsevier Inc., 360 Park Avenue South, New York, New York, 10010-1710; Tel.: +1-212-633-3874; Fax: +1-212-633-3820, and E-mail: reprints@elsevier.com.

Neurologic Clinics is also published in Spanish by Nueva Editorial Interamericana S.A., Mexico City, Mexico.

Neurologic Clinics is covered in *Current Contents/Clinical Medicine, MEDLINE/PubMed (Index Medicus), EMBASE/Excerpta Medica,* and *PsycINFO,* and *ISI/BIOMED.*

Contributors

CONSULTING EDITOR

RANDOLPH W. EVANS, MD
Clinical Professor, Department of Neurology, Baylor College of Medicine, Houston, Texas, USA

EDITORS

VANJA C. DOUGLAS, MD
Professor of Neurology, Sara & Evan Williams Foundation Endowed Neurohospitalist Chair, Chief, Neurohospitalist Division, Department of Neurology, Weill Institute for Neurosciences, University of California, San Francisco, California, USA

MAULIK P. SHAH, MD, MHS
Associate Professor of Neurology, Medical Director, Inpatient Neurology and UCSF Integrated Transfer Center, Department of Neurology, Weill Institute for Neurosciences, University of California, San Francisco, San Francisco, California, USA

AUTHORS

ERIC BERNIER, MSN, RN
Stanford Health Care, Stanford, California, USA

RACHEL J. BYSTRITSKY, MD
Assistant Professor, Department of Medicine, University of California, San Francisco, San Francisco, California, USA

FELICIA C. CHOW, MD, MAS
Assistant Professor, Departments of Neurology and Medicine, University of California, San Francisco, San Francisco, California, USA

CLAIRE J. CREUTZFELDT, MD
Associate Professor, Department of Neurology, University of Washington, Seattle, Washington, USA

ANNE G. DOUGLAS, MD
Department of Neurology, Perelman School of Medicine, University of Pennsylvania, Philadelphia, Pennsylvania, USA

VANJA C. DOUGLAS, MD
Professor of Neurology, Sara & Evan Williams Foundation Endowed Neurohospitalist Chair, Chief, Neurohospitalist Division, Department of Neurology, Weill Institute for Neurosciences, University of California, San Francisco, California, USA

JOLINE M. FAN, MD
Clinical Fellow, Department of Neurology, University of California, San Francisco, Weill Institute for Neurosciences, San Francisco, California, USA

CARL A. GOLD, MD, MS
Neurohospitalist Program, Department of Neurology and Neurological Sciences, Stanford University School of Medicine, Stanford, California, USA

ADELINE L. GOSS, MD
Neurohospitalist Fellow, Department of Neurology, University of California, San Francisco, San Francisco, California, USA

ELAN L. GUTERMAN, MD
Assistant Professor, Department of Neurology, University of California, San Francisco, Weill Institute for Neurosciences, San Francisco, California, USA

CATHRA HALABI, MD
Assistant Professor of Neurology, Director, Neurorecovery Clinic, Department of Neurology, Division of Neurovascular, University of California, San Francisco, Weill Institute for Neuroscience, San Francisco, California, USA

JOSHUA P. KLEIN, MD, PhD
Department of Neurology, Brigham and Women's Hospital, Harvard Medical School, Boston, Massachusetts, USA

KATHRYN A. KVAM, MD
Neurohospitalist Program, Department of Neurology and Neurological Sciences, Stanford University School of Medicine, Stanford, California, USA

SARA C. LAHUE, MD
Assistant Professor of Clinical Neurology, Department of Neurology, School of Medicine, University of California, San Francisco, Department of Neurology, Weill Institute for Neurosciences, California, USA

STEPHANIE LYDEN, MD
Assistant Professor, Department of Neurology, University of Utah School of Medicine, Salt Lake City, Utah, USA

ALEXANDRA MUCCILLI, MD, MEd, FRCPC
Department of Medicine, Division of Neurology, St. Michael's Hospital University of Toronto, Toronto, Canada

LAUREN PATRICK, MD
Assistant Professor of Neurology, Associate Program Director, Vascular Neurology Fellowship, Department of Neurology, Division of Neurovascular, University of California, San Francisco, Weill Institute for Neuroscience, San Francisco, California, USA

MEGAN B. RICHIE, MD
Associate Professor, Glenn J. Bingle and David A. Josephson Endowed Professor, Department of Neurology, University of California San Francisco, San Francisco, California, USA

NICOLE ROSENDALE, MD
Assistant Professor of Neurology, Neurohospitalist Division, Department of Neurology, University of California, San Francisco, San Francisco, California, USA

LAURA ROSOW, MD
Associate Professor of Neurology, University of California, San Francisco, San Francisco, California, USA

MAULIK P. SHAH, MD, MHS
Associate Professor of Neurology, Medical Director, Inpatient Neurology and UCSF Integrated Transfer Center, Department of Neurology, Weill Institute for Neurosciences University of California, San Francisco

NEEL S. SINGHAL, MD, PhD
Assistant Professor, Department of Neurology, University of California, San Francisco, Weill Institute for Neurosciences, San Francisco, California, USA

DANIEL TALMASOV, MD
Department of Neurology, NYU Grossman School of Medicine, New York, New York, USA

MARK TERRELONGE Jr., MD, MPH
Assistant Professor of Neurology, University of California, San Francisco, San Francisco, California, USA

LAHOUD TOUMA, MD
Department of Neurosciences, University of Montreal, Centre Hospitalier de l'Université de Montréal, Montreal, Quebec, Canada

ARUN S. VARADHACHARY, MD, PhD
Associate Professor, Department of Neurology, Washington University in St. Louis, St Louis, Missouri, USA

JANA WOLD, MD
Associate Professor, Department of Neurology, University of Utah School of Medicine, Salt Lake City, Utah, USA

DENISE J. XU, MD
Department of Neurology, Perelman School of Medicine, University of Pennsylvania, Philadelphia, Pennsylvania, USA

Contents

Status epilepticus (SE) is a neurologic emergency requiring immediate time-sensitive treatment to minimize neuronal injury and systemic complications. Minimizing time to administration of first- and second-line therapy is necessary to optimize the chances of successful seizure termination in generalized convulsive SE (GCSE). The approach to refractory and super-refractory GCSE is less well defined. Multiple agents with differing complementary actions that facilitate seizure termination are recommended. Nonconvulsive SE (NCSE) has a wide range of presentations and approaches to treatment. Continuous electroencephalography is critical to the management of both GCSE and NCSE, while its use for patients without seizure continues to expand.

Ischemic stroke affects 2.5% of the population of the United States and is the leading cause of disability. This article outlines the evidence to support intravenous thrombolysis with alteplase and tenecteplase, thrombolysis in the setting of DWI/flair mismatch, endovascular treatment in the 6-hour and 6- to 24-hour window, and the use of telemedicine in acute stroke. Current controversies and ongoing trials within endovascular treatment are also detailed. Case presentations are included to provide clinical context and the application of data to practice.

This article focuses on the inpatient evaluation and management of ischemic stroke and transient ischemic attack (TIA). We describe foundational principles including quality metrics, TIA, and stroke as emergencies, TIA/minor stroke management, and standard assessments before discussing tailored evaluation and management strategies by stroke type.

Altered mental status is a nonspecific phenotype that encompasses a wide spectrum of disease and is frequently cited as a reason for both hospital admission and inpatient neurologic consultation. There are numerous etiologies of altered mental status, and so although many are facile with the workup of this potentially life-threatening entity, it can nevertheless be overwhelming. Our goal was to provide a practical framework embedded in a current, comprehensive review of the epidemiology, clinical evaluation, and management of undifferentiated altered mental status. We pay particular attention to the management of a critical yet underdiagnosed subtype of altered mental status: delirium.

Adeline L. Goss and Claire J. Creutzfeldt

Research advances in recent years have shown that some individuals with vegetative state or minimally conscious state can emerge to higher states of consciousness even years after injury. A minority of behaviorally unresponsive patients with vegetative state have also been shown to follow commands, or even communicate, using neuroimaging or electrophysiological techniques. These advances raise ethical questions that have important implications for clinical care. In this article, the authors argue that adopting a neuropalliative care approach can help clinicians provide ethical, compassionate care to these patients and their caregivers.

Rachel J. Bystritsky and Felicia C. Chow

Infectious meningitis and encephalitis are associated with significant morbidity and mortality worldwide. Acute bacterial meningitis is rapidly fatal and early recognition and institution of therapy are imperative. Viral meningitis is typically a benign self-limited illness. Chronic meningitis (defined as presenting with >4 weeks of symptoms) is most often caused by tuberculosis and fungal infection. Because the diagnostic testing for tuberculous meningitis is insensitive and cultures often take weeks to grow, therapy is often initiated empirically when the diagnosis is suspected. Human simplex virus encephalitis is the most common cause of encephalitis and requires prompt treatment with intravenous acyclovir.

Megan B. Richie

Meningitis and encephalitis are inflammatory syndromes of the meninges and brain parenchyma, respectively. Evaluation requires simultaneous consideration of autoimmune, infectious, and neoplastic causes. When considering autoimmune causes, an important diagnostic question is whether a specific neural autoantibody syndrome is likely. If so, clinicians should pursue thorough autoantibody and neoplastic workup, awaiting results before pursuing brain biopsy, potentially providing empiric IVIG or plasmapheresis in deteriorating patients but withholding corticosteroids pending definitive diagnosis. In patients unlikely to have an autoantibody, brain or systemic biopsy is often warranted. Once a specific diagnosis is identified, systemic corticosteroids and disease-specific treatment is initiated.

The spectrum of demyelinating diseases affecting the central nervous system is broad. Although many have a chronic course, neuroinflammatory conditions often present with acute to subacute onset symptoms requiring hospitalization when severe. This article reviews the acute phase assessment and management of these disorders, with a particular focus on multiple sclerosis, neuromyelitis optica spectrum disorder, myelin oligodendrocyte glycoprotein antibody disorder, and several atypical demyelinating diseases.

Myelopathy can present acutely or more insidiously and has a broad differential diagnosis. In addition to the clinical history and neurologic examination, diagnostic testing, including MRI and cerebrospinal fluid analysis, as well as thorough review of patient comorbidities, risk factors, and potential toxic exposures, can help neurohospitalists distinguish between various causes and potentially start appropriate empiric therapy while awaiting definitive testing. This article focuses on how imaging can help in determining the most likely cause of myelopathy and highlights a range of causes, including compressive, vascular, metabolic and toxic, infectious, autoimmune, neoplastic, and paraneoplastic causes of spinal cord dysfunction.

Acute neuromuscular disorders represent an important subset of neurologic consultation requests in the inpatient setting. Although most neuromuscular disorders are subacute to chronic, hospital-based neurologists encounter neuromuscular disorders presenting with rapidly progressive or severe weakness affecting limb movement, respiratory, and bulbar function. Recalling fundamentals of neurologic localization assists in prompt recognition and diagnosis. Despite the differing localizations and the causal diagnoses, the initial management principles of acute myopathies, neuropathies, and neuromuscular junction disorders are similar.

Neuropathies are a common problem encountered by neurologist in the hospitalized setting. Nerve injury may occur secondary to compression, stretch, and direct trauma, among other causes. Common focal neuropathies include the ulnar, median, and radial nerve in the upper extremities and sciatic, peroneal, and femoral nerve in the lower extremities. Surgical and obstetric risk factors are especially important considerations in evaluation of patients with focal neuropathies. Treatment is either conservative therapy or surgery depending on the mechanism of injury and extent of recovery.

NEUROLOGIC CLINICS

ISSUES OF RELATED INTEREST

Neurosurgery Clinics
https://www.neurosurgery.theclinics.com/
Neuroimaging Clinics
https://www.neuroimaging.theclinics.com/
Psychiatric Clinics
https://www.psych.theclinics.com/
Child and Adolescent Psychiatric Clinics
https://www.childpsych.theclinics.com/

THE CLINICS ARE AVAILABLE ONLINE!
Access your subscription at:
www.theclinics.com

Preface

Hospital Neurology

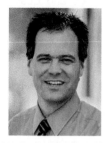
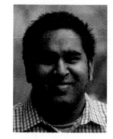

Vanja C. Douglas, MD   Maulik P. Shah, MD, MHS
Editors

How can the best neurologic care be delivered to hospitalized patients? Neurohospitalists are one model of care increasingly used by health systems around the United States to address this question.

There is no doubt neurohospitalists improve access to neurologic care. Not only are dedicated inpatient neurologists more available than neurologists who are simultaneously beholden to an outpatient clinic schedule but neurohospitalists can also fill a void for hospitals that otherwise have no access to neurologic consultation. Those of us who have had the experience of consulting in a hospital where there was previously no neurologist available are often left wondering: how were these neurologic problems addressed before I arrived?

The conditions neurohospitalists treat most frequently—stroke, seizure, and delirium—demand immediate access to experienced clinicians. Patients, too, demand access to consultants in an increasingly competitive hospital landscape. Neurohospitalists, as a result, are a rapidly growing neurologic subspecialty.

From the perspective of diagnosis and management, neurohospitalists must be familiar with the full range of neurologic diseases, albeit in the acute setting. In this issue of *Neurologic Clinics*, we cover a broad range of topics with practical updates for neurologists seeing patients in the hospital. We address the most frequently encountered conditions: stroke, seizure, and delirium. We also address those less frequently encountered: myelopathy, demyelinating disease, encephalitis, and neuromuscular emergencies. We also address perioperative consultation and frequently encountered focal neuropathies in surgical and obstetric patients.

In addition to providing access to neurologic expertise, neurohospitalists also provide value to health care systems through their familiarity with quality metrics and quality improvement, as well as through their facility with systems-based practice topics commonly encountered in the inpatient setting. In perhaps no other setting than the hospital are social determinants of health more important, when patients are at their

Neurol Clin 40 (2022) xiii–xiv
https://doi.org/10.1016/j.ncl.2021.09.001
0733-8619/22/© 2021 Published by Elsevier Inc.   **neurologic.theclinics.com**

most vulnerable and in need of the most caregiving support. As such, neurohospitalists must have a deep understanding of these in order to provide holistic care and achieve the best outcomes. Ethics of neuroprognostication in disorders of consciousness are becoming ever more complex as life-sustaining treatments advance, along with the ability to investigate brain activity using functional neuroimaging. In this issue, we address these topics with updates on inpatient quality metrics and quality improvement, social determinants of health, and ethical considerations in disorders of consciousness.

We hope you enjoy this collection of articles from leading experts in neurohospitalist neurology and find them of value in your daily practice. Happy rounding!

Vanja C. Douglas, MD
Professor of Neurology
Sara & Evan Williams Foundation Endowed
Neurohospitalist Chair
Chief, Neurohospitalist Division
Department of Neurology
Weill Institute for Neurosciences
University of California, San Francisco

Maulik P. Shah, MD, MHS
Associate Professor of Neurology
Medical Director, Inpatient Neurology and
UCSF Integrated Transfer Center
Department of Neurology
Weill Institute for Neurosciences
University of California, San Francisco

E-mail addresses:
Vanja.Douglas@ucsf.edu (V.C. Douglas)
maulik.shah@ucsf.edu (M.P. Shah)

Management of Status Epilepticus and Indications for Inpatient Electroencephalography Monitoring

Joline M. Fan, MD[a,b,*], Neel S. Singhal, MD, PhD[a,b],
Elan L. Guterman, MD[a,b]

KEYWORDS

- Status epilepticus • Refractory • Continuous EEG • Convulsive • Non-convulsive

KEY POINTS

- Status epilepticus is a neurologic emergency with severe neurologic and systemic complications.
- Immediate time-sensitive treatment of prolonged seizures will minimize risk of long-term morbidity.
- Nonconvulsive status epilepticus should be considered in critically ill patients with and without a history of epilepsy who have unexplained alteration of consciousness.
- In addition to monitoring for seizures, continuous electroencephalography has a broad range of indications, including monitoring for cerebral ischemia, aiding in neurologic prognosis after cardiac arrest, and providing adjunctive evidence of brain death.

INTRODUCTION

Status epilepticus (SE) is a state of failed seizure termination, leading to considerable morbidity and mortality. The incidence of SE is estimated to be 8 to 60 per 100,000 person-years with a mortality of 8% to 20%, yielding up to 40,000 deaths per year in the United States.[1–3] The treatment of SE requires prompt diagnosis and medical therapy. In this review, the authors first outline the current definitions, treatment paradigms, and potential complications of SE. They then discuss the role of

[a] Department of Neurology, University of California, San Francisco, 505 Parnassus Avenue, M798 Box 0114, San Francisco, CA 94143, USA; [b] Weill Institute for Neurosciences, University of California, San Francisco, San Francisco, CA 94143, USA
* Corresponding author.
E-mail address: Joline.Fan@ucsf.edu

Neurol Clin 40 (2022) 1–16
https://doi.org/10.1016/j.ncl.2021.08.001
0733-8619/22/© 2021 Elsevier Inc. All rights reserved.

electroencephalography (EEG) monitoring in the management of seizure as well as additional indications for EEG monitoring aside from seizure.

PART 1. MANAGEMENT OF STATUS EPILEPTICUS
Defining the Spectrum of Status Epilepticus

Seizure
A seizure is a paroxysmal event of aberrant, hypersynchronous neuronal activity in the brain, which is often but not necessarily accompanied by behavioral changes. Seizures are self-limited, and as such, require an onset and clear offset.[4] Seizures have intrinsic mechanisms of termination that typically facilitate their cessation within 5 minutes.[5]

Status epilepticus
SE occurs when mechanisms that terminate a seizure fail or mechanisms that initiate a seizure are continuously activated, resulting in abnormal seizure prolongation.[6] The International League Against Epilepsy (ILAE) defines SE by 2 specific time points: (1) when a seizure is unlikely to terminate spontaneously, thereby warranting emergent medical treatment; and (2) when long-term neuronal injury is likely.[6] In the case of generalized convulsive seizure activity, seizures are unlikely to terminate if seizure activity persists for more than 5 minutes (continuously or 2 or more seizures occur without return to baseline mental status), and long-term neuronal injury occurs at 30 minutes.[6–8] Therefore, the Neurocritical Care Society and ILAE have supported a definition that defines generalized convulsive status epilepticus (GCSE) as seizures lasting more than 5 minutes.[9] For other seizure types, the time points are defined differently to reflect differences in their associated morbidity.[6] In the case of focal SE with impairment of awareness, seizures are unlikely to terminate after 10 minutes of seizure activity and neuronal injury is thought to occur at 60 minutes.[6] In the case of absence SE, seizures are unlikely to terminate after 10 to 15 minutes of seizure activity and the second timepoint is unknown.[6] In the case of other seizure types, there is a lack of consensus about the standards.

The classification of different forms of SE is based on differences in the clinical and electrographic manifestation of seizure. For instance, nonconvulsive status epilepticus (NCSE) does not have prominent motor symptoms of GCSE and instead presents as waxing-and-waning language impairment, impaired consciousness, subtle eyelid, facial, or finger twitching, or eye deviation. Nevertheless, like GCSE, NCSE can lead to long-term consequences, such as neuronal injury, neuronal death, or restructuring of the neuronal network.[10,11] Despite the prevalence and potential risk of prolonged NCSE, most of the current treatment algorithms are based on studies of the treatment of GCSE. No formal time-based definitions have been established for NCSE, and the appropriate urgency and approach to treating NCSE remain similarly undefined. Thus, the treatment pathway discussed in this article primarily applies to GCSE rather than NCSE and other types of SE, which each involve their own treatment approach.

Refractory status epilepticus
Refractory status epilepticus (RSE) is defined as persistent SE, despite first-line treatment with benzodiazepines and an adequate dose of 1 second-line antiseizure medication (ASM).[12,13] RSE occurs in approximately 20% to 30% of patients presenting in SE.[14,15]

Super-refractory status epilepticus
Super-refractory status epilepticus (SRSE) is defined as SE that persists for 24 hours or recurs as therapies are weaned despite receiving treatment with first-line

benzodiasepines, at least 1 second-line ASM, and third-line therapy (typically anesthetic medications).[16] Mortality increases with progression along the spectrum from SE to SRSE, with an associated mortality as high as 50% for SRSE.[17] The mechanisms underlying SRSE are unknown, but possibilities include acute cellular responses to SE, such as a reduction of GABA receptors, overexpression of glutamatergic receptors, and mitochondrial failure, which can perpetuate hyperexcitability.[16]

Status Epilepticus Treatment

The guiding principle of SE treatment is that early seizure termination improves neurologic outcomes and reduces systemic complications. In part, this is because the longer treatment is delayed, the greater the risk that seizures become refractory to pharmacologic treatment and self-sustained.[11,18] Delayed seizure termination also increases the risk of cardiopulmonary complications. Thus, treatment should be delivered emergently.[19] This involves rapid therapy with benzodiazepines followed by initiation and escalation of ASMs to terminate clinical and electrographic seizure activity. In parallel with pharmacologic treatment, it is imperative that the medical team screens for systemic drivers and complications and provides supportive care as necessary.

Stage 1: Benzodiazepines

First-line therapy for prolonged seizure activity is benzodiazepine administration (**Table 1**). Consensus-based guidelines supported by high-quality randomized clinical trials recommend treatment with intravenous (IV) lorazepam, intramuscular (IM) midazolam, or IV diazepam.[19–22] If IV access is already established, IV lorazepam is the preferred agent.[23] Lorazepam should be administered as a single 4-mg dose for any person weighing more than 40 kg, and at a dose of 0.1 mg/kg for those who weigh less. This dose should be repeated once for ongoing seizure activity. If IV access is not available, IM midazolam is preferred to avoid the delay imposed by establishing IV access for medication administration. IM midazolam should be administered as a single 10-mg dose for any person weighing more than 40 kg and a single 5-mg dose for any person weighing less than 40 kg.[19–22] Adverse effects of benzodiazepines include hypotension and respiratory depression, although evidence suggests the respiratory risks of undertreated SE and recurrent seizures are greater, and appropriate dosing of benzodiazepines should not be withheld.[24] In addition, IV thiamine should be given before any dextrose is administered to avoid precipitating acute Wernicke encephalopathy, particularly for patients with a history of heavy alcohol use and others who are at increased risk of this complication.

Stage 2: Non-benzodiazepine intravenous antiseizure medications

Treatment with second-line therapy should follow benzodiazepine administration for all patients with SE, except for patients with alcohol withdrawal for whom benzodiazepines are the treatment of choice along with phenobarbital and propofol. Randomized controlled trials have established treatment with IV fosphenytoin, IV valproic acid, and IV levetiracetam as equivalent.[25] These medications represent the standard of care for second-line therapy (see **Table 1**) and should be administered using an IV loading dose to rapidly achieve a therapeutic serum level followed by maintenance dosing. If SE has been terminated with benzodiazepine therapy, ongoing treatment to maintain a therapeutic serum level is still required for longer-term seizure control, unless a provoking factor has been identified and addressed.[26] Deciding between fosphenytoin, valproic acid, and levetiracetam is often a matter of physician preference

Table 1
Medication treatment escalation for convulsive status epilepticus

Medication	Initial Dose[12,13,29]	Maintenance Dose	Notes/Pearls
First-line agents (<20 min)			
Benzodiazepines			
Lorazepam	4 mg IV		May repeat dose once if seizure persists
Midazolam	10 mg IM		May repeat dose once if seizure persists
Diazepam	10 mg IV		
Second-line agents (20–40 min)			
Antiseizure medications (ASMs)			
Fosphenytoin/phenytoin	20 PE/kg IV	100 mg IV q8h	Check serum level 2 h after load and administer partial load if level is subtherapeutic (goal level 10–20, corrected for albumin level). Adverse effects include cardiac arrhythmias and hypotension. Avoid in myoclonic or absence SE. Fosphenytoin is preferred over phenytoin because rapid peripheral infusion of phenytoin carries a risk of purple glove syndrome
Valproic acid[a]	40 mg/kg IV	500–750 mg IV q8h	Goal serum level 70–120 mg/L. Adverse effects include hepatotoxicity, thrombocytopenia
Levetiracetam[a]	60 mg/kg IV (maximum 4 g)	1500 mg IV q12h	Minimal drug-drug interactions. May be added as an adjunctive agent if fosphenytoin or valproic acid is used as primary agent

Adjunctive agents			
Lacosamide	200–400 mg IV	200 mg IV q12h	Minimal drug-drug interactions; excellent adjunctive agent given IV formulation
Phenobarbital	20 mg/kg IV	50–100 mg IV q12h	Goal level 20–50 µg/mL. IV formulation contains propylene glycol and is thus not compatible with ketogenic diet
Topiramate[a]	200 mg PO	200 mg PO q12h	Offers multiple alternative mechanisms of actions
Oxcarbazepine	300 mg PO	300–600 mg PO q12h	Monitor for hyponatremia, particularly in patients with intracranial lesions
Clobazam[a]	10 mg PO	10–20 mg PO q12h	Minimal drug-drug interactions; may cause excess sedation
Alternative adjunctive ASMs include pregabalin, zonisamide, carbamazepine, brivaracetam			
Third-line agents (40–60 min)			
IV anesthetics			
Midazolam	0.2 mg/kg IV	0.05–2 mg/kg/h with uptitration to maximum	Longer half-life than propofol; tachyphylaxis after prolonged use
Propofol	2 mg/kg IV	1–10 mg/kg/h with uptitration to maximum	Monitor triglycerides for propofol infusion syndrome; short half-life
Pentobarbital	5–15 mg/kg IV	1–10 mg/kg/h	May cause significant hemodynamic instability

[a] Broad spectrum IV ASMs, implying that they can be used for both generalized and focal epilepsies.

with some consideration to negative side effects of the loading dose. Important considerations include hemodynamic instability for fosphenytoin and hepatic dysfunction or blood dyscrasias for valproic acid as well as patient comorbidities and drug interactions. Valproic acid should also be avoided in a person with childbearing potential, as the medication has increased risk of teratogenicity. Fosphenytoin is a phenytoin prodrug, which is preferred over phenytoin because it carries a lower risk of thrombophlebitis and purple glove syndrome, a rare complication of rapidly infusing IV phenytoin that presents with pain, edema, and discoloration.[27] For patients who have absence or myoclonic SE, fosphenytoin can worsen seizures; thus, valproic acid or levetiracetam should be used in these cases.[28]

Stage 3: IV anesthetics

When SE persists despite benzodiazepine and nonbenzodiazepine IV ASM therapy, the patient has developed RSE, and treatment should progress to third-line therapy. Appropriate management of patients with RSE includes EEG monitoring to guide titration of third-line anesthetic agents and to monitor for recurrent subclinical seizures. Usually, IV midazolam and propofol are first-choice agents. Barbiturates, including IV pentobarbital and thiopental, are also accepted agents, but are more likely to cause hypotension and depressed cardiac contractility and often require adjunctive pressor agents.

The primary mechanism of action for midazolam, propofol, and barbiturates is through modulation of $GABA_A$ receptors. These agents should be administered with an IV loading dose followed by a continuous infusion. Increases in the dose of the continuous infusion should be preceded by an additional loading dose.[12,13,29]

The standard of care for patients with RSE is to titrate anesthetic infusions to burst suppression on continuous EEG monitoring. The optimal depth or duration of burst suppression is unknown[30]; often treatment is targeted toward burst suppression with an interburst interval of 10 seconds for 24 to 48 hours while initiating treatment with additional ASMs.[12] The infusion is then weaned gradually (over 24 hours) with adjustment and potential reinitiation of burst suppression for recurrent seizures or SE. When continuous EEG monitoring is not available and there is concern for RSE, the authors recommend urgent transfer to a facility that can provide EEG monitoring.

There is limited guidance for the management of RSE when the patient has forms of SE different from GCSE. In these circumstances, the degree of neuronal injury associated with prolonged seizure and importance of early therapy are not as well established. Thus, treatment should initially focus on increasing the number of ASMs and not the induction of burst suppression with anesthetic agents.[31] Some groups have developed clinical scores and proposed using them to provide guidance on early therapy, but at present, adequate data to use them to inform real-world treatment decisions are lacking.[32,33] For instance, the appropriate time to pursue burst suppression for patients presenting with NCSE remains of great debate,[34] and guidelines dictating when to make this treatment decision for these patients continue to be lacking.[26]

Stage 4: Super-refractory status epilepticus therapies

SRSE is highly morbid, and its treatment is less well studied.[35] Management is guided by expert opinion and involves increasing the number of ASMs, increasing the number of anesthetic infusions, and trialing additional alternative therapies.[16] Additional ASMs should be selected in an effort to activate multiple different mechanisms of seizure termination.

Table 2
Pharmacologic options for management of superrefractory status epilepticus

	Name	Dosing	Notes/Pearls
Pharmacologic	IV anesthetics	As above	
	Ketamine[a]	Optimal dosing not yet defined[68]	NMDA receptor antagonist, may be helpful in late SE where NMDA receptor overexpression is reported.[10] Consider for hypotensive patients
	Magnesium	Load 2–6 g IV Maintenance 2 g tid IV × 2–7 d[69]	First line for seizures in eclampsia
	Pyridoxine	200 mg/d	Consider for empiric treatment of pyridoxine-dependent seizures
	Inhaled anesthetics (desflurane, isoflurane)		GABA agonists; requires closed loop anesthetic system; risk of hypotension, ileus, and rarely, neurotoxicity
	Immune modulation		Consider for empiric treatment of immune-mediated causes of RSE
	Steroids	Methylprednisolone: 1 g IV × 3–5 d	Cannot be used with ketogenic diet
	IV immunoglobulin	0.4 g/kg/d × 5 d	Adverse risks include thrombosis, fluid overload, cardiac failure, aseptic meningitis
	Plasma exchange	Daily or every other day × 5–7 d	Avoid in patients with hemodynamic instability
Nonpharmacologic	Ketogenic diet	24–48 h fasting followed by transition onto 4:1 ratio of fat: carbohydrates + protein in grams over 2 d, then maintain	Perform in consultation with a dietician. Requires monitoring blood beta-hydroxybutyrate to target level of 3–6 mmol/L, or if unavailable, monitoring urine ketones to target level of 80–160 mmol/L.[70] Concurrent monitoring of glucose, pH, and CO_2 recommended

(continued on next page)

	Name	Dosing	Notes/Pearls
Table 2 (*continued*)			
	Electroconvulsive therapy		Use governed by state law and requires judicial approval
	Transcranial magnetic stimulation	Typically <1 Hz repetitive stimulation[71]	Appears to be more effective if applied to defined ictal focus. Risk profile not well characterized
	Emergent surgery		Multiple approaches including subpial transections, resection, and corpus callosotomy in appropriately selected, severely refractory cases

[a] The quality of the evidence supporting the use of these drugs is based on small case series.

Various alternative pharmacologic and nonpharmacologic therapies have been used in SRSE but have weak evidence of benefit. Alternative pharmacologic therapies include ketamine and inhaled anesthetics, which have limited and conflicting data on efficacy (**Table 2**). Ketamine acts as an NMDA receptor antagonist[36] and has been associated with 50% or greater reduction of seizure burden in up to 50% to 80% of patients.[37] Alternative nonpharmacologic therapies include the ketogenic diet, electroconvulsive therapy,[38] transcranial magnetic stimulation,[39] vagus nerve stimulation, and emergency neurosurgery (see **Table 2**). Of these, the ketogenic diet has the strongest supportive data in SE and should be initiated in consultation with an experienced dietician.[40] Surgery can also be effective in select patients with a single seizure focus that can be resected.[41] Therapies such as allopregnanolone and therapeutic hypothermia are even less well supported by the literature.

Empiric therapies for rare disorders that may underlie refractory SE should also be considered and include pyridoxine supplementation for pyridoxine-dependent epilepsy,[42] vitamin supplementation for possible underlying mitochondrial disease, and immunotherapy. Empiric immunotherapy includes corticosteroids, IV immunoglobulin, and plasmapheresis and addresses the high incidence of immune-mediated encephalitis identified among cases of new-onset refractory status epilepticus. IV magnesium is the standard of care for controlling seizures in eclampsia but may also have benefit in epilepsy related to the mitochondrial polymerase gamma (*POLG*) gene.[43]

Management of Systemic Consequences

There are multiple systemic consequences of SE and its treatment. SE can lead to cardiac arrhythmias, pulmonary edema, autonomic instability, and respiratory failure as well as a peripheral leukocytosis and cerebrospinal fluid (CSF) pleocytosis. GCSE can lead to rhabdomyolysis and subsequent renal injury.[44,45] Medications used in the treatment of SE also have important side effects that include respiratory depression, sedation, hypotension, ileus, and cardiac arrhythmias (see **Table 1**). For these reasons, management of patients with SE should involve close monitoring by experienced neurologists and often requires admission to a specialized neurocritical care setting when SE is prolonged.

Evaluation to Determine Cause of Status Epilepticus

Any condition that can lead to seizure can also cause SE, SE may present in a patient with known epilepsy, or, in 12% to 30% of adults with epilepsy, SE will be their initial presentation.[8] Chronic conditions that may lead to SE include primary epilepsy syndromes and intracranial lesions, such as prior stroke, severe head trauma, tumors, or vascular malformations. Acute conditions associated with SE include central nervous system (CNS) infection, immune-mediated encephalitis, drug toxicity or withdrawal, metabolic derangements, and acute CNS injury, such as from hypertensive emergency, posterior reversible encephalopathy syndrome, trauma, hypoxia, or stroke.

In evaluating a patient with SE, careful review of their medical history and medications is crucial. A common cause of SE in patients with epilepsy is subtherapeutic ASM levels owing to medication nonadherence, medication changes, or inadequate dosing.[46] Obtaining serum ASM drug levels is important, particularly if it is unclear whether the patient has been taking their medication regularly or the dose is adequate. Initial serum testing should also assess for common provoking factors, such as hypomagnesemia, hypoglycemia and hyperglycemia, hyponatremia and hypernatremia, hypocalcemia and hypercalcemia, acute liver and kidney injury, systemic infection, and stimulant use. Patients should undergo brain imaging if presenting with their first lifetime seizure. There is not a clear cause identified from the initial evaluation, RSE develops, or the patient has a persistently abnormal neurologic examination after SE cessation. Although computed tomography (CT) is frequently performed, magnetic resonance has increased sensitivity for many acute causes of SE and should follow or replace CT in most circumstances. Patients without a clear cause for SE should also undergo urgent lumbar puncture to evaluate for infectious or immune-mediated encephalitis. Although seizures can lead to a mild CSF pleocytosis, patients should receive empiric antibacterial and acyclovir treatment for any CSF pleocytosis or if there is other clinical suspicion for meningoencephalitis, which can be discontinued if follow-up testing lowers suspicion for infection.

Summary

SE is a neurologic emergency requiring acute therapy to minimize neuronal injury and systemic complications. The treatment pathway focuses on supportive care and EEG monitoring while quickly escalating benzodiazepines and ASMs for longer-term control. SE and its pharmacologic treatments have multiple systemic consequences that require close monitoring and treatment. For patients without known epilepsy, the identification of provoking factors is critical to treating SE.

PART 2. INDICATIONS FOR INPATIENT ELECTROENCEPHALOGRAPHY MONITORING
Electroencephalography Monitoring in the Seizure Patient

EEG monitoring has 4 common uses in the management of patients with seizure and SE: (1) evaluate for subclinical seizures, (2) titrate therapy to achieve burst suppression, (3) determine whether an event is epileptic or nonepileptic, and (4) determine a patient's risk of recurrent seizure. Aside from the last indication, continuous rather than routine EEG monitoring is recommended.

Subclinical seizures are common and should be considered in any patient with unexplained alterations of consciousness, unilateral motor or sensory deficit, or aphasia, particularly if there are subtle abnormal movements in the eyelid, face, or finger, as can occur in NCSE. The Critical Care Continuous EEG Task Force of American Clinical Neurophysiology Study recommends EEG monitoring in groups that are at increased risk of subclinical seizure.[31] This includes patients with GCSE who do not return to their baseline mental status within 60 minutes of their presenting seizure, patients with acute intracranial injury and mental status alterations that are out of proportion to their intracranial insult, critically ill patients with inappropriately severe or prolonged encephalopathy, and patients with high-risk epileptiform features on routine EEG.[47,48] Studies demonstrate that after resolution of convulsive activity in patients presenting with GCSE, up to 50% of patients have persistent or recurrent electrographic seizures or NCSE.[49] Furthermore, NCSE occurs in 10% to 20% of patients with critical illness and unexplained encephalopathy as well as in patients with acute CNS injury, such as aneurysmal subarachnoid hemorrhage (SAH), intracerebral hemorrhage, trauma, and CNS infection.[50–53]

The appropriate duration of EEG monitoring when evaluating for NCSE and intermittent subclinical seizures is debated. For patients with a high risk of seizure, EEG monitoring for at least 24 hours is recommended[54]; however, EEG monitoring for a shorter period may have reasonable sensitivity and specificity. A retrospective analysis of 625 critically ill patients who underwent prolonged continuous EEG monitoring found that 27% of patients had detectable seizures and 58% of these seizures began within the first 30 minutes of recording.[55] Recently, a risk-stratification tool named the 2HELPS2B Score was developed to quantify a patient's risk of seizure based on clinical data and a 1-hour EEG recording. The score incorporates whether there is a history of epilepsy and whether the EEG study contains any of 5 EEG features to provide guidance on the optimal duration of EEG monitoring.[56]

It is also important to be mindful of EEG patterns that are difficult to interpret. One such example is the ictal-interictal continuum, which represents rhythmic, periodic epileptiform discharges that approach but do not definitively meet the electrographic criteria for NCSE[57] (Fig. 1). Monitoring the clinical and electrographic response to a single dose of ASM or treatment for a defined period can be helpful in determining how aggressively to treat patients with this EEG pattern. Another EEG pattern commonly confused for seizure is generalized periodic discharges with triphasic wave morphology, or triphasic waves, owing to toxic or metabolic derangements (see Fig. 1). These are frequently misinterpreted as epileptiform, and treatment should focus on the reversal of the underlying cause of encephalopathy.

Electroencephalography Monitoring in the Intensive Care Unit

Additional indications for continuous EEG monitoring are highlighted in later discussion to demonstrate the range of uses of EEG monitoring in an inpatient setting. The use of EEG to facilitate early detection of neural injuries and inform prognosis in acute brain injuries is an active and rapidly advancing area of research; thus, indications for EEG monitoring are likely to increase over time.[58,59]

Electroencephalography in critically ill patients without brain injury

Continuous EEG is indicated in critically ill patients with unexplained alterations in consciousness or neurologic symptoms because of the high prevalence of seizures in this patient population. NCSE or subclinical seizures occur in 10% to 20% of critically ill patients with encephalopathy and can develop in the absence of acute brain injury.[50,52,53,60] Precipitating factors include sepsis, hepatic dysfunction, or renal failure. EEG should also be considered in patients undergoing pharmacologic paralysis

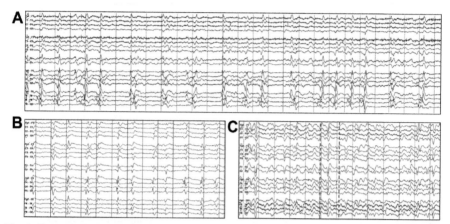

Fig. 1. Example EEG recordings. (*A*) A 57-year-old man with HSV-1 encephalitis and altered mental status. EEG with waxing-and-waning 1- to 2-Hz LPDs+ that lie on the interictal-ictal continuum. (*B*) A 70-year-old woman with rapid cognitive decline consistent with CJD. EEG reveals 1-Hz GPDs with a subtle right hemispheric predominance. (*C*) A 54-year-old woman presenting with altered mental status secondary to baclofen toxicity. Red dotted box represents a typical triphasic wave. Each vertical grid line represents 1 second. CJD, Creutzfeld-Jakob disease.

(ie, for treatment of refractory acute respiratory distress syndrome) whereby adequate monitoring of patient neurologic examination is no longer possible.[31]

Detection of ischemia in subarachnoid hemorrhage

Continuous EEG monitoring can be used an adjunctive tool for the detection of delayed cerebral ischemia after SAH.[59,61] Reduced cerebral blood flow or ischemia has been associated with a decrease in faster frequencies and increase in slower frequencies on EEG.[62,63] Upon infarction, an EEG may reveal even slower frequencies and suppression. Quantitative EEG, which provides frequency-based metrics, such as the alpha/delta ratio, relative alpha variability, and total power and asymmetry measures, has been increasingly used in this population to support earlier and more sensitive detection of delayed cerebral ischemia.[61]

Prognostication after cardiac arrest

Early EEG monitoring is recommended in all patients with coma after cardiac arrest.[64] EEG monitoring is used to detect seizures and as part of a multimodal approach to prognostication, providing information about the severity of brain injury and a patient's capacity for neurologic recovery. EEG patterns can be classified as highly malignant, malignant, or benign. Highly malignant EEG features include a suppressed background without discharges, suppressed background with continuous periodic discharges, or burst-suppression with or without discharges occurring after rewarming. The presence of at least 1 highly malignant EEG feature was found to have 100% specificity for predicting poor neurologic outcome.[65] Malignant EEG features include seizures, abundant rhythmic discharges, and discontinuous or absent background activity. The presence of 2 or more malignant EEG features was also found to have a high specificity (96%) for predicting poor neurologic outcome.[65] Benign EEG patterns lack malignant features and demonstrate reactivity to auditory or painful stimuli and are suggestive of a good neurologic outcome.[65,66] There is ongoing research to determine whether EEG can be used to guide treatments that improve outcomes for survivors of cardiac arrest.[65]

Table 3
Electroencephalography signatures in special populations

Special Population	Hallmark EEG Findings
Creutzfeldt-Jakob disease	Early stage: lateralized periodic discharges (LPDs) Late stage: generalized periodic discharges (GPDs) occurring at 0.5–2 Hz with biphasic or triphasic morphology, which is not necessarily time-locked to myoclonic twitches
NMDA encephalitis	Delta brushes, manifested as generalized rhythmic delta waves with overriding beta activity
Herpes simplex virus (HSV) encephalitis	Most commonly, LPDs with or without evolution into an ictal pattern
Subacute sclerosing panencephalitis	High-amplitude GPDs (200–500 mV) occurring at a frequency of 4- to 10-s intervals
Catatonia	Normal EEG
Posterior reversible encephalopathy syndrome	Focal slowing or LPDs typically occurring in a posterior distribution
Metabolic/toxic (ie, hepatic encephalopathy, medications, including cephalosporins)	Triphasic waves

Brain death

Diagnosing brain death requires a bedside neurologic examination in which the patient is normothermic, and the confounding effect of medications and metabolic abnormalities have been removed to confirm the presence of coma and cessation of brainstem function. Although it is often not necessary, EEG can be an important ancillary test in brain death determination when the clinical context precludes a definitive examination. An EEG in a patient with brain death reveals electrocerebral silence, which is the absence of cerebral electrical activity greater than 2 uV for at least 30 minutes, using scalp electrodes that are placed at least 10 cm apart.[67] Specific criteria must be met for the EEG set up, including complete montage coverage, thresholds for electrode impedance, and electrode integrity.[67] Extreme care must be taken to identify and limit sources of artifact in EEG recordings for cases of suspected brain death.

Electroencephalography Monitoring in Special Populations

In addition to its use in the critically ill patient, EEG monitoring is helpful in the evaluation of other inpatient populations. **Table 3** summarizes unique scenarios wherein EEG monitoring offers supplementary data to aid in the diagnosis of specific conditions, and **Fig. 1** provides several example EEG patterns.

Summary

Inpatient EEG monitoring has multiple uses in patients with and without SE. Most commonly, it is used to direct management of patients with seizure or seizure-like events as well as to evaluate for NCSE, which may have serious neurologic complications despite its seemingly benign clinical presentation. Outside of treating and monitoring for seizures, EEG is increasingly used in other populations, including patients with SAH to monitor for cerebral ischemia, patients with cardiac arrest to inform neurologic prognostication, patients with potential brain death, and as an ancillary diagnostic tool in specific populations commonly evaluated in the inpatient neurologic setting.

DISCLOSURE

J.M. Fan receives funding from the National Center for Advancing Translational Sciences of the NIH (5TL1TR001871-05). N.S. Singhal receives funding from the American Heart Association (18CDA34030443) and the Hellman Family Foundation. E.L. Guterman receives funding from the National Institute of Neurological Disorders and Stroke (1K23NS116128-01) and the National Institute on Aging (5R01AG056715), American Academy of Neurology, as well as consulting fees from Marinus Pharmaceuticals, Inc.

REFERENCES

1. Dham BS, Hunter K, Rincon F. The epidemiology of status epilepticus in the United States. Neurocrit Care 2014;20(3):476–83.
2. Leitinger M, Trinka E, Giovannini G, et al. Epidemiology of status epilepticus in adults: a population-based study on incidence, causes, and outcomes. Epilepsia 2019;60(1):53–62.
3. Wu YW, Shek DW, Garcia PA, et al. Incidence and mortality of generalized convulsive status epilepticus in California. Neurology 2002;58(7):1070–6.
4. Gotman J. A few thoughts on "What is a seizure? Epilepsy Behav 2011; 22(SUPPL. 1):S2.
5. Lado FA, Moshé SL. How do seizures stop? Epilepsia 2008;49(10):1651–64.
6. Trinka E, Cock H, Hesdorffer D, et al. A definition and classification of status epilepticus - report of the ILAE Task Force on Classification of Status Epilepticus. Epilepsia 2015;56(10):1515–23.
7. Jenssen S, Gracely EJ, Sperling MR. How long do most seizures last? A systematic comparison of seizures recorded in the epilepsy monitoring unit. Epilepsia 2006;47(9):1499–503.
8. Lowenstein DH, Alldredge BK. Status epilepticus. N Engl J Med 1998;338(14): 970–6.
9. Brophy GM, Bell R, Claassen J, et al. Guidelines for the evaluation and management of status epilepticus. Neurocrit Care 2012;17(1):3–23.
10. Chen JWY, Wasterlain CG. Status epilepticus: pathophysiology and management in adults. Lancet Neurol 2006;5(3):246–56.
11. Goodkin HP, Yeh JL, Kapur J. Status epilepticus increases the intracellular accumulation of GABA A receptors. J Neurosci 2005;25(23):5511–20.
12. Rossetti AO, Lowenstein DH. Management of refractory status epilepticus in adults: still more questions than answers. Lancet Neurol 2011;10(10):922–30.
13. Holtkamp M. Treatment strategies for refractory status epilepticus. Curr Opin Crit Care 2011;17(2):94–100.
14. Towne AR, Pellock JM, Ko D, et al. Determinants of mortality in status epilepticus. Epilepsia 1994;35(1):27–34.
15. Novy J, Logroscino G, Rossetti AO. Refractory status epilepticus: a prospective observational study. Epilepsia 2010;51(2):251–6.
16. Shorvon S, Ferlisi M. The treatment of super-refractory status epilepticus: a critical review of available therapies and a clinical treatment protocol. Brain 2011; 134(10):2802–18.

17. Alvarez V, Drislane FW. Is favorable outcome possible after prolonged refractory status epilepticus? J Clin Neurophysiol 2016;33(1):32–41.

18. Lowenstein DH, Alldredge BK. Status epilepticus at an urban public hospital in the 1980s. Neurology 1993;43(3):483–8.

19. Alldredge BK, Gelb AM, Isaacs SM, et al. A comparison of lorazepam, diazepam, and placebo for the treatment of out-of-hospital status epilepticus. N Engl J Med 2001;345(9):631–7.

20. Lowenstein DH, Alldredge BK, Allen F, et al. The Prehospital Treatment of Status Epilepticus (PHTSE) study: design and methodology. Control Clin Trials 2001; 22(3):290–309.

21. Treiman DM, Meyers PD, Walton NY, et al. A comparison of four treatments for generalized convulsive status epilepticus. N Engl J Med 1998;339(12):792–8.

22. Silbergleit R, Durkalski V, Lowenstein D, et al. Intramuscular versus intravenous therapy for prehospital status epilepticus. N Engl J Med 2012;366(7):591–600.

23. Leppik LE, Derivan AT, Homan RW, et al. Double-blind study of lorazepam and diazepam in status epilepticus. JAMA 1983;249(11):1452–4.

24. Guterman EL, Sanford JK, Betjemann JP, et al. Prehospital midazolam use and outcomes among patients with out-of-hospital status epilepticus. Neurology 2020;95(24):e3203–12.

25. Kapur J, Elm J, Chamberlain JM, et al. Randomized trial of three anticonvulsant medications for status epilepticus. N Engl J Med 2019;381(22):2103–13.

26. Glauser T, Shinnar S, Gloss D, et al. Evidence-based guideline: treatment of convulsive status epilepticus in children and adults: report of the guideline committee of the American Epilepsy Society. Epilepsy Curr 2016;16(1):48–61.

27. O'Brien TJ, Cascino GD, So EL, et al. Incidence and clinical consequence of the purple glove syndrome in patients receiving intravenous phenytoin. Neurology 1998;51(4):1034–9.

28. Guerrini R, Dravet C, Genton P, et al. Lamotrigine and seizure aggravation in severe myoclonic epilepsy. Epilepsia 1998;39(5):508–12.

29. Rossetti AO. Which anesthetic should be used in the treatment of refractory status epilepticus? Epilepsia 2007;48(s8):52–5.

30. Perry MS. Flat out unnecessary: burst characteristics, not duration of interburst intervals, predict successful anesthetic wean in refractory status epilepticus. Epilepsy Curr 2017;17(3):153–4.

31. Herman ST, Abend NS, Bleck TP, et al. Consensus statement on continuous EEG in critically ill adults and children, part I: indications. J Clin Neurophysiol 2015; 32(2):87–95.

32. Rossetti AO, Logroscino G, Bromfield EB. A clinical score for prognosis of status epilepticus in adults. Neurology 2006;66(11):1736–8.

33. Rossetti AO, Logroscino G, Milligan TA, et al. Status Epilepticus Severity Score (STESS): a tool to orient early treatment strategy. J Neurol 2008;255(10):1561–6.

34. Jordan KG, Hirsch LJ. In nonconvulsive status epilepticus (NCSE), treat to burst-suppression: pro and con. Epilepsia 2006;47(SUPPL. 1):41–5.

35. Kantanen AM, Reinikainen M, Parviainen I, et al. Incidence and mortality of super-refractory status epilepticus in adults. Epilepsy Behav 2015;49:131–4.

36. Borris DJ, Bertram EH, Kapur J. Ketamine controls prolonged status epilepticus. Epilepsy Res 2000;42(2–3):117–22.

37. Alkhachroum A, Der-Nigoghossian CA, Mathews E, et al. Ketamine to treat super-refractory status epilepticus. Neurology 2020;95(16):e2286–94.

38. Zeiler FA, Matuszczak M, Teitelbaum J, et al. Electroconvulsive therapy for refractory status epilepticus: a systematic review. Seizure 2016;35:23–32.

39. Zeiler FA, Matuszczak M, Teitelbaum J, et al. Transcranial magnetic stimulation for status epilepticus. Epilepsy Res Treat 2015;2015:1–10.
40. Thakur KT, Probasco JC, Hocker SE, et al. Ketogenic diet for adults in super-refractory status epilepticus. Neurology 2014;82(8):665–70.
41. Winkler PA. Surgical treatment of status epilepticus: a palliative approach. Epilepsia 2013;54(SUPPL. 6):68–71.
42. Goutières F, Aicardi J. Atypical presentations of pyridoxine-dependent seizures: a treatable cause of intractable epilepsy in infants. Ann Neurol 1985;17(2):117–20.
43. Visser NA, Braun KPJ, Leijten FSS, et al. Magnesium treatment for patients with refractory status epilepticus due to POLG1-mutations. J Neurol 2011;258(2):218–22.
44. Barry E, Hauser WA. Pleocytosis after status epilepticus. Arch Neurol 1994;51(2):190–3.
45. Aminoff MJ, Simon RP. Status epilepticus: causes, clinical features and consequences in 98 patients. Am J Med 1980;69(5):657–66.
46. Lie IA, Hoggen I, Samsonsen C, et al. Treatment non-adherence as a trigger for status epilepticus: an observational, retrospective study based on therapeutic drug monitoring. Epilepsy Res 2015;113:28–33.
47. Claassen J, Taccone FS, Horn P, et al. Recommendations on the use of EEG monitoring in critically ill patients: consensus statement from the neurointensive care section of the ESICM. Intensive Care Med 2013;39(8):1337–51.
48. Fagan KJ, Lee SI. Prolonged confusion following convulsions due to generalized nonconvulsive status epilepticus. Neurology 1990;40(11):1689–94.
49. Yuan F, Yang F, Li W, et al. Nonconvulsive status epilepticus after convulsive status epilepticus: clinical features, outcomes, and prognostic factors. Epilepsy Res 2018;142:53–7.
50. Claassen J, Mayer SA. Continuous electroencephalographic monitoring in neurocritical care. Curr Neurol Neurosci Rep 2002;2(6):534–40.
51. Claassen J, Mayer SA, Kowalski RG, et al. Detection of electrographic seizures with continuous EEG monitoring in critically ill patients. Neurology 2004;62(10):1743–8.
52. Oddo M, Carrera E, Claassen J, et al. Continuous electroencephalography in the medical intensive care unit. Crit Care Med 2009;37(6):2051–6.
53. Kamel H, Betjemann JP, Navi BB, et al. Diagnostic yield of electroencephalography in the medical and surgical intensive care unit. Neurocrit Care 2013;19(3):336–41.
54. Caricato A, Melchionda I, Antonelli M. Continuous electroencephalography monitoring in adults in the intensive care unit. Crit Care 2018;22(1):75.
55. Westover MB, Shafi MM, Bianchi MT, et al. The probability of seizures during EEG monitoring in critically ill adults. Clin Neurophysiol 2015;126(3):463–71.
56. Struck AF, Tabaeizadeh M, Schmitt SE, et al. Assessment of the validity of the 2HELPS2B Score for inpatient seizure risk prediction. JAMA Neurol 2020;77:500–7.
57. Kaplan PW. EEG criteria for nonconvulsive status epilepticus. Epilepsia 2007;48(s8):39–41.
58. Claassen J, Doyle K, Matory A, et al. Detection of brain activation in unresponsive patients with acute brain injury. N Engl J Med 2019;380(26):2497–505.
59. Rosenthal ES, Biswal S, Zafar SF, et al. Continuous electroencephalography predicts delayed cerebral ischemia after subarachnoid hemorrhage: a prospective study of diagnostic accuracy. Ann Neurol 2018;83(5):958–69.

60. Towne AR, Waterhouse EJ, Boggs JG, et al. Prevalence of nonconvulsive status epilepticus in comatose patients. Neurology 2000;54(2):340–5.
61. Foreman B, Claassen J. Quantitative EEG for the detection of brain ischemia. Crit Care 2012;16(2):216.
62. Hossmann K-A. Viability thresholds and the penumbra of focal ischemia. Ann Neurol 1994;36(4):557–65.
63. Jordan K. Emergency EEG and continuous EEG monitoring in acute ischemic stroke. J Clin Neurophysiol 2004;21(5):341–52.
64. Panchal AR, Bartos JA, Cabañas JG, et al. Part 3: adult basic and advanced life support; 2020 American Heart Association Guidelines for Cardiopulmonary Resuscitation and Emergency Cardiovascular Care. Circulation 2020;142(16 2): S366–468.
65. Westhall E, Rossetti AO, Van Rootselaar AF, et al. Standardized EEG interpretation accurately predicts prognosis after cardiac arrest. Neurology 2016;86(16): 1482–90.
66. Admiraal MM, Horn J, Hofmeijer J, et al. EEG reactivity testing for prediction of good outcome in patients after cardiac arrest. Neurology 2020;95(6):e653–61.
67. Stecker MM, Sabau D, Sullivan L, et al. American Clinical Neurophysiology Society guideline 6: minimum technical standards for EEG recording in suspected cerebral death. J Clin Neurophysiol 2016;33(4):324–7.
68. Gaspard N, Foreman B, Judd LM, et al. Intravenous ketamine for the treatment of refractory status epilepticus: a retrospective multicenter study. Epilepsia 2013; 54(8):1498–503.
69. Zeiler FA, Matuszczak M, Teitelbaum J, et al. Magnesium sulfate for non-eclamptic status epilepticus. Seizure 2015;32:100–8.
70. Gilbert DL, Pyzik PL, Freeman JM. The ketogenic diet: seizure control correlates better with serum β-hydroxybutyrate than with urine ketones. J Child Neurol 2000; 15(12):787–90.
71. Pereira LS, Müller VT, da Mota Gomes M, et al. Safety of repetitive transcranial magnetic stimulation in patients with epilepsy: a systematic review. Epilepsy Behav 2016;57:167–76.

Acute Treatment of Ischemic Stroke

Stephanie Lyden, MD, Jana Wold, MD*

KEYWORDS

- Acute ischemic stroke • Thrombolysis • Endovascular treatment

KEY POINTS

- Intravenous alteplase is safe and effective when given within 4.5 hours of stroke symptom onset.
- Endovascular treatment within 6 hours is safe and effective for acute ischemic stroke due to anterior circulation proximal large vessel occlusion with aspects ≥6.
- Endovascular treatment within 6 to 24 hours from symptom onset is safe and effective in patients who meet dawn or defuse-3 trial criteria.
- Further research is needed in the area of endovascular treatment in patients with low NIHSS, large core infarction, and middle vessel occlusions.

INTRODUCTION

Every year close to 700,000 people experience a new or recurrent ischemic stroke in the United States, and 3% of the total US population is affected by stroke. Stroke is the leading cause of severe disability and the fifth leading cause of death in the nation. Owing to the widespread impact of stroke in patients' individual lives and the tremendous financial cost on the economy, there are many efforts to improve stroke care. Acute therapies are available to decrease the morbidity associated with ischemic stroke and include intravenous thrombolysis and endovascular treatment.

INTRAVENOUS THROMBOLYSIS

Intravenous (IV) recombinant tissue-type plasminogen activator (alteplase) has been approved by the United States Food and Drug Administration (USFDA) for the treatment of acute ischemic stroke within 3 hours of witnessed symptom onset or last known well since 1996.[1] Patients older than 18 years are eligible to receive this treatment if they have a disabling deficit, which is often quantified using the National Institutes of Stroke Severity Scale (NIHSS), and those deficits are presumed to be due to an ischemic stroke with no evidence of an acute hemorrhage on a noncontrast head

Department of Neurology, University of Utah School of Medicine, 175 North Medical Drive, Salt Lake City, UT 84132, USA
* Corresponding author.
E-mail address: jana.wold@hsc.utah.edu

Neurol Clin 40 (2022) 17–32
https://doi.org/10.1016/j.ncl.2021.08.002
0733-8619/22/Published by Elsevier Inc.

computed tomography (CT). This includes patients with rapidly improving symptoms who continue to have deficits, seizure at onset with disabling symptoms not due to a postictal state, large NIHSS scores, and age more than 80 years. Blood pressure must be kept less than 185/110 before and during the infusion and less than 180/105 for 24 hours after the infusion. Blood pressure parameters may be achieved however the treating physician sees fit, though labetalol, nicardipine, and clevidipine are commonly used agents. Patients treated with alteplase have been shown to be 30% more likely to have minimal or no disability at 3 months compared to patients treated with placebo.[2] This favorable outcome helped lead to widespread practice implementation.

Extended Window for Intravenous Alteplase

Intravenous alteplase can also be given within 3 to 4.5 hours of witnessed symptom onset or last known well, although the odds ratio for a favorable outcome compared with placebo during this time frame is 1.28, and its use during this time frame is not approved by the USFDA.[3,4] The European Cooperative Acute Stroke Study (ECASS) III trial showed that alteplase was safe and effective in this time window with strict inclusion criteria that included patients ≤80 years of age, without a history of both diabetes mellitus and prior stroke, with an NIHSS score ≤25, not taking any oral anticoagulation, and without imaging evidence of ischemic injury involving more than one-third of the middle cerebral artery (MCA) territory.[3] Further published data indicate that not all these exclusion criteria are justified. The 2019 American Heart Association/American Stroke Association (AHA/ASA) guideline for the early management of acute ischemic stroke states that alteplase treatment in the 3- to 4.5-hour window may be safe and reasonable in patients who are older than 80 years, or have a history of diabetes mellitus and stroke, or are on warfarin with an international normalized ratio (INR) less than 1.7.[4] However, the benefit remains uncertain in patients with an NIHSS greater than 25.

Current Evidence and Guidelines for Intravenous Alteplase Thrombolysis

Although the original National Institute of Neurologic Disorders and Stroke (NINDS) trial had an extensive list of exclusion criteria, the AHA/ASA committees have revised this list based on documented scientific evidence of harm or lack of benefit with the use of data repositories and clinical expertise. A list of contraindications, based on either a benefit of treatment that equals the risk of treatment or a greater risk of treatment than benefit, are provided in a bulleted list below.[2]

In patients without a known coagulopathy, IV alteplase can be begun before the availability of the platelet count, INR, activated partial thromboplastin time (aPTT), or prothrombin time (PT). This is due to the overall low rates of unsuspected abnormal platelet counts or coagulation studies in the population of acute stroke patients.[5,6] However, if the platelet count returns and is less than 100,000/mm^3 or the INR is greater than 1.7 or the PT is abnormally elevated, alteplase should be discontinued.[7] In addition, if a patient is on a direct thrombin inhibitor or a direct factor Xa inhibitor, and the appropriate laboratory test such as aPTT, INR, ecarin clotting time, thrombin time, or direct factor Xa activity assay is normal, alteplase could be considered. Obtaining these additional coagulation tests may cause delays, so practitioners should be aware of the availability of and the time required to obtain results at their institution.

There is an important emphasis on whether a patient's symptoms are disabling. If a patient presents within 4.5 hours of last known well and has a mild deficit that is judged by the examiner to be disabling, then treatment with IV alteplase is recommended, regardless of a "low" NIHSS score. This assessment should be based on the impact the deficit has on the patient's livelihood and lifestyle. For example, if a patient scores a 1 for aphasia on the NIHSS and is a reporter, they may be judged to have a disabling deficit despite a low NIHSS. However, if a patient presents within 4.5 hours from last known well and has mild, *non-disabling* deficits, treatment with IV alteplase is not recommended. The Potential of tPA for Ischemic Strokes with Mild Symptoms (PRISMS) trial affirmed this recommendation. It randomized patients with mild symptoms, defined as an NIHSS 0 to 5, where the neurologic deficits were not felt to interfere with activities of daily living or prevent return to work, to aspirin and IV alteplase, and found no benefit from treatment with IV alteplase.[8]

It is also important to understand limitations of the NIHSS. The scoring paradigm is heavily weighted toward left MCA infarcts. A patient can have a disabling posterior circulation stroke, but have a low score because the NIHSS does not quantify symptoms of posterior circulation strokes such as axial ataxia, dysphagia, and diplopia.

Intravenous alteplase contraindications

- Mild *non-disabling* symptoms (NIHSS 0–5)
- Head CT with extensive regions of hypoattenuation
- Prior ischemic stroke within 3 months
- Head CT with acute intracranial hemorrhage
- Subarachnoid hemorrhage
- Intra-axial intracranial neoplasm
- Intraspinal or intracranial surgery or serious head trauma within 3 months
- History of intracranial hemorrhage
- Gastrointestinal malignancy or gastrointestinal bleed within 21 days
- Known coagulopathy, including platelets less than 100,000/mm^3, INR greater than 1.7, aPTT greater than 40s, or PT greater than 15s
- Low-molecular-weight heparin full treatment dose received within 24 hours
- Current use of direct thrombin inhibitors or direct factor Xa inhibitors within 48 hours
- Infective endocarditis
- Aortic arch dissection

Expanded inclusion criteria
Although patients with the following conditions were historically excluded from receiving alteplase, further evidence has shown that IV alteplase is reasonable in patients with[9]:

- Extracranial arterial dissection
- Unruptured intracranial aneurysm ≤10 mm
- 1 to 10 cerebral microbleeds demonstrated on a prior MRI
- Menstruating women without a history of menorrhagia
- Extra-axial intracranial neoplasms
- Acute myocardial infarction
- Non-ST-segment myocardial infarction (STEMI) and STEMI involving the right or inferior myocardium within 3 months
- Acute ischemic stroke as a complication of cardiac or cerebral angiographic procedures
- History of diabetic hemorrhagic retinopathy or other hemorrhagic ophthalmic condition while weighing the potential increased risk of visual loss against the benefit of treatment
- Suspected stroke mimic but obtaining additional confirmatory studies would delay treatment

- Illicit drug use
- Sickle cell anemia

Intravenous alteplase may be considered, with careful weighing of the risks and benefits, in individuals with disabling acute stroke symptoms and the following known conditions[2]:

- Initial blood glucose values less than 50 or greater than 400 that have normalized, yet clinical deficits remain
- Dural puncture in the previous 7 days
- Major nonhead trauma within the previous 14 days
- Major surgery in the previous 14 days
- History of previous (greater than 21 days prior) gastrointestinal or genitourinary bleeding
- Active menstruation with a history of menorrhagia without anemia or hypotension
- Pre-existing dementia
- Warfarin use and an INR ≤1.7 or a PT less than 15 seconds
- Myocardial infarction within 3 months involving the left anterior myocardium
- Acute pericarditis and stroke symptoms likely to produce severe disability (cardiology consultation is recommended)
- Left atrial or ventricular thrombus and stroke symptoms likely to produce severe disability
- Cardiac myxoma or papillary fibroelastoma and stroke symptoms likely to produce severe disability
- Pregnancy and moderate to severe stroke
- Pre-existing disability with a modified Rankin score ≥2
- Systemic malignancy and reasonable (>6 months) life expectancy

Patient conditions where the benefit of and risk associated with intravenous alteplase remain uncertain are[2]:

- Arterial puncture at a noncompressible site in the previous 7 days
- Intracranial arterial dissection
- Giant unruptured intracranial aneurysms
- Unruptured, untreated intracranial vascular malformations
- High burden (>10) of cerebral microbleeds on a previous MRI
- Acute pericarditis and stroke symptoms likely to produce mild disability
- Left atrial or ventricular thrombus and stroke symptoms likely to produce mild disability
- Early postpartum period (<14 days after delivery)
- History of bleeding diathesis or coagulopathy

Complications of Treatment

Life-threatening complications of intravenous alteplase therapy include orolingual angioedema and symptomatic intracerebral hemorrhage. **Box 1** includes treatment algorithms for orolingual angioedema management and alteplase reversal in patients with a symptomatic intracranial hemorrhage.

Further Expansion of Treatment with Intravenous Thrombolysis: Fluid-Attenuated Inversion Recovery/Diffusion Weighted Imaging Mismatch

Approximately, 30% of acute ischemic stroke patients who present to the emergency department have an unclear stroke symptom onset time,[10] making it difficult to determine intravenous thrombolysis eligibility. The WAKE-UP and MR WITNESS trials

---

Box 1
Management of IV alteplase complications

A. Orolingual Edema
  1. Maintain airway
    a. Intubation may not be necessary if the edema is limited to the anterior tongue and lips
    b. Edema involving larynx, palate, floor of mouth, or oropharynx with rapid progression within 30 minutes may require intubation
    c. Awake fiberoptic intubation is optimal as nasal-tracheal intubation my pose risk of epistaxis post-IV alteplase.
  2. Discontinue IV alteplase infusion and hold any angiotensin-converting enzyme inhibitors
  3. Administer IV methylprednisolone 125 mg x1
  4. Administer IV diphenhydramine 50 mg x1
  5. Administer famotidine 20 mg IV x1
  6. If there is further increase in angioedema:
    a. Administer epinephrine 1 mg/mL 0.3 mL intramuscular injection x1 OR racemic epinephrine 2.25% orally inhaled solution 0.5 mL nebulization x1
    b. Plasma-derived C1 esterase inhibitor (Berinert) 20 international units/kg IV infusion may be considered in refractory cases

B. Symptomatic Intracranial Bleeding within 12 hours of IV Alteplase
  1. Stop alteplase infusion
  2. Obtain CBC, PT (INR), aPTT, fibrinogen level, and type and cross-match
  3. Obtain an emergent nonenhanced head CT
  4. If intracranial hemorrhage is confirmed:
    a. Cryoprecipitate (includes factor VIII): 10 U infused over 10 to 30 minutes (onset in 1 hour, peaks in 12 hours); administer an additional dose for fibrinogen level of less than 200 mg/dL
    b. Consider Tranexamic acid 1000 mg IV infused over 10 minutes OR ε-aminocaproic acid 4 to 5 g over 1 hour, followed by 1 g IV/h if cryoprecipitate is unavailable, or other blood products are contraindicated
  5. Supportive care to include blood pressure, intracranial pressure, cerebral perfusion pressure, and mean arterial pressure management

Abbreviations: aPTT, activated partial thromboplastin time; CBC, complete blood count; CT, computed tomography; INR, international normalized ratio; IV, intravenous; PT, prothrombin time.

---

enrolled 503 patients and 80 patients, respectively, between the ages of 18 and 85 years, who either awoke with stroke symptoms or had unclear time of symptom onset, but remained within 4.5 hours of symptom recognition. These trials enrolled patients in whom MRI demonstrated ischemia on diffusion-weighted imaging (DWI) but no visible change on fluid-attenuated inversion recovery (FLAIR), thereby identifying patients with recent stroke onset. Patients were excluded if there was a DWI lesion larger than one-third of the MCA territory, NIHSS greater than 25, contraindication to treatment with alteplase, or if thrombectomy was planned.[11,12]

In MR WITNESS, which was an observational study in which all subjects were treated with IV alteplase, rates of symptomatic hemorrhage were similar to those in the ECASS III trial. This helped to establish that the use of intravenous alteplase in patients with unwitnessed stroke that have a DWI-FLAIR mismatch is safe.[11] The WAKE-UP trial helped establish a functional outcome benefit in patients who receive alteplase. More specifically, the primary end-point of a modified Rankin scale (mRS; **Box 2**) of 0 to 1 at 90 days was achieved in 53.3% of patients in the alteplase arm as compared to 41.8% in the placebo arm ($P = .02$).[12] The median NIHSS was 7 in MR WITNESS and 6 in WAKE-UP, exhibiting that the majority of patients had minor strokes compared to the median NIHSS of 16 to 17 seen in landmark endovascular studies. Wake-up strokes accounted for 94% of the WAKE-UP study population. As a result, their study

Box 2
Modified Rankin scale (mRS)

0—No symptoms

1—No significant disability, despite symptoms; able to perform all usual duties and activities

2—Slight disability; unable to perform all previous activities but able to look after own affairs without assistance

3—Moderate disability; requires some help, but able to walk without assistance

4—Moderately severe disability; unable to walk without assistance and unable to attend to own bodily needs without assistance

5—Severe disability; bedridden, incontinent, and requires constant nursing care and attention

6—Death

population was a representative sample and, ultimately, helped expand treatment options to patients with unclear symptom onset.

Following these trials, the 2019 AHA/ASA Acute Ischemic Stroke Guideline stated that intravenous alteplase treatment in this patient population can be beneficial.[9] Consequently, some institutions have created rapid MRI protocols with limited

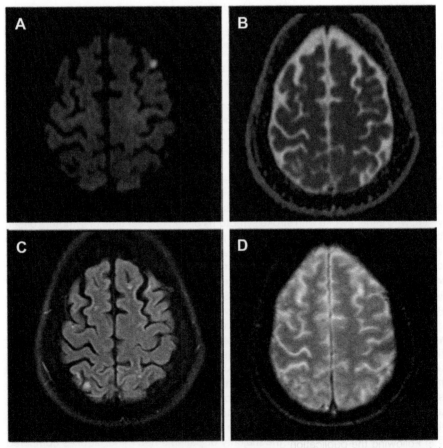

Fig. 1. MRI brain without contrast shows an area of restricted diffusion on DWI sequence (*A*) in the left frontal lobe with apparent diffusion coefficient correlate (*B*) and no evidence of correlating hyperintensity on FLAIR sequence (*C*), suggesting an acute infarct. Gradient echo sequence (*D*) was negative for acute hemorrhage.

sequences, such as DWI, FLAIR, apparent diffusion coefficient and gradient echo, or susceptibility-weighted imaging, to rapidly assess this patient demographic for thrombolysis candidacy. **Fig. 1** provides an illustrative case with a radiographic example.

Case presentation

A 62-year-old male with type II diabetes, hypertension, and hyperlipidemia awoke with expressive aphasia and impaired executive function. NIHSS was 1 for aphasia. He reported concern that his deficits would impair his ability to work as a contractor and operate heavy machinery. He was taken for rapid MRI brain—completed in 8 minutes—with the limited sequences shown below. After informed consent, the patient was treated with IV alteplase based on DWI-FLAIR mismatch and his concern for disabling symptoms. The following day his symptoms had improved with an NIHSS of 0.

Current Evidence for Tenecteplase Thrombolysis

Although intravenous alteplase is currently the only agent approved by the USFDA for the treatment of acute ischemic stroke, a second fibrinolytic, tenecteplase, may be as effective. Tenecteplase is a variant of alteplase bioengineered to have higher fibrin specificity and increased resistance to plasminogen activator inhibitor-1, and is administered via a single intravenous bolus. In the largest trial comparing tenecteplase to alteplase in minor stroke patients (median NIHSS 4) without a major intracranial occlusion, tenecteplase at 0.4 mg/kg failed to demonstrate superiority, but had a safety and efficacy profile similar to that of alteplase.[13] Current guidelines recommended that tenecteplase may be considered as an alternative treatment for patients with a minor stroke without a large vessel occlusion at a class IIb level recommendation.[9] A more recent meta-analysis of 5 tenecteplase stroke trials demonstrated that tenecteplase has noninferior safety and efficacy relative to alteplase for the primary endpoint of freedom from disability (mRS of 0–1) at 3 months.[14] Because of the shorter time to prepare and administer tenecteplase and the lack of requirement for an IV infusion pump during interfacility transfer, some institutions have adopted its use.[15]

ENDOVASCULAR MANAGEMENT OF ACUTE ISCHEMIC STROKE WITH LARGE VESSEL OCCLUSION

Proximal occlusion of a major intracranial vessel accounts for roughly one-third of all anterior circulation acute ischemic strokes. Unfortunately, intravenous alteplase is successful at recanalization of these occluded arteries only one-third of the time.[16] Before 2015, randomized thrombectomy trials in this patient population used inefficacious thrombectomy devices and had long delays from onset to treatment, leading to poor outcomes and lack of support for this treatment modality. In 2015, 5 clinical trials using newer devices were published showing clear benefit of endovascular therapy in the treatment of acute ischemic stroke with a large vessel occlusion from 0 to 6 hours from symptom onset.[17–21] In these studies, patients eligible for IV alteplase before embolectomy were still treated with thrombolysis. The Highly Effective Reperfusion Using Multiple Endovascular Devices (HERMES) meta-analysis published in 2016 included patient-level data from these 5 trials for a total of 1287 patients.[22] For the primary outcome of mRS score reduction by 1 point at 90 days, the authors found a common odds ratio of 2.49 favoring intervention.[22] This equated to a number needed to treat of 2.6. Following the publication of these studies, endovascular treatment became the standard of care for this patient population. **Box 3** outlines the inclusion criteria for such treatment when initiated within 6 hours from symptom onset.

Imaging studies required to determine eligibility for endovascular therapy include a noncontrast head CT and CT angiogram of the head and neck. CT perfusion (CTP) is not required. Some institutions may use MRI and magnetic resonance angiography (MRA) based on their local accessibility to such imaging. The ASPECTS is a 10-point topographic score used to assess early ischemic stroke changes on noncontrast CT scans in patients with MCA occlusions. As noted in **Box 3**, it is used as part of the inclusion criteria for endovascular therapy up to 6 hours from symptom onset. Because hypoattenuation on CT indicates infarcted tissue and injury that is more likely irreversible, treatment is no longer beneficial with lower ASPECTS. To calculate this score, 10 segmental areas in the MCA territory are each given 1 point, as visualized in **Fig. 2**. One point is subtracted from the total of 10 for each area that exhibits early ischemic changes with loss of gray-white differentiation.

Tenecteplase Before Endovascular Therapy

The Tenecteplase Versus Alteplase Before Endovascular Therapy for Ischemic Stroke (EXTEND-IA TNK) trial investigated intravenous tenecteplase, 0.25 mg/kg as a single bolus, versus intravenous alteplase at standard dosing in patients presenting within 4.5 hours of symptom onset and eligible for endovascular therapy.[23] The primary outcome was reperfusion of greater than 50% of the involved ischemic territory or an absence of retrieval thrombus at the time of the initial angiographic assessment. This primary outcome was reached in 22% of the tenecteplase treated patients versus 10% of those treated with alteplase ($P = .002$ for noninferiority, $P = .03$ for superiority).[23] The tenecteplase group had a median mRS of 2 at 90 days versus a median mRS of 3 in the alteplase group ($P = .04$). An obvious critique of this trial is that the primary outcome was a radiologic outcome and not a clinical one. Regardless, the 2019 AHA/ASA guideline for the early management of acute ischemic stroke states that it may be reasonable to choose tenecteplase over alteplase in patients without contraindications for IV fibrinolysis who are eligible for mechanical thrombectomy.[9] A follow-up open-label trial comparing 2 doses of tenecteplase (0.4 mg/kg and 0.25 mg/kg) in patients with ischemic stroke due to large vessel occlusion did not find a radiographic or clinical advantage of the higher dose.[24]

Basilar Occlusion

Basilar artery occlusion carries very high fatality rates.[25] Treatment approaches to basilar artery occlusion have been heterogeneous, and the pivotal endovascular trials

---

Box 3
Inclusion criteria for endovascular therapy from 0 to 6 hours from symptom onset

Prestroke mRS of 0 to 1

Causative occlusion of the internal carotid artery or MCA segment 1 (M1)[a]

Age ≥18 years

NIHSS score of ≥6

Alberta Stroke Program Early Computed Tomography Score (ASPECTS) of ≥6

Treatment (groin puncture) can be initiated within 6 hours of symptom onset

[a]M1 is defined as the horizontal or sphenoidal segment of the MCA from the internal carotid terminus until the bifurcation.

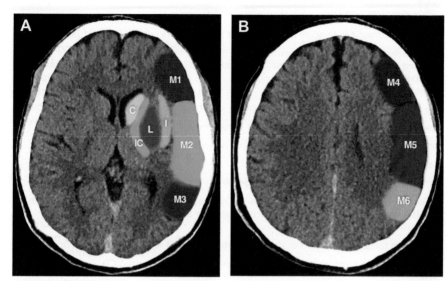

Fig. 2. (A) C = caudate, L = lentiform nucleus, IC = internal capsule, I = insular cortex, M1 = anterior MCA cortex, M2 = MCA cortex lateral to insular ribbon, M3 = posterior MCA cortex. (B) M4 = anterior MCA territory immediately superior to M1, M5 = lateral MCA territory immediately superior to M2, M6 = posterior MCA territory immediately superior to M3.

from 2015 included only small numbers of patients with basilar occlusion.[17–21] Despite the lack of evidence, due to the near-universal poor outcome in the absence of thrombectomy,[26] many institutions include basilar artery occlusion in their endovascular treatment protocol up to 24 hours from symptom onset.

Thrombectomy Beyond 6 Hours

Eligibility for mechanical thrombectomy was broadened beyond 6 hours in 2018 following the publication of the DWI or CTP Assessment with Clinical Mismatch in the Triage of Wake-Up and Late Presenting Strokes Undergoing Neurointervention with Trevo (DAWN) and Endovascular Therapy Following Imaging Evaluation for Ischemic Stroke (DEFUSE 3) trials. Each of these trials used different methods to identify patients with a mismatch between infarcted tissue and ischemic penumbra, selecting patients most likely to benefit from late endovascular therapy. The DAWN trial evaluated patients with a high NIHSS relative to a small infarct core (using CTP or DWI) in the setting of a proximal MCA or internal carotid artery occlusion, who presented between 6 and 24 hours from last known well. The primary outcome of an mRS score 0 to 2 at 90 days was seen in 49% of the thrombectomy group versus 13% in the standard medical group, which reached statistical significance and corresponds to a number needed to treat of 2.8. The rate of symptomatic intracranial hemorrhage and mortality did not differ between the 2 groups.[27] **Box 4** includes the DAWN eligibility criteria.

The DEFUSE 3 trial differed in that it selected patients with a proximal MCA or internal carotid artery occlusion who presented 6 to 16 hours from last known well with a perfusion-core mismatch ratio greater than 1.8 and maximum core size less than 70 mL. Specialized perfusion imaging software is required to assess infarct-perfusion mismatch. A core infarct area is usually depicted by reduction in cerebral

> **Box 4**
> **DAWN eligibility criteria**
>
> Symptoms attributable to acute ischemic stroke
>
> Patient belongs to one of the following:
> a. Failed IV t-PA therapy (defined as a confirmed persistent occlusion 60 min after administration)
> b. Contraindication for IV t-PA
>
> Age ≥18 years
>
> Baseline NIHSS ≥10 (assessed within 1 hour before measuring core infarct volume)
>
> Patient randomization could occur within 6 to 24 hours after time last known well
>
> Prestroke mRS of 0 or 1
>
> Anticipated life expectancy of at least 6 months
>
> Patients receiving heparin or low-molecular-weight heparin or an intravenous direct thrombin inhibitor within the last 24 hours from screening were eligible to participate if their coagulation profile was acceptable
>
> Subjects on factor Xa inhibitors or direct thrombin inhibitors were eligible for participation
>
> Less than 1/3 MCA territory involved, as evidenced using noncontrasted CTH or DWI sequence on MRI
>
> Occlusion of the intracranial ICA and/or MCA-M1, as evidenced by MRA or CTA
>
> Achievement of one of the following measures of Clinical-Imaging Mismatch on CTP or MRI
> a. 0 to 20 cc core infarct and NIHSS ≥ 10 (and age ≥ 80 years)
> b. 0 to 30 cc core infarct and NIHSS ≥ 10 (and age < 80 years)
> c. 31 cc to less than 50 cc core infarct and NIHSS ≥ 20 (and age < 80 years)
>
> *Data from* Nogueira RG, Jadhav AP, Haussen DC, et al. Thrombectomy 6 to 24 Hours after Stroke with a Mismatch between Deficit and Infarct. N Engl J Med. 2018;378(1):11-21. https://doi.org/10.1056/NEJMoa1706442.

blood flow (CBF) less than 30% of normal. Hypoperfused brain is a brain that is at risk for progression to infarction and could be salvageable with reperfusion. It is depicted by the prolonged or delayed time it takes for contrast to reach areas of the brain. There are different thresholds with the most common being a time to maximum (Tmax) greater than 6 seconds. Tmax and CBF are the main parameters to determine core and penumbra. A penumbra or mismatch volume can be calculated by subtracting the infarct core volume from the total area of hypoperfused brain.

At 90 days, an mRS score of 0 to 2 was seen in 44.6% of the thrombectomy group versus 16.7% in the standard medical therapy group ($P < .0001$). The endovascular group was also found to have a favorable mortality rate at 14% compared to 26%, and there was no significant difference in the frequency of intracranial hemorrhage.[28] **Box 5** includes a detailed list of the DEFUSE 3 eligibility criteria.

As these are the only 2 randomized controlled trials that have demonstrated safety and efficacy for thrombectomy greater than 6 hours from symptom onset, only patients who meet the eligibility criteria for either DAWN or DEFUSE 3 should receive mechanical thrombectomy in this time window.[9] **Fig. 3** describes a case using RAPID© software to help assess for the radiographic Target Mismatch Profile.

CONTROVERSIES AND ONGOING CLINICAL TRIALS IN ENDOVASCULAR THERAPY
Large Core

It is unclear if patients with medium to large core infarctions could benefit from thrombectomy, as patients with large baseline ischemic infarctions (ASPECTS ≤6 and 7)

Box 5
DEFUSE 3 eligibility criteria

Symptoms attributable to acute ischemic stroke

Age 18 to 90 years

NIHSS score of ≥ 6

Treatment (groin puncture) within 6 to 16 hours after time last known well

Prestroke mRS of 0, 1, or 2

Occlusion of the intracranial ICA and/or MCA-M1, as evidenced by MRA or CTA

Achievement of all of the following radiographic measures (Target Mismatch Profile) on CTP or MRI
a. Ischemic core volume is < 70 mL
b. Mismatch ratio is ≥ 1.8
c. Mismatch volume[a] is $\geq$ 15 mL)

[a]Alternative neuroimaging inclusion criteria if perfusion imaging or CTA/MRA was technically inadequate:

a. If CTA (or MRA) was technically inadequate:
   • Tmax>6s perfusion deficit consistent with an ICA or MCA-M1 occlusion AND Target Mismatch Profile was met

b. If MRP was technically inadequate:
   • Occlusion of the intracranial ICA and/or MCA-M1 by MRA (or CTA, if MRA was technically inadequate and a CTA was performed within 60 minutes before the MRI) AND DWI lesion volume less than 25 mL

c. If CTP was technically inadequate:
   • Patient could be screened with MRI and randomized if Target Mismatch Profile was met.

Data from Albers GW, Marks MP, Kemp S, et al. Thrombectomy for Stroke at 6 to 16 Hours with Selection by Perfusion Imaging. N Engl J Med. 2018;378(8):708-718. https://doi.org/10.1056/NEJMoa1713973.

---

have been excluded from many of the thrombectomy clinical trials.[18–21] These patients were excluded based on prior evidence that large initial infarct volume was an independent predictor of poor outcome, mortality, and hemorrhagic transformation.[22,29–34] Subgroup analyses and meta-analyses have attempted to address this question. A subgroup analysis within the MR CLEAN trial failed to show benefit with thrombectomy in patients with an ASPECTS of 0 to 4.[17] However, this subgroup represented only 6% of the study population and was likely underpowered. Another meta-analysis assessed the impact of thrombectomy in patients with pretreatment ASPECTS 0 to 6 and found that 30.1% of patients achieved an mRS of 0 to 2 in the thrombectomy arm as compared to 3.2% in the medical management. On further subdivision, patients with an ASPECTS 5 and 6 achieved good outcome (33% and 38%, respectively) as compared to patients with ASPECTS of 0 to 4 (17%).[35] The HERMES meta-analysis also found that only 25% of the 126 patients with an ASPECTS 0 to 4 achieved an mRS of 0 to 2 at 90 days following thrombectomy.[22] Several clinical trials are currently planned to determine if endovascular thrombectomy is efficacious in these patients.[36–38]

Low National Institutes of Stroke Severity Scale

Currently, there is insufficient data to help with decision-making in patients with low NIHSS and proximal large vessel occlusions. Consequently, there are ongoing trials

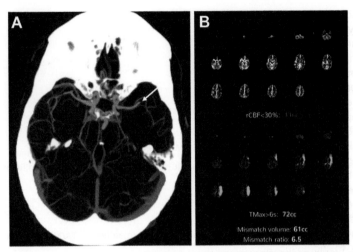

Fig. 3. Case presentation: A 31-year-old male with a prior left hemispheric stroke and alcohol use disorder presented to the emergency department 7 hours from last known well after he awoke with aphasia and right-sided hemiparesis. NIHSS was 15. CT angiogram of the head and neck showed an occlusion of the left middle cerebral artery at the M2 segment (*A*). CT perfusion showed a large perfusion deficit (*B*). Patient's imaging was felt to be favorable, given the core size of 11 cc was less than 70 cc, the mismatch ratio at 6.5 was above 1.8, and the mismatch volume at 61 cc was above 15 cc, meeting the radiographic parameters of the DEFUSE 3 trial. Consequently, the patient was taken for mechanical thrombectomy in the extended time window. A TICI 3 revascularization was achieved. Patient's NIHSS at 90 days was 1 for aphasia with an mRS of 1. The arrow is pointing to the occluded left middle cerebral artery.

investigating the efficacy of endovascular thrombectomy in these patients.[39,40] Some argue that the low NIHSS reflects sufficient collateral vascular supply to perfuse the ischemic territory, but others report cases where patients have robust, acute collateral compensation that later fails, leading to increased infarction. It is difficult to understand the appropriate intervention given these factors, thus necessitating further clinical trials.

Medium Vessel Occlusions

For patients with an occlusion of the MCA segment 2 (M2), the direction of treatment effect has been found to be positive, but not statistically significant.[22] The 2019 AHA/ASA Acute Ischemic Stroke Guidelines[9] state the benefits are uncertain in this patient population but treatment may be reasonable. Inadequate numbers of patients with MCA segment 3 (M3), anterior cerebral, vertebral, basilar, and posterior cerebral artery occlusions have been enrolled in clinical trials of endovascular therapy, so benefit in this patient population is also uncertain, yet may be reasonable in carefully selected patients. Further clinical trials are needed to assess patients presenting with medium vessel occlusions.

Telemedicine

Telemedicine has become a major tool for care delivery during the COVID-19 pandemic. However, telemedicine utilization in stroke care has been in place for many years before 2020.

The STRokEDOC trial assessed the efficacy of telemedicine versus telephone consultation regarding treatment decisions with IV alteplase. This prospective trial randomized patients to telemedicine or telephone consultation with a primary outcome of correct thrombolytic decision making. Secondary outcomes included IV alteplase use-rate, 90-day functional outcomes, postalteplase hemorrhage, and technical complications. It found that an accurate alteplase decision was made in 98.2% of telemedicine consultations versus 82% of telephone consultations (OR 10.9; 95% CI 2.7–44.6; $P = .0009$). No difference was found in 90-day functional outcomes, mortality, or post-tPA hemorrhage. There was an increase in alteplase use rate in the telemedicine group compared to the telephone consultation group (28% vs 23%, respectively; OR 1.3; 95% CI 0.7–2.5; $P = .4248$). Low technical complications and favorable assessment time were also found in the telemedicine group. This trial was pivotal in providing an evidence-based foundation for telemedicine implementation within stroke neurology.[41]

Use of telemedicine to direct thrombolysis treatment has also been shown to have similar complication rates as those reported in the National Institute of Neurologic Disorders and Stroke Trial,[1,42] helping to assert the safety of using telemedicine in this capacity. Telemedicine stroke care networks are also a means to increase the use of thrombolysis in rural and underserved areas.[43] Improved treatment rates have been attributed to increased access to neurologic expertise. It is presumed that with increased use of thrombolysis in appropriately selected candidates, there would be a positive effect on patient outcomes. However, further clinical trials are needed to formally assess the use of telestroke and outcome.

SUMMARY

There are many therapies available to reduce disability after acute ischemic stroke. When approaching a patient with symptoms consistent with acute ischemic stroke, the first step is to obtain a last known well time, an onset of symptoms time, and an NIHSS as the patient is taken for imaging. If the patient was last known well less than 6 hours before presentation, obtain a noncontrasted head CT to rule out intracranial hemorrhage, and CTA head and neck to assess for a large vessel occlusion. If the patient has a disabling deficit, normal glucose, and a last known well less than 4.5 hours, assess for alteplase candidacy. If the patient has disabling deficits, symptom onset time is unknown and has no contraindication to alteplase, obtain a rapid MRI brain to determine if there is a DWI-FLAIR mismatch and no hemorrhage to determine alteplase candidacy. If the patient is found to have a proximal large vessel occlusion, has an ASPECTS score ≥ 6 and an NIHSS ≥ 6, proceed to endovascular intervention. If, however, the patient is eligible for both alteplase and endovascular reperfusion, treat with alteplase first if it does not delay endovascular intervention. In patients with a last known well greater than 6 hours and less than 24 hours, obtain a noncontrasted head CT, CTA head and neck, and CT perfusion or rapid MRI brain with MRA head and neck to determine if a patient has a large vessel occlusion and is an endovascular candidate using the DAWN or DEFUSE-3 inclusion criteria.

DISCLOSURE

The authors have nothing to disclose.

REFERENCE

1. Tissue plasminogen activator for acute ischemic stroke. N Engl J Med 1995; 333(24):1581–7.

2. Ingall TJ, O'Fallon WM, Asplund K, et al. Findings from the reanalysis of the NINDS tissue plasminogen activator for acute ischemic stroke treatment trial. Stroke 2004;35(10):2418–24.

3. Hacke W, Kaste M, Bluhmki E, et al. Thrombolysis with alteplase 3 to 4.5 hours after acute ischemic stroke. N Engl J Med 2008;359(13):1317–29.

4. Demaerschalk BM, Kleindorfer DO, Adeoye OM, et al. Scientific rationale for the inclusion and exclusion criteria for intravenous alteplase in acute ischemic stroke. Stroke 2016;47(2):581–641.

5. Cucchiara BL, Jackson B, Weiner M, et al. Usefulness of checking platelet count before thrombolysis in acute ischemic stroke. Stroke 2007;38(5):1639–40.

6. Saposnik G, Fang J, Kapral MK, et al. The iScore predicts effectiveness of thrombolytic therapy for acute ischemic stroke. Stroke 2012;43(5):1315–22.

7. Jauch EC, Saver JL, Adams HP Jr, et al. Guidelines for the early management of patients with acute ischemic stroke: a guideline for healthcare professionals from the American Heart Association/American Stroke Association. Stroke 2013;44(3):870–947.

8. Khatri P, Kleindorfer DO, Devlin T, et al. Effect of alteplase vs aspirin on functional outcome for patients with acute ischemic stroke and minor nondisabling neurologic deficits: the PRISMS randomized clinical trial. JAMA 2018;320(2):156–66.

9. Powers WJ, Rabinstein AA, Ackerson T, et al. Guidelines for the early management of patients with acute ischemic stroke: 2019 update to the 2018 guidelines for the early management of acute ischemic stroke: a guideline for healthcare professionals from the American Heart Association/American Stroke Association. Stroke 2019;50(12):e344–418.

10. Rimmele DL, Thomalla G. Wake-up stroke: clinical characteristics, imaging findings, and treatment option - an update. Front Neurol 2014;5:35.

11. Schwamm LH, Wu O, Song SS, et al. Intravenous thrombolysis in unwitnessed stroke onset: MR WITNESS trial results. Ann Neurol 2018;83(5):980–93.

12. Thomalla G, Simonsen CZ, Boutitie F, et al. MRI-guided thrombolysis for stroke with unknown time of onset. N Engl J Med 2018;379(7):611–22.

13. Logallo N, Novotny V, Assmus J, et al. Tenecteplase versus alteplase for management of acute ischaemic stroke (NORTEST): a phase 3, randomised, open-label, blinded endpoint trial. Lancet Neurol 2017;16:781–8.

14. Burgos AM, Saver JL. Evidence that tenecteplase is noninferior to alteplase for acute ischemic stroke: meta-analysis of 5 randomized trials. Stroke 2019;50(8):2156–62.

15. Warach SJ, Saver JL. Stroke thrombolysis with tenecteplase to reduce emergency department spread of coronavirus disease 2019 and shortages of alteplase. JAMA 2020. https://doi.org/10.1001/jamaneurol.2020.2396.

16. Christou I, Burgin WS, Alexandrov AV, et al. Arterial status after intravenous TPA therapy for ischaemic stroke. A need for further interventions. Int Angiol 2001;20(3):208–13.

17. Berkhemer OA, Fransen PS, Beumer D, et al. A randomized trial of intraarterial treatment for acute ischemic stroke. N Engl J Med 2015;372(1):11–20.

18. Goyal M, Demchuk AM, Menon BK, et al. Randomized assessment of rapid endovascular treatment of ischemic stroke. N Engl J Med 2015;372(11):1019–30.

19. Saver JL, Goyal M, Bonafe A, et al. Stent-retriever thrombectomy after intravenous t-PA vs. t-PA alone in stroke. N Engl J Med 2015;372(24):2285–95.

20. Campbell BCV, Mitchell PJ, Kleinig TJ, et al. Endovascular therapy for ischemic stroke with perfusion-imaging selection. New Engl J Med 2015;372(11):1009–18.

21. Jovin TG, Chamorro A, Cobo E, et al. Thrombectomy within 8 hours after symptom onset in ischemic stroke. New Engl J Med 2015;372(24):2296–306.

22. Goyal M, Menon BK, van Zwam WH, et al. Endovascular thrombectomy after large-vessel ischaemic stroke: a meta-analysis of individual patient data from five randomised trials. Lancet 2016;387(10029):1723–31.

23. Campbell BCV, Mitchell PJ, Churilov L, et al, EXTEND-IA TNK Investigators. Tenecteplase versus alteplase before thrombectomy for ischemic stroke. N Engl J Med 2018;378:1573–82.

24. Campbell BCV, Mitchell PJ, Churilov L, et al. Effect of intravenous tenecteplase dose on cerebral reperfusion before thrombectomy in patients with large vessel occlusion ischemic stroke: the EXTEND-IA TNK part 2 randomized clinical trial. JAMA 2020;323(13):1257–65.

25. Baird TA, Muir KW, Bone I. Basilar artery occlusion. Neurocrit Care 2004;1: 319–29.

26. Schonewille W, Algra A, Serena J, et al. Outcome in patients with basilar artery occlusion treated conventionally. J Neurol Neurosurg Psychiatry 2005;76: 1238–41.

27. Nogueira RG, Jadhav AP, Haussen DC, et al. Thrombectomy 6 to 24 hours after stroke with a mismatch between deficit and infarct. N Engl J Med 2018;378(1): 11–21.

28. Albers GW, Marks MP, Kemp S, et al. Thrombectomy for stroke at 6 to 16 hours with selection by perfusion imaging. New Engl J Med 2018;378(8):708–18.

29. Thijs VN, Lansberg MG, Beaulieu C, et al. Is early ischemic lesion volume on diffusion-weighted imaging an independent predictor of stroke outcome? A multivariable analysis. Stroke 2000;31(11):2597–602.

30. Lansberg MG, Thijs VN, Bammer R, et al. Risk factors of symptomatic intracerebral hemorrhage after tPA therapy for acute stroke. Stroke 2007;38(8):2275–8.

31. Kimura K, Iguchi Y, Shibazaki K, et al. Large ischemic lesions on diffusion-weighted imaging done before intravenous tissue plasminogen activator thrombolysis predicts a poor outcome in patients with acute stroke. Stroke 2008; 39(8):2388–91.

32. Nezu T, Koga M, Kimura K, et al. Pretreatment ASPECTS on DWI predicts 3-month outcome following rt-PA: SAMURAI rt-PA Registry. Neurology 2010;75(6): 555–61.

33. Albers GW, Thijs VN, Wechsler L, et al. Magnetic resonance imaging profiles predict clinical response to early reperfusion: the diffusion and perfusion imaging evaluation for understanding stroke evolution (DEFUSE) study. Ann Neurol 2006;60(5):508–17.

34. Mlynash M, Lansberg MG, De Silva DA, et al. Refining the definition of the malignant profile: insights from the DEFUSE-EPITHET pooled data set. Stroke 2011; 42(5):1270–5.

35. Cagnazzo F, Derraz I, Dargazanli C, et al. Mechanical thrombectomy in patients with acute ischemic stroke and ASPECTS ≤6: a meta-analysis. J Neurointerv Surg 2020;12(4):350–5.

36. Bendszus M. Efficacy and safety of thrombectomy in stroke with extended lesion and extended time window (tension). NIH U.S. National Library of Medicine. ClinicalTrials.gov. Available at: https://clinicaltrials.gov/ct2/show/NCT03094715. Accessed April 16, 2021.

37. Zaidat OO. The TESLA trial: thrombectomy for emergent salvage of large anterior circulation ischemic stroke (TESLA). NIH U.S. National Library of Medicine.

ClinicalTrials.gov. Available at: https://clinicaltrials.gov/ct2/show/NCT03805308. Accessed April 16, 2021.

38. Large stroke therapy evaluation (LASTE). NIH U.S. National Library of Medicine. ClinicalTrials.gov. Available at: https://clinicaltrials.gov/ct2/show/NCT03811769. Accessed April 16, 2021.

39. Nogueira RG. Endovascular therapy for low nihss ischemic strokes (ENDOLOW). NIH U.S. National Library of Medicine. ClinicalTrials.gov. Available at: https://clinicaltrials.gov/ct2/show/NCT04167527. Accessed April 16, 2021.

40. Minor stroke therapy evaluation (MOSTE). NIH U.S. National Library of Medicine. ClinicalTrials.gov. Available at: https://clinicaltrials.gov/ct2/show/NCT03796468. Accessed April 16, 2021.

41. Meyer BC, Raman R, Hemmen T, et al. Efficacy of site-independent telemedicine in the STRokE DOC trial: a randomised, blinded, prospective study. Lancet Neurol 2008;7(9):787–95.

42. Audebert HJ, Kukla C, Claranau SCv, et al. Telemedicine for safe and extended use of thrombolysis in stroke. Stroke 2005;36(2):287–91.

43. Amorim E, Shih MM, Koehler SA, et al. Impact of telemedicine implementation in thrombolytic use for acute ischemic stroke: the University of Pittsburgh Medical Center telestroke network experience. J Stroke Cerebrovasc Dis 2013;22(4): 527–31.

Inpatient Management of Acute Stroke and Transient Ischemic Attack

Lauren Patrick, MD[a,b], Cathra Halabi, MD[a,b,*]

KEYWORDS

- Acute ischemic stroke • Transient ischemic attack • Antithrombotics
- Quality metrics

KEY POINTS

- Quality metrics standardize inpatient management of acute stroke to improve stroke care and related outcomes.
- TIA and stroke are medical emergencies that require prompt diagnostic evaluation and therapeutic intervention.
- Evaluation and management are guided by suspected etiology.
- Short-term dual antiplatelet therapy is indicated in very specific clinical situations.

FOUNDATIONAL PRINCIPLES
Quality Metrics and Performance Measures

Stroke is a condition with evidence-based diagnostic and treatment strategies. To improve adherence to clinical practice guidelines, numerous organizations in the United States developed initiatives to endorse hospital-based quality metrics; some metrics are additionally endorsed as performance measures for institutional feedback.[1-3] Organizations such as the American Heart Association (AHA)/American Stroke Association (ASA) Get With The Guidelines (GWTG) registry, The Joint Commission, Centers for Disease Control, National Quality Forum, and the Centers for Medicare & Medicaid Services routinely evaluate scientific evidence to reassess quality metric endorsements.

As one example, GWTG is a national registry program that standardizes stroke care. Participating institutions report structured information for each hospitalized patient with a stroke-related diagnosis including demographics, stroke etiology (modeled after Trial of Org 10,172 in Acute Stroke Treatment, or TOAST, subtypes), and

The authors have no financial conflicts of interest to disclose.

[a] Department of Neurology, Division of Neurovascular, University of California San Francisco, 505 Parnassus Avenue, M-830, San Francisco, CA 94143, USA; [b] Weill Institute for Neuroscience, San Francisco, CA, USA

* Corresponding author. UCSF Weill Institute for Neuroscience, 1651 4th Street, San Francisco, CA 94143.

E-mail address: cathra.halabi@ucsf.edu

Neurol Clin 40 (2022) 33–43
https://doi.org/10.1016/j.ncl.2021.08.003
0733-8619/22/© 2021 Elsevier Inc. All rights reserved.

neurologic.theclinics.com

prespecified quality metrics and performance measures. Harmonized metrics within GWTG and other initiatives include reducing time to intravenous thrombolysis, early antithrombotic initiation, venous thromboembolism prophylaxis, dysphagia screening, antithrombotics prescribed at discharge, intensive statin initiation, smoking cessation counseling, stroke education, and assessment for rehabilitation.[3] Participation in a data repository is additionally endorsed by practice guidelines.[4]

The Importance of Urgent Evaluation for Cerebrovascular Ischemic Events

The primary objectives in acute stroke and TIA care are to identify etiology while initiating treatment to reduce the risk of recurrence. The highest risk period following TIA is within 48 hours; rapid evaluation and treatment are associated with reduced risk of stroke.[5] TIA and stroke are therefore both neurologic emergencies. Patients with TIA should be evaluated and treated emergently; a standard evaluation must be completed definitively within 24 to 48 hours to identify intervenable etiologies. Hospital observation for high-risk TIA patients allows for emergent interventions if symptoms recur or worsen.[5] Most other patients diagnosed with stroke will require hospital admission for structured evaluation and management aligned with quality and performance measures known to improve outcomes.

Stroke Classification Schemes

The TOAST criteria were developed to categorize ischemic stroke into 5 major etiologies[6]: large artery atherosclerosis, cardioembolism, small vessel occlusion (lacune), stroke of other determined etiology, and stroke of undetermined etiology (now cryptogenic stroke, of which half are embolic stroke of undetermined source). Other classification schemes exist, but convenience and moderate interobserver reliability has sustained TOAST as a common research and clinical classification mechanism,[7] including for data registries such as GWTG. Diagnostic methodology improvements are now more likely to identify an etiology in cases that would previously have been categorized as undetermined.

Transient Ischemic Attack and Minor Ischemic Stroke

Transient ischemic attack is transient neurologic dysfunction caused by brain, spinal cord, or retinal ischemia in a vascular distribution without radiographic evidence of infarct. This tissue-based definition is more accurate than time-based endpoints (symptoms lasting <24 hours) in predicting the risk of stroke.[8] The widely used ABCD^2 stroke risk calculator was originally intended to identify high-risk patients for hospitalization. ABCD^2 has suboptimal predictive performance as its score omits intervenable, high-risk features including atrial fibrillation, carotid stenosis, and infarct. Newer iterations (ABCD^2-I, ABCD^3-I) include acute infarct in risk estimates[9] though ABCD^2 remains ubiquitous in stroke study design for harmonization with prior work. We emphasize that disposition following TIA should be determined clinically given the notable limitations of the ABCD^2 score.

Minor stroke is defined as infarct with NIHSS less than 5 and nondisabling deficits.[10] The Platelet-Oriented Inhibition in New TIA and Minor Ischemic Stroke (POINT) trial showed decreased risk of recurrent ischemic events with a short course of dual antiplatelet therapy (DAPT) in patients with TIA and minor stroke (defined in POINT as NIHSS $\leq$3) without apparent cardioembolic or carotid disease[11]; subsequent analysis revealed the benefit of DAPT was maximal in the first 21 days.[12] In a higher risk population, the Acute Stroke or Transient Ischemic Attack Treated with Ticagrelor and Acetylsalicylic Acid for Prevention of Stroke and Death (THALES) trial showed short-course DAPT with ticagrelor with aspirin improved stroke risk reduction in TIA/minor stroke but with higher rates hemorrhage in the DAPT group.[13] Patients with TIA/minor stroke with NIHSS $\leq$3 and ABCD^2 $\geq$4 presenting early may be treated with a loading dose of clopidogrel (600 mg) followed by 75 mg daily for 21 days in addition to aspirin 81 mg daily indefinitely. DAPT is used only if there are no other identifiable etiologies with specific treatment strategies (carotid stenosis, atrial fibrillation) and if thrombolysis is not administered acutely. Treatment should be implemented as early as possible in addition to other medical therapy described below.

Standard Stroke Evaluation

Evaluation must include brain imaging with computed tomography (CT) or MRI; MR diffusion-weighted imaging is more sensitive than CT for small and/or early infarcts and may be preferred for delayed presentations.[14] Noninvasive vascular imaging of the cervicocephalic vessels via CT or MR angiography or Doppler ultrasound is indicated to query symptomatic stenosis. A 12-lead electrocardiogram, transthoracic echocardiogram (TTE) with shunt evaluation, and telemetry monitoring (with extended cardiac rhythm monitor for 30 days) are indicated to query cardioembolic etiology such as atrial fibrillation or paradoxic embolism. Treating hypertension, insulin resistance, dyslipidemia, and tobacco use is also indicated.[5,14] Evaluation is expanded for patients with cryptogenic stroke, young patients, or patients with atypical presentations suggestive of a genetic disorder or secondary hypercoagulable state.

Prevention of Secondary Brain Injury

Hypoglycemia exacerbates energy failure and hyperglycemia is associated with worse outcomes after stroke.[15,16] Fever is also associated with worse outcomes after stroke and normothermia should be maintained with surface cooling and antipyretics.[17] Following the hyperacute period, blood pressure parameters require additional research; in general, hypovolemia and hypoperfusion are avoided to minimize further ischemia of penumbral tissue, and extreme hypertension with pressures $\geq$220/120 may be lowered cautiously. Antihypertensive treatment for pressures less than 220/120 within the first 48 to 72 hours is not recommended unless there is another indication to do so. Comorbid conditions must be considered when setting blood pressure goals for an individual patient.

Secondary Stroke Prevention

Core strategies to reduce stroke risk include antithrombotic, cholesterol-lowering, and antihypertensive therapies, plus insulin resistance treatment and lifestyle modifications (collectively referred to as medical management herein). Specific antithrombotic strategies will be discussed by stroke etiology below. Long-term blood pressure reduction is a critical modifiable risk factor; for every 10/5 mm Hg reduction, relative risk of stroke is reduced by nearly 30%.[18] Blood pressure can be lowered in the hospital after the 48- to 72-hour acute period with a plan to meet an outpatient target of less than 130/80 over days to weeks. Dyslipidemia therapy includes high-intensity statin with target LDL of less than 70 mg/dL.[19] One quantitative modeling study using stroke prevention strategies revealed relative risk reduction of second stroke by 80% over 5 years with the combination of lifestyle modifications plus aspirin, statin, and antihypertensive treatment.[20] Stroke prevention strategies may require adjustments based on diagnostic study results. Initiating secondary prevention during the hospitalization aligns with required quality metrics and performance measures.

EVALUATION AND MANAGEMENT BY STROKE ETIOLOGY
Intracranial and Extracranial Large Vessel Disease

Important causes of large vessel disease of the intracranial and extracranial arteries include atherosclerosis and dissection. Stroke from in-situ thrombosis or parent vessel thromboembolic events is strongly suspected when there is greater than 50% atherosclerosis in the culprit vascular territory; large vessel atherosclerosis accounts for 15% of stroke.[14] Intensive medical therapy is recommended for all patients with large vessel stroke or TIA. Revascularization may be indicated for some patients with extracranial atherosclerotic disease.

Diagnostic considerations

Digital subtraction catheter angiography is the gold standard for the evaluation of vessel stenosis and other features like collateral hemodynamics. In clinical practice, CT and MR angiography are preferred first-line studies. They are noninvasive with high sensitivity and specificity for stenosis. Carotid Doppler ultrasonography also has high specificity for severe carotid stenosis.[14] More recent revascularization trials (eg, Carotid Revascularization Endarterectomy vs Stenting Trial/CREST series) use noninvasive angiography. The North American Symptomatic Carotid Endarterectomy Trial (NASCET) criteria are used in the United States to measure carotid stenosis through invasive and noninvasive angiography. Diagnostic evaluation for nonatherosclerotic large vessel disease is tailored to the suspected etiology and may include central or systemic evaluation and is not discussed in detail here.

Management

Extracranial large artery atherosclerosis. Extracranial large artery atherosclerosis may affect the carotid and vertebral arteries and intensive medical management is indicated. Patients with carotid disease may be candidates for procedural revascularization with carotid endarterectomy (CEA) or endovascular carotid artery stenting (CAS). Medical management *without* carotid revascularization is preferred in men with symptomatic stenosis but luminal narrowing measuring less than 50% and women with symptomatic carotid stenosis but luminal narrowing measuring less than 70%.[21] Additional contraindications to carotid revascularization include severe medical comorbidities precluding safe procedural intervention, ipsilateral stroke with persistent disabling neurologic deficits, and total or near-total occlusion of the culprit carotid artery.[21] The decision to recommend revascularization should account for baseline stroke risk as well as risks and benefits of the intervention. Intervention should be performed by providers with less than 6% rate of periprocedural morbidity and mortality, between 2 and 14 days of last symptomatic event and ideally during index hospitalization.[22] Benefit of vertebral artery revascularization by any mechanism is not established and not recommended.[23]

Carotid endarterectomy. CEA is indicated in most patients with TIA or nondisabling stroke and severe stenosis (70%–99%) with a surgically accessible lesion, as supported by meta-analysis of the original NASCET, European Carotid Surgery Trial (ECST), and VA CEA trials.[24] CEA should also be considered in men with moderate (50%–69%) stenosis. Patients older than 70 years should undergo CEA over CAS. Contraindications include medical comorbidities that increase risk of perioperative adverse events, prior ipsilateral CEA, and life expectancy less than 5 years.[14,21] Early trials enrolled participants within 2 weeks of the index events, yielding current threshold for intervention during this period. Analysis of 4 randomized controlled trials (RCTs) showed that CEA was associated with lower rates of procedural complications compared to CAS when treatment was performed within 1 week.[25] Medical management with antiplatelet monotherapy remains indicated.

Carotid artery stenting. CAS is considered if the carotid lesion is not surgically accessible, the patient is not a surgical candidate, there is history of radiation-induced stenosis, or if the contralateral ICA is completely occluded.[21] Prior RCTs comparing CAS to CEA in symptomatic patients (International Carotid Stenting Study/ICSS, Endarterectomy vs Angioplasty in Patients with Symptomatic Severe Carotid Stenosis Trial/EVA-3S, CREST) demonstrated an increased risk of endpoints (stroke and death) with CAS at 30 days and long-term follow-up.[26–29] The Stenting and Angioplasty with Protection in Patients at High Risk for Endarterectomy (SAPPHIRE) trial suggested that CAS was not inferior to CEA but included mostly asymptomatic patients.[30] CREST long-term follow-up analysis revealed similar 10-year endpoints between CAS and CEA; prior subanalyses in symptomatic patients revealed higher rates of 30-day endpoints with CAS, especially in patients aged 70 years or older.[31]

Transcarotid artery revascularization (TCAR) is a hybrid procedure combining surgical exposure of the common carotid artery with stent deployment and concurrent flow reversal to prevent distal embolization. The TCAR surveillance project tracks outcomes, and studies thus far include registry analyses and single-arm safety and efficacy trials.[32] TCAR has not been directly compared to medical management or to CEA in randomized trials but registry analyses suggest comparative risk/benefit profiles to CAS. TCAR may be considered in patients who are not surgical candidates who also have severe vascular or cardiac disease precluding safe catheter angiography.[33] A course of DAPT is indicated for stenting procedures followed subsequently by antiplatelet monotherapy.

Intracranial large artery atherosclerosis. Intensive medical management and specifically daily aspirin 325 mg and systolic blood pressure goal of less than 140 are endorsed by recent guidelines for stroke prevention when the etiology is moderate to severe ICAS (50%–99% stenosis).[14] The Warfarin-Aspirin Symptomatic Intracranial Disease (WASID) trial compared warfarin to aspirin and revealed higher rate of hemorrhage and death with warfarin despite similar rates of stroke.[34] For patients with severe intracranial atherosclerosis (ICAS) (70%–99% stenosis) and related stroke or TIA, Stenting and Aggressive Medical Management for Preventing Recurrent Stroke in Intracranial Stenosis (SAMMPRIS) showed reduced risk of stroke and death in the medical treatment arm compared to intracranial artery stenting.[35] Medical treatment included daily aspirin 325 mg indefinitely and clopidogrel 75 mg for 90 days. Specific DAPT regimens have not been compared with each other.

Angioplasty and stenting in the absence of intensive medical management is not recommended; there is equipoise for patients with rapid clinical deterioration despite medical management. In summary, aspirin 325 mg daily is indicated for moderate to severe ICAS causing stroke or TIA. For patients with severe ICAS presenting within 30 days of the index event, the addition of clopidogrel 75 mg daily for 90 days is likely of benefit in preventing stroke recurrence.[14]

Cervical vessel dissection. The most common etiology of stroke from nonatherosclerotic large artery disease is arterial dissection. Antithrombotic therapy is indicated for secondary prevention after stroke or TIA.[36] The Cervical Artery Dissection In Stroke Study (CADISS) trial randomized patients with extracranial carotid and vertebral artery dissection and stroke or TIA to anticoagulation or antiplatelet therapy; there was no significant difference in ipsilateral stroke or death within 3 months, and anticoagulation was associated with increased bleeding risk.[36] Recently, the Biomarkers and Antithrombotic Treatment in Cervical Artery Dissection (TREAT-CAD) trial was designed to test noninferiority of aspirin to vitamin K antagonists in patients with cervical artery dissection.[37] Results did not confirm noninferiority of aspirin. Based on expert consensus, current guidelines recommend antithrombotics for at least 3 months after TIA or stroke from dissection with either aspirin or warfarin.[14]

Small Vessel Disease

Lacunar infarcts (<15 mm in diameter) occur in subcortical structures from occlusion of penetrating arteries and comprise 20% to 30% of ischemic infarcts.[38] Mechanisms for small vessel disease and lacunar infarcts include hypertension-related microangiopathy and microatheroma.[39] Risk factors for small vessel ischemic disease include hypertension, diabetes, dyslipidemia, and tobacco use.

Diagnostic considerations

Classic lacunar syndromes are diagnosed via clinical features, neuroanatomical localization, and presence of vascular risk factors. The standard stroke evaluation is recommended as a minority of subcortical infarcts may be due to cardioembolic or large artery thromboembolism, and early endarterectomy trials included patients with ipsilateral subcortical infarcts (thus identifying ipsilateral carotid stenosis remains of value).

Management

Treatment involves medical management.[40] A common pharmacologic regimen includes aspirin or clopidogrel monotherapy in addition to statin and antihypertensives. Aggressive small vessel risk factor control is important for stroke prevention but also prevention of cognitive impairment and vascular dementia.

Cardioembolism

Proximal sources of embolism account for 20% of ischemic strokes, largely from high-risk conditions of the cardiac structures.[41] Common examples of high-risk conditions include atrial fibrillation or flutter, left atrial thrombus, left ventricular thrombus, valvular vegetations (marantic or infectious), or prosthetic valves (bioprosthetic or mechanical).

Diagnostic considerations

Studies have demonstrated higher rates of atrial fibrillation detection with a longer duration of monitoring.[42,43] TTE is cost-effective and typically sufficient to diagnose significant structural and functional heart disease and some atrial septal defects. Contrast-enhanced echocardiography increases the sensitivity of TTE to identify left ventricular thrombus. Transesophageal echocardiography (TEE) may be useful for patients with cryptogenic stroke or young patients. TEE is used to identify left atrial thrombus, valve disease, and aortic atheromatous disease, and TEE can better characterize atrial septal defects.[14,44]

Management

Many cardioembolic sources of stroke or TIA have indications for anticoagulation, notably atrial fibrillation or flutter. Infarct size and hemorrhagic transformation guide timing of initiation. For small infarcts, anticoagulation can be started 2 days after acute thrombolysis therapy; for TIA due to atrial fibrillation, anticoagulation may be started immediately.[14] Larger infarcts or infarcts with hemorrhagic transformation may necessitate delaying anticoagulation therapy by at least 1 to 2 weeks.[45] Aspirin monotherapy is used until anticoagulation is initiated. Management strategies for select proximal sources of stroke and TIA are discussed below.

Atrial fibrillation or atrial flutter. For nonvalvular atrial fibrillation and atrial flutter, anticoagulants such as direct oral anticoagulants (DOACs) and warfarin are recommended for stroke secondary prevention. In this case, DOACs are as effective or better than warfarin with improved safety profiles including fewer rates of intracranial hemorrhage.[46] Patients who are unable to maintain therapeutic INR with warfarin should instead be prescribed a DOAC. DOAC dose adjustment or an alternative agent may be necessary for patients older than 80 years, with low weight, and renal impairment based on initial study design and renal clearance of these agents.

Valvular disease. Aspirin is indicated in patients with stroke or TIA who have aortic or nonrheumatic mitral valve disease. Patients with bioprosthetic aortic or mitral valves and history of stroke or TIA are also treated with aspirin following short-term anticoagulation during and after valve replacement. Patients with a history of stroke or TIA and mechanical mitral valve are treated with aspirin plus warfarin with a higher INR target of 3.

Cryptogenic Stroke Including Embolic Stroke of Undetermined Source

Approximately 25% of ischemic strokes do not have a determined etiology despite standard evaluation and are subsequently deemed "cryptogenic."[14] A proportion of cryptogenic strokes meet criteria for embolic stroke of undetermined source (ESUS), or nonlacunar infarct, without $\geq$ 50% stenosis of a parent vessel or high-risk source of proximal embolism and without another specific cause.[47]

Diagnostic evaluation

Standard and expanded diagnostic strategies may help diagnose etiology. CTA and MRA may identify large artery vasculopathy or subclinical atherosclerotic plaques. Transcranial Doppler with emboli detection may detect asymptomatic microemboli from large arteries or cardioembolic sources. TEE often follows nondiagnostic TTE, especially in patients younger than 60 years without vascular risk factors.[44] Extended cardiac event monitoring is indicated.[42] Depending on clinical context, hypercoagulable states from genetic, autoimmune, inflammatory, infectious, or occult malignant causes are considered. Systemic imaging may be useful, and serum studies may include inflammatory markers (ESR, CRP), genetic disorders (protein C/S deficiency, prothrombin gene mutation, factor V Leiden, antithrombin III deficiency[48]), hemoglobinopathies (eg, sickle cell), and other studies indicative of autoimmune (eg, APLS), inflammatory, neoplastic, or infectious states.[14] CSF evaluation can exclude inflammatory or infectious etiologies. Rarely, with recurrent or fulminant presentations despite exhaustive evaluation and intensive medical therapy, brain biopsy is indicated to exclude vasculitis, intravascular lymphoma, and certain infectious diseases.[49]

Management

Antithrombotic therapy. Secondary prevention of cryptogenic stroke may evolve with diagnostic study results. Medical management remains important given similar recurrence rates to established stroke subtypes.[50] Regarding ESUS, the New Approach Rivaroxaban Inhibition of Factor Xa in a Global Trial versus Acetylsalicylic Acid to Prevent Embolism in ESUS (NAVIGATE ESUS) trial and the Randomized, Double-Blind, Evaluation in Secondary Stroke Prevention Comparing the Efficacy and Safety of the Oral Thrombin Inhibitor Dabigatran Etexilate versus Acetylsalicylic Acid in Patients with ESUS (RE-SPECT ESUS) trial did not reveal reduction in stroke recurrence rates with DOACs against antiplatelet use[51,52] and DOACs are specifically not recommended for secondary prevention. A single antiplatelet agent (except ticagrelor) is indicated for secondary stroke prevention.[40] Diagnosis of an alternative condition such as occult malignancy or autoimmune condition warrants treatment of the underlying condition and possible adjustments to antithrombotic regimen (eg, anticoagulation for malignancy-associated hypercoagulable state and stroke).

Patent foramen ovale closure. Patients with ESUS and high-risk PFO without alternative etiology of stroke may be diagnosed with PFO-associated stroke. In specific patients, and following interdisciplinary shared decision making, PFO closure can reduce the risk of recurrent stroke at the expense of 4.9% rate of periprocedural complications and atrial fibrillation. Patients must be younger than 60 years with embolic-appearing stroke without alternative stroke etiology.[53] Patients with a PFO closure device require antiplatelet therapy.[14] Patients who do not meet the criteria for PFO closure should still be treated with antiplatelets.[51,54,55] If the patient has a PFO and evidence of other venous thromboembolism, anticoagulation is indicated and duration is dictated by treatment of the venous thromboembolism.

SUMMARY

Stroke and TIA are medical emergencies and emergent evaluation is indicated to improve outcomes. National quality metrics and stroke registries improve adherence to evidence-based clinical practice guidelines. All patients should receive standard diagnostic studies to determine etiology and guide selection of optimal secondary prevention strategies. Core evidence-based strategies always include antithrombotics, statin, antihypertensives if needed, diabetes treatment, smoking cessation, and other lifestyle modifications. Collectively, core strategies may significantly reduce the risk of stroke. Evaluation and management in the hospital setting with tailored secondary prevention strategies can profoundly reduce the risk of stroke recurrence.

CLINICS CARE POINTS

- Stroke and TIA are medical emergencies. Goals of early evaluation include determining etiology and initiating appropriate secondary prevention strategies.
- Risk of stroke after TIA is highest within 48 hours. Disposition following evaluation and treatment initiation should be determined clinically and not by ABCD2 criteria.
- Dual antiplatelet therapy is indicated in very specific conditions such as TIA (not attributed to specific cause like carotid stenosis or atrial fibrillation), and stroke or TIA due to severe intracranial atherosclerotic disease. The dual antiplatelet treatment course is for a prescribed time and followed by single antiplatelet therapy thereafter.
- Long-term blood pressure management is an extremely valuable modifiable risk factor for stroke and TIA of any etiology. Blood pressure reduction to a goal of <130/80 in most cases reduces risk of secondary events significantly.
- Patients < 60 years of age with ESUS and high-risk PFO may be candidates for PFO closure following shared decision making with the patient and interdisciplinary team.

REFERENCES

1. Association AH. Get with the guidelines stroke. Available at: https://www.heart.org/en/professional/quality-improvement/get-with-the-guidelines/get-with-the-guidelines-stroke.
2. Poisson SN, Josephson SA. Quality measures in stroke. Neurohospitalist 2011; 1(2):71–7.
3. Smith EE, Saver JL, Alexander DN, et al. Clinical performance measures for adults hospitalized with acute ischemic stroke: performance measures for healthcare professionals from the American Heart Association/American Stroke Association. Stroke 2014;45(11):3472–98.
4. Powers WJ, Rabinstein AA, Ackerson T, et al. Guidelines for the early management of patients with acute ischemic stroke: 2019 update to the 2018 guidelines for the early management of acute ischemic stroke: a guideline for healthcare

professionals from the American Heart Association/American Stroke Association. Stroke 2019;50(12):e344–418.

5. Easton JD, Saver JL, Albers GW, et al. Definition and evaluation of transient ischemic attack: a scientific statement for healthcare professionals from the American Heart Association/American Stroke Association Stroke Council; Council on Cardiovascular Surgery and Anesthesia; Council on Cardiovascular Radiology and Intervention; Council on Cardiovascular Nursing; and the Interdisciplinary Council on Peripheral Vascular Disease. The American Academy of Neurology affirms the value of this statement as an educational tool for neurologists. Stroke 2009;40(6):2276–93.

6. Adams HP Jr, Bendixen BH, Kappelle LJ, et al. Classification of subtype of acute ischemic stroke. Definitions for use in a multicenter clinical trial. TOAST. Trial of Org 10172 in Acute Stroke Treatment. Stroke 1993;24(1):35–41.

7. Radu RA, Terecoasă EO, Băjenaru OA, et al. Etiologic classification of ischemic stroke: where do we stand? Clin Neurol Neurosurg 2017;159:93–106.

8. Sacco RL, Kasner SE, Broderick JP, et al. An updated definition of stroke for the 21st century: a statement for healthcare professionals from the American Heart Association/American Stroke Association. Stroke 2013;44(7):2064–89.

9. Mayer L, Ferrari J, Krebs S, et al. ABCD3-I score and the risk of early or 3-month stroke recurrence in tissue- and time-based definitions of TIA and minor stroke. J Neurol 2018;265(3):530–4.

10. Levine SR, Khatri P, Broderick JP, et al. Review, historical context, and clarifications of the NINDS rt-PA stroke trials exclusion criteria: part 1: rapidly improving stroke symptoms. Stroke 2013;44(9):2500–5.

11. Johnston SC, Easton JD, Farrant M, et al. Clopidogrel and aspirin in acute ischemic stroke and high-risk TIA. N Engl J Med 2018;379(3):215–25.

12. Johnston SC, Elm JJ, Easton JD, et al. Time course for benefit and risk of clopidogrel and aspirin after acute transient ischemic attack and minor ischemic stroke. Circulation 2019;140(8):658–64.

13. Amarenco P, Denison H, Evans SR, et al. Ticagrelor added to aspirin in acute ischemic stroke or transient ischemic attack in prevention of disabling stroke: a randomized clinical trial. JAMA Neurol 2020;78(2):1–9.

14. Kleindorfer DO, Towfighi A, Chaturvedi S, et al. 2021 guideline for the prevention of stroke in patients with stroke and transient ischemic attack: a guideline from the American Heart Association/American Stroke Association. Stroke 2021;52(7):e364–467.

15. Godoy DA, Di Napoli M, Rabinstein AA. Treating hyperglycemia in neurocritical patients: benefits and perils. Neurocrit Care 2010;13(3):425–38.

16. Johnston KC, Bruno A, Pauls Q, et al. Intensive vs standard treatment of hyperglycemia and functional outcome in patients with acute ischemic stroke: the SHINE randomized clinical trial. JAMA 2019;322(4):326–35.

17. den Hertog HM, van der Worp HB, van Gemert HM, et al. The Paracetamol (Acetaminophen) in stroke (PAIS) trial: a multicentre, randomised, placebo-controlled, phase III trial. Lancet Neurol 2009;8(5):434–40.

18. Lawes CM, Bennett DA, Feigin VL, et al. Blood pressure and stroke: an overview of published reviews. Stroke 2004;35(3):776–85.

19. Amarenco P, Kim JS, Labreuche J, et al. A comparison of two LDL cholesterol targets after ischemic stroke. N Engl J Med 2020;382(1):9.

20. Hackam DG, Spence JD. Combining multiple approaches for the secondary prevention of vascular events after stroke: a quantitative modeling study. Stroke 2007;38(6):1881–5.

21. Brott TG, Halperin JL, Abbara S, et al. 2011 ASA/ACCF/AHA/AANN/AANS/ACR/ ASNR/CNS/SAIP/SCAI/SIR/SNIS/SVM/SVS guideline on the management of

patients with extracranial carotid and vertebral artery disease: executive summary: a report of the American College of Cardiology Foundation/American Heart Association Task Force on Practice Guidelines, and the American Stroke Association, American Association of Neuroscience Nurses, American Association of Neurological Surgeons, American College of Radiology, American Society of Neuroradiology, Congress of Neurological Surgeons, Society of Atherosclerosis Imaging and Prevention, Society for Cardiovascular Angiography and Interventions, Society of Interventional Radiology, Society of NeuroInterventional Surgery, Society for Vascular Medicine, and Society for Vascular Surgery. Developed in collaboration with the American Academy of Neurology and Society of Cardiovascular Computed Tomography. Catheter Cardiovasc Interv 2013;81(1):E76–123.

22. Vasconcelos V, Cassola N, da Silva EM, et al. Immediate versus delayed treatment for recently symptomatic carotid artery stenosis. Cochrane Database Syst Rev 2016;9(9):Cd011401.

23. Markus HS, Harshfield EL, Compter A, et al. Stenting for symptomatic vertebral artery stenosis: a preplanned pooled individual patient data analysis. Lancet Neurol 2019;18(7):666–73.

24. Rothwell PM, Eliasziw M, Gutnikov SA, et al. Analysis of pooled data from the randomised controlled trials of endarterectomy for symptomatic carotid stenosis. Lancet 2003;361(9352):107–16.

25. Rantner B, Kollerits B, Roubin GS, et al. Early endarterectomy carries a lower procedural risk than early stenting in patients with symptomatic stenosis of the internal carotid artery: results from 4 randomized controlled trials. Stroke 2017;48(6):1580–7.

26. Bonati LH, Dobson J, Featherstone RL, et al. Long-term outcomes after stenting versus endarterectomy for treatment of symptomatic carotid stenosis: the International Carotid Stenting Study (ICSS) randomised trial. Lancet 2015;385(9967):529–38.

27. Brott TG, Hobson RW 2nd, Howard G, et al. Stenting versus endarterectomy for treatment of carotid-artery stenosis. N Engl J Med 2010;363(1):11–23.

28. Mas JL, Trinquart L, Leys D, et al. Endarterectomy versus angioplasty in patients with symptomatic severe carotid stenosis (EVA-3S) trial: results up to 4 years from a randomised, multicentre trial. Lancet Neurol 2008;7(10):885–92.

29. Silver FL, Mackey A, Clark WM, et al. Safety of stenting and endarterectomy by symptomatic status in the Carotid Revascularization Endarterectomy Versus Stenting Trial (CREST). Stroke 2011;42(3):675–80.

30. Yadav JS, Wholey MH, Kuntz RE, et al. Protected carotid-artery stenting versus endarterectomy in high-risk patients. N Engl J Med 2004;351(15):1493–501.

31. Lichtman JH, Jones MR, Leifheit EC, et al. Carotid endarterectomy and carotid artery stenting in the US medicare population, 1999-2014. JAMA 2017;318(11):1035–46.

32. Malas MB, Dakour-Aridi H, Kashyap VS, et al. TransCarotid Revascularization with dynamic flow reversal versus carotid endarterectomy in the vascular quality initiative surveillance project. Ann Surg 2020.

33. Malas MB, Dakour-Aridi H, Wang GJ, et al. Transcarotid artery revascularization versus transfemoral carotid artery stenting in the Society for Vascular Surgery Vascular Quality Initiative. J Vasc Surg 2019;69(1):92–103.e2.

34. Chimowitz MI, Lynn MJ, Howlett-Smith H, et al. Comparison of warfarin and aspirin for symptomatic intracranial arterial stenosis. N Engl J Med 2005;352(13):1305–16.

35. Chimowitz MI, Lynn MJ, Derdeyn CP, et al. Stenting versus aggressive medical therapy for intracranial arterial stenosis. N Engl J Med 2011;365(11):993–1003.

36. Markus HS, Hayter E, Levi C, et al. Antiplatelet treatment compared with anticoagulation treatment for cervical artery dissection (CADISS): a randomised trial. Lancet Neurol 2015;14(4):361–7.

37. Engelter ST, Traenka C, Gensicke H, et al. Aspirin versus anticoagulation in cervical artery dissection (TREAT-CAD): an open-label, randomised, non-inferiority trial. Lancet Neurol 2021;20(5):341–50.

38. Moran C, Phan TG, Srikanth VK. Cerebral small vessel disease: a review of clinical, radiological, and histopathological phenotypes. Int J Stroke 2012;7(1):36–46.

39. Regenhardt RW, Das AS, Lo EH, et al. Advances in Understanding the Pathophysiology of Lacunar Stroke: A Review. JAMA Neurol 2018;75(10):1273–81.

40. Kernan WN, Ovbiagele B, Black HR, et al. Guidelines for the prevention of stroke in patients with stroke and transient ischemic attack: a guideline for healthcare professionals from the American Heart Association/American Stroke Association. Stroke 2014;45(7):2160–236.

41. Doufekias E, Segal AZ, Kizer JR. Cardiogenic and aortogenic brain embolism. J Am Coll Cardiol 2008;51(11):1049–59.

42. Gladstone DJ, Spring M, Dorian P, et al. Atrial fibrillation in patients with cryptogenic stroke. N Engl J Med 2014;370(26):2467–77.

43. Sanna T, Diener HC, Passman RS, et al. Cryptogenic stroke and underlying atrial fibrillation. N Engl J Med 2014;370(26):2478–86.

44. Katsanos AH, Bhole R, Frogoudaki A, et al. The value of transesophageal echocardiography for embolic strokes of undetermined source. Neurology 2016; 87(10):988–95.

45. Seiffge DJ, Werring DJ, Paciaroni M, et al. Timing of anticoagulation after recent ischaemic stroke in patients with atrial fibrillation. Lancet Neurol 2019;18(1):117–26.

46. Ruff CT, Giugliano RP, Braunwald E, et al. Comparison of the efficacy and safety of new oral anticoagulants with warfarin in patients with atrial fibrillation: a meta-analysis of randomised trials. Lancet 2014;383(9921):955–62.

47. Kamel H, Merkler AE, Iadecola C, et al. Tailoring the approach to embolic stroke of undetermined source: a review. JAMA Neurol 2019;76(7):855–61.

48. Chiasakul T, De Jesus E, Tong J, et al. Inherited thrombophilia and the risk of arterial ischemic stroke: a systematic review and meta-analysis. J Am Heart Assoc 2019;8(19):e012877.

49. Saver JL. CLINICAL PRACTICE. Cryptogenic stroke. N Engl J Med 2016;374(21): 2065–74.

50. Li L, Yiin GS, Geraghty OC, et al. Incidence, outcome, risk factors, and long-term prognosis of cryptogenic transient ischaemic attack and ischaemic stroke: a population-based study. Lancet Neurol 2015;14(9):903–13.

51. Diener HC, Sacco RL, Easton JD, et al. Dabigatran for prevention of stroke after embolic stroke of undetermined source. N Engl J Med 2019;380(20):1906–17.

52. Hart RG, Sharma M, Mundl H, et al. Rivaroxaban for stroke prevention after embolic stroke of undetermined source. N Engl J Med 2018;378(23):2191–201.

53. Shah R, Nayyar M, Jovin IS, et al. Device closure versus medical therapy alone for patent foramen ovale in patients with cryptogenic stroke: a systematic review and meta-analysis. Ann Intern Med 2018;168(5):335–42.

54. Kasner SE, Swaminathan B, Lavados P, et al. Rivaroxaban or aspirin for patent foramen ovale and embolic stroke of undetermined source: a prespecified subgroup analysis from the NAVIGATE ESUS trial. Lancet Neurol 2018;17(12):1053–60.

55. Kent DM, Dahabreh IJ, Ruthazer R, et al. Anticoagulant vs. antiplatelet therapy in patients with cryptogenic stroke and patent foramen ovale: an individual participant data meta-analysis. Eur Heart J 2015;36(35):2381–9.

Approach to Altered Mental Status and Inpatient Delirium

Sara C. LaHue, MD[a,b,*], Vanja C. Douglas, MD[a,b,1]

KEYWORDS

- Altered mental status • Delirium • Encephalopathy • Inattention • Elderly
- Postoperative • Hospitalized • Inpatient

KEY POINTS

- Altered mental status is a common occurrence in patients who present to the emergency department or who are hospitalized, and is associated with increased mortality.
- Altered mental status is descriptor, not a diagnosis, which requires a prompt and careful evaluation to exclude life-threatening precipitants.
- A thorough neurologic examination should be performed to exclude a focal deficit in someone with altered mental status.
- Delirium is not inevitable for older adults or those with cognitive impairment; rather, it can be prevented in 30% to 40% of cases by using multicomponent delirium prevention pathways.
- Delirium prevention and management should center on nonpharmacologic measures with reservation of medications (eg, antipsychotics) only to those who are at risk of harming themselves or others.

INTRODUCTION

Altered mental status describes a nonspecific change in baseline level of awareness, cognition, attention, or consciousness. There are many synonyms for altered mental status, and its imprecision can complicate both communication across providers and review of the literature for workup or management recommendations. Common synonyms for altered mental status include "acute confusional state" or "confusion," "acute brain failure," "encephalopathy," and "disorientation."[1,2] Although often used as a synonym, delirium is a more specific descriptor for an acute, usually fluctuating

[a] Department of Neurology, School of Medicine, University of California, San Francisco, CA, USA; [b] Department of Neurology, Weill Institute for Neurosciences, University of California, San Francisco, CA, USA

[1] Present address. 505 Parnassus Avenue, S784, San Francisco, CA 94143-0114.

* Corresponding author. UCSF Department of Clinical Neurology, Box 0114, 505 Parnassus Avenue, S784, San Francisco, CA 94143.

E-mail address: Sara.LaHue@ucsf.edu

Neurol Clin 40 (2022) 45–57
https://doi.org/10.1016/j.ncl.2021.08.004
0733-8619/22/© 2021 Elsevier Inc. All rights reserved.

neurologic.theclinics.com

altered mental status characterized by a decline in attention, and an additional cognitive deficit or altered level of arousal.[3] Both altered mental status and delirium serve as important phenotypes but are not in themselves diagnoses. Rather, they are symptoms resulting from a host of illnesses with varying time courses and levels of severity. The differential diagnosis of altered mental status includes conditions that are both life-threatening and reversible, and so a prompt systematic approach to the patient is key. This article provides an advanced overview for the neurologist evaluating and managing hospitalized adults with altered mental status.

EPIDEMIOLOGY

Altered mental status is commonly observed in hospitalized adults. Approximately 5% to 10% of adults presenting to the emergency department exhibit altered mental status, especially older adults, although some studies describe a bimodal age distribution with a high incidence also observed in very young children.[4,5] Altered mental status is a common reason for hospital admission and is associated with poor outcomes, including mortality in approximately 10% of patients.[6] The substantial adverse outcomes associated with altered mental status are best characterized in studies of older adults with inpatient delirium, which is present in an estimated 10% to 23% of patients admitted to a general medical service, 15% to 50% of postoperative patients, and as many as 85% of patients in the intensive care unit.[7-11] However, unless there is a standardized screening protocol, most recognized cases will exhibit agitation, as opposed to hypoactivity, which is a cause for underdiagnosis. Like altered mental status, delirium has traditionally been viewed as a transient condition with a benign prognosis. However, there is a strong body of literature documenting both the protracted course and significant clinical consequences experienced by many with delirium. Delirium is associated with prolonged hospital stay and readmission, loss of independence, and new or accelerated cognitive impairment.[12-18] Although delirium may result in a significant physical and psychological cost, it is also associated with a substantial economic burden, with an estimated attributable cost of $38 billion to $152 billion annually in the United States alone, or more than $182 billion annually in a combined population of 18 European countries.[9,19]

Although the need for swift identification and management of altered mental status is clear, complete understanding of its epidemiology is limited due to underdiagnosis by both physicians and nurses.[20,21] For instance, delirium may be unrecognized because of lack of screening, its overlap with cognitive impairment, its fluctuating course, and the expectation that this may be normal behavior for a hospitalized older adult.[22] As neurologists, we have the opportunity to identify altered mental status in our patients, especially in patients for whom we are consulted about an issue other than altered mental status, by performing a careful neurologic assessment.

INITIAL EVALUATION

The evaluation of a patient with altered mental status begins with a focused history (Table 1). As the patient may be unable to provide a history, it will likely be necessary to collect collateral information from family, friends, or the primary medical team. The first step is to determine the timeline for the mental status change, and the circumstances surrounding it, such as medication/drug use or trauma. An acute alteration in mental status is a medical emergency that requires a prompt, standardized evaluation. Airway, breathing, and circulation ("ABC's") should be assessed in tandem with an updated set of complete vital signs and finger-stick blood glucose. Tachycardia may be a sign of systemic infection, pulmonary embolism, or atrial fibrillation with rapid

Table 1	
Initial approach to altered mental status	
Initial evaluation	Vital signs; airway, breathing, and circulation
	Blood glucose level
	Consider naloxone
	Electrolyte panel, including sodium, potassium, chloride, bicarbonate, calcium, magnesium, phosphorus
	Complete blood count
	Urine toxicology
	Renal function tests
	Liver function tests including albumin
	Urine analysis with culture
	Chest radiograph
	Focused history: baseline cognitive function, time course
	Physical examination, looking especially for focal neurologic deficits
Subsequent evaluation	Brain imaging with computed tomography (CT) and/or MRI
	Lumbar puncture (performed after CT; should be performed initially if high suspicion for infection)
	Serum ammonia, thyroid function tests, vitamin B12
	Autoimmune serologies
	Blood cultures
	Electroencephalography (should be performed initially if high suspicion of status epilepticus)

ventricular rate. Hypoxemia and fever can each result in altered mental status and both shape the differential. Naloxone should be administered if there is a high index of suspicion for opiate overdose, which should not be overlooked in postoperative and hospitalized patients. If hypoglycemic, glucose should be administered, but only after thiamine supplementation to reduce the risk for developing Wernicke encephalopathy.

A focused neurologic examination, discussed in more detail later in this article, may reveal a focal finding that will guide initial management. An adult with acute altered mental status will frequently present as a stroke activation, in which case a National Institutes of Health Stroke Scale will be performed followed by a decision regarding acute stroke management. However, a general physical examination and detailed neurologic examination should follow, as described later in this article.

Additional tests should be obtained in tandem with the initial assessment. These include a complete blood count and comprehensive metabolic panel to look for aberrances in electrolytes, especially sodium, calcium, and magnesium, as well as renal and liver function. An arterial blood gas may be necessary if there is concern for hypoxemia or hypercarbia. Troponin and electrocardiogram should be considered to rule out myocardial infarction. Human immunodeficiency virus may be tested early to stratify immune status. Urine should be collected to look for infection and recreational substances; a postvoid residual can be measured if there is concern for urinary retention. A nasopharyngeal swab for Severe Acute Respiratory Syndrome Coronavirus 2 infection and a chest radiograph may be helpful if there is concern for lung infection.

History

Additional pieces of the history can be collected once the patient is stabilized. In addition to timeline, it is important to understand the patient's baseline cognitive function and the trajectory of the altered mental status; for example, does the mental status fluctuate (and if so, are there periods when the patient is close to baseline), or is the patient persistently altered? A fluctuating mental status oscillating between being altered and being at baseline may be more likely to be due to sleep deprivation or medications, whereas persistently altered mental status that may fluctuate but not return to baseline, may represent a more static process, such as an infection or stroke. Premorbid cognitive dysfunction is an important risk factor for the development of altered mental status, especially delirium, and may consist of features that can mimic delirium, such as hallucinations in Lewy body dementia. A wide array of comorbid medical conditions may also contribute to altered mental status, including epilepsy, known structural brain abnormalities (eq, tumor, ventriculoperitoneal shunt), chronic kidney disease, and liver disease. Immune status should be investigated both in medical history and medication review. New or recently discontinued medications or herbal supplements, and recreational substance use may also provide clues to the cause of altered mental status. A detailed review of systems should focus on symptoms referable to a systemic infection, such as headache, stiff neck, fever, cough, shortness of breath, or dysuria. Because history and review of systems may be limited, a through physical examination, in addition to a targeted battery of laboratory tests or imaging, will likely be warranted.

Physical Examination

The systematic general physical examination may offer clues to non-neurological causes of altered mental status and is crucial for guiding a targeted workup. One should examine the head and neck for evidence of trauma, tenderness, and meningismus. The cardiac examination should include a volume status assessment with inspection of jugular venous pulsations and extremities, and auscultation of the heart to assess for murmurs that may hint at endocarditis. Auscultation of the lungs may reveal evidence of volume overload or infection. Palpation of the back may cause point tenderness over the spinous processes, as in epidural abscesses, or over the kidneys, as in pyelonephritis. An abdominal examination may demonstrate ascites or tenderness. A careful skin examination may reveal stigmata of injection drug use or liver disease, or rash.

The primary goal of the neurologic evaluation is to assess for focal abnormalities. The mental status examination begins during the initial assessment of the patient, which may reveal the patient's level of alertness, attention, and thought organization through the course of obtaining the history and initial general physical examination. Although altered mental status may be viewed as a global cerebral dysfunction, the neurologist can identify underlying focal pathology that may be missed by the non-neurologist. Focal lesions, such as from stroke or tumor, may result in Wernicke aphasia (dominant superior temporal gyrus), abulia (frontal lobe, anterior cingulate cortex, basal ganglia), agitation (nondominant parietal lobe), and coma (reticular activating system). Lesions in these locations often produce colocalizing signs, such as a homonymous hemianopsia, pyramidal weakness, neglect, or loss of brainstem reflexes, respectively. Although most patients with acute altered mental status do not have stroke, altered mental status is common in patients with stroke: one recent meta-analysis found that delirium occurred in 25% of patients within 6 weeks of a stroke.[23]

The mental status examination may result in a clinical diagnosis of delirium, although the remainder of the examination and workup must be completed to uncover its etiology. The mental status examination may include targeted delirium assessments using validated scales. The "gold standard" research criteria for a diagnosis of delirium are found in the *Diagnostic and Statistical Manual of Mental Disorders, Fifth Edition* (DSM-5).[24] One of the most widely used and validated, and simpler, scales is the Confusion

Assessment Method (CAM), which includes 4 fundamental features of delirium: (1) acute onset and fluctuating course, (2) inattention, and either (3) disorganized thinking, or (4) altered level of consciousness.[25] Compared with the DSM, this scale has a high specificity for delirium diagnosis, is relatively efficient, and can be administered by a variety of health care professionals. The CAM has several adaptations, including for intensive care unit (ICU) patients (CAM-ICU).[14] Additional commonly used scales for non-ICU patients include the Delirium Rating Scale, Delirium Observation Screening Scale, and the Nursing Delirium Screening Scale.[26,27] Each scale has advantages and disadvantages, including complexity and requirement for training.[28] One recently developed delirium screening instrument that is brief and does not require additional training is the 4AT, which assesses for alertness, acute/fluctuating course, orientation, and attention (reciting the months of the year backward).[29] Not only are these scales useful to confirm the phenotype of delirium, they can also be used as daily screening tests for all hospitalized patients.

In the process of completing a thorough neurologic examination on a patient with altered mental status, one should remain vigilant for several key features associated with altered mental status. Thiamine deficiency may result in gaze palsies, nystagmus, and ataxia. Myoclonus or asterixis may be caused by uremia, hyperammonemia, or an offending medication (eg, cefepime, benzodiazepines). One should also evaluate for evidence of parkinsonism, which may suggest an underlying neurodegenerative disease such as Parkinson disease or Lewy body dementia. Identifying a focal deficit will guide subsequent management, which must include neuroimaging if a focal deficit is found, as well as consideration of blood tests, lumbar puncture, and/or electroencephalogram (EEG).

SUBSEQUENT EVALUATION

If the cause of altered mental status is not found with the initial workup, additional testing may be warranted. Mnemonics exist to organize the many causes of altered mental status, such as "AEIOU TIPS," and "VITAMIN E." Here, we will focus on the latter, which stands for: vascular, infectious, traumatic/toxic, autoimmune, metabolic, iatrogenic, neoplastic/neurodegenerative, and epileptic (**Table 2**).[30] As the differential for altered mental status is extensive, the workup can feel like an expensive, potentially harmful fishing expedition. For this reason, a focused algorithmic approach based on clinical suspicion is key.

The next step should be to obtain neuroimaging, especially if there is a focal finding on examination. A noncontrast computed tomography (CT) scan of the brain is an appropriate screen for intracranial hemorrhage, hydrocephalus, or a large mass, and vascular imaging of the head and neck can be included if there is concern for stroke. If the CT does not reveal an obvious precipitant for the altered mental status, then MRI brain with gadolinium should be pursued.

The utility of a lumbar puncture as part of an altered mental status workup is a common question for consulting neurologists. A head CT should be obtained before lumbar puncture in patients with altered mental status.[31] As nosocomial meningitis is uncommon, a lumbar puncture is most useful in patients who present to the emergency department with altered mental status, although it should still be considered in hospitalized patients with recent neurosurgery or skull fracture, medical devices or surgical hardware implanted in the central nervous system, or immunocompromise.[32] It is reasonable to have a low threshold to start empiric treatment for bacterial and viral meningitis given their high morbidity and mortality. In the setting of infection, cerebrospinal fluid (CSF) may be only mildly abnormal within 24 hours of symptom

Table 2 Common precipitants of altered mental status ("VITAMIN E")	
Vascular	Stroke (ischemic or hemorrhagic) Subarachnoid hemorrhage Hypertensive emergency and posterior reversible encephalopathy syndrome (PRES) Cerebral amyloid angiopathy (CAA) Vasculitis
Infectious	Urinary tract infection Pneumonia Encephalitis, meningitis Sepsis
Traumatic	Posttraumatic encephalopathy Subdural hemorrhage
Toxic	Intoxication or overdose Withdrawal Medications (prescription, over-the-counter, supplements)
Autoimmune	Vasculitis Systemic lupus erythematosus or Sjogren syndrome Steroid-responsive encephalopathy with autoimmune thyroiditis (SREAT), or Hashimoto encephalitis Acute disseminated encephalomyelitis Autoimmune limbic encephalitis

Metabolic	Electrolyte abnormalities (eg, hypo/hypernatremia,
	  hypercalcemia, hypermagnesemia)
	Endocrine abnormalities (eg, hypo/hyperglycemia,
	  hypo/hyperthyroidism, adrenal crisis, Cushing syndrome)
	Uremic encephalopathy
	Hepatic encephalopathy
	Thiamine or cobalamin deficiency
	Hypoxia, hypercarbia

Iatrogenic	Day/night dysregulation, sleep deprivation
	Sensory deprivation
	Limited mobility (use of restraints, urinary catheters)
	Surgery
	Untreated pain
	Polypharmacy, especially with certain medications
	  (eg, anticholinergics, antihistamines, benzodiazepines,
	  steroids, fluoroquinolone and cephalosporin antibiotics)

Neoplastic	Intracranial neoplasm (primary or metastatic) Paraneoplastic encephalitis Carcinomatous meningitis
Neurodegenerative	Alzheimer disease Lewy body dementia Prion disease
Epileptic	Nonconvulsive status epilepticus Postictal state

onset, or even normal, as can be seen in herpes simplex virus encephalitis.[33,34] For this reason, if one has a high suspicion for meningitis or encephalitis, the lumbar puncture should be repeated 72 hours later. CSF testing should be especially broad in those who are immunocompromised, including for fungal (especially *Cryptococcus*) and other viral (eg, cytomegalovirus) etiologies.

Abnormal CSF may also point toward autoimmune, paraneoplastic, or neoplastic etiologies. The detection of autoimmune encephalitis is increasing over time with more frequent testing and identification of new autoantibodies. Indeed, the prevalence and incidence of autoimmune encephalitis is similar to that of infectious encephalitis.[35] It can be helpful to test for oligoclonal bands and immunoglobulin G index (both in CSF and serum), as this may point to inflammation even if there is no pleocytosis; CSF protein may also be elevated in these cases. Additional workup with systemic imaging (CT chest, abdomen, and pelvis) and testing for autoantibodies on serum and CSF should be considered if inflammation is found. Carcinomatous meningitis is also a consideration, which may present with focal findings, such as cranial nerve deficits and ataxia, and is more likely to be found in patients with lymphoma, leukemia, melanoma, or lung and breast cancer.[36] Although MRI may show abnormal enhancement, including of the cranial nerves or nerve roots, obtaining both CSF cytology and flow cytometry increases the sensitivity of detection, especially if repeated.[37] The treatment of malignancy with chimeric antigen receptor T-cell immunotherapy or check point inhibitors may also result in meningitis or encephalitis, either as an adverse event from the medication or due to susceptibility to infection, and so testing is often warranted if altered mental status develops in these patients.[38,39]

Focal seizures with impaired awareness must be ruled out with EEG in every patient with altered mental status without a clear etiology, as the yield is high in patients with unexplained altered mental status on general medical wards.[40] Risk factors for seizure include history of prior seizure, mass, and infection, and so it is very reasonable to obtain EEG in patients with altered mental status.[41]

Additional serum studies beyond those described previously are warranted in certain clinical contexts. A comprehensive/extended toxicology screen may helpful but is time-sensitive. If there is a history of liver disease, presence of liver enzyme abnormalities, or use of hepatically cleared medications such as valproic acid, then an ammonia should be checked; hyperammonemia of unclear etiology may be due to a portal-systemic shunt.[42] In addition to the initial workup, other metabolic abnormalities, such as hypo/hypernatremia (especially if rapidly fluctuating), and vitamin B12 deficiency, should be considered. Endocrinopathies, such as hypo/hyperthyroidism, and autoimmune diseases, such as steroid-responsive encephalopathy with autoimmune thyroiditis (SREAT), or Hashimoto encephalitis, should be considered if antithyroid antibodies are present in the right clinical context. Additional autoimmune diseases such as systemic lupus erythematosus or Sjogren syndrome, can present with altered mental status; in those with an existing diagnosis of systemic lupus erythematosus, the presence of active disease should be screened for with antinuclear antibodies, double-stranded DNA, and complement levels.[41]

EVALUATION AND MANAGEMENT OF DELIRIUM

More extensive testing may not be necessary for a patient with a nonfocal neurologic examination, a clinical diagnosis of delirium, and clear risk factor(s) for delirium (**Box 1**). Delirium should improve once the precipitant is removed; if the patient does not improve, then additional workup is warranted. Once the diagnosis of delirium is established, the goals of the neurologic evaluation are to identify both risk factors (underlying vulnerabilities) and inciting events, which will then frame management recommendations. Some of the most common risk factors for delirium include advanced age, cognitive impairment, and hearing and vision impairments.[10,43–48] Indeed, in one prospective study, older adults with known dementia were 40% more likely to develop delirium; for general medicine service patients, those with dementia are 2.3 to 4.7

> **Box 1**
> **Delirium risk factors**
>
> Age >65
>
> Cognitive impairment or dementia
>
> Prior history of delirium
>
> Sensory impairment (vision, hearing)
>
> Immobility
>
> Impairment in activities of daily living
>
> Dehydration
>
> Malnutrition
>
> History of alcohol use or substance use disorder
>
> Multiple comorbid conditions

times more likely to develop delirium compared with those without dementia.[9,10] Given this association, older adults without a known diagnosis of cognitive impairment who develop delirium while hospitalized should undergo an outpatient neurocognitive evaluation. There are many precipitants for delirium, which, in addition to the causes of altered mental status discussed previously, include immobility (eg, physical restraints), dehydration, polypharmacy (especially the use of narcotics, benzodiazepines, or anticholinergics), bladder catheters, and surgery.[43,48,49] The postoperative period features several risk factors that exemplify the delicate balance of clinical care in older adults who are susceptible to delirium. For instance, both postoperative pain medication use, and inadequate pain management, are associated with the development of delirium.[50]

Once considered an inevitability for older adults in the hospital, clinical studies conducted over the past 30 years have demonstrated improved clinical outcomes, including a reduction in incident delirium by as much as 30% to 40% in both non-ICU medical and surgical patients through implementation of largely nonpharmacologic, clinical pathways (**Fig. 1**).[51–55] The first multicomponent delirium prevention pathway used several nursing interventions to mitigate delirium risk factors and provokers, including cognitive impairment (through cognitive stimulation, frequent reorientation), immobility, hearing impairment (through providing amplification devices), and making fluids more available to avoid dehydration. This protocol was inexpensive and was associated with a reduction of delirium incidence.[53] Similar evidence-based protocols are increasingly used in a variety of hospital settings with excellent results. Indeed, one Cochrane systematic review of 39 trials encompassing 16,082 patients found that multicomponent delirium interventions reduced delirium incidence when compared with usual care in both medical and surgical populations.[56] These protocols include both screening for delirium, as discussed previously, as well as calculating delirium risk on admission. The AWOL score, which incorporates age, spelling "world" backward (or serial 7s in non-English speakers), orientation, and illness severity, is an example of an efficient, validated delirium prediction scale for people admitted to the hospital from the emergency department.[57] Use of delirium risk prediction scores are especially helpful in settings in which delirium prevention resources are limited.

Pharmacology has largely been unhelpful, and at times harmful, when applied to delirium management. Indeed, a key intervention in the prevention and management

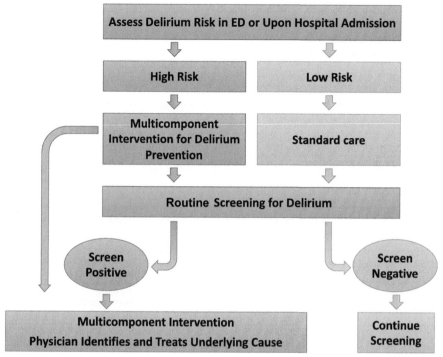

Fig. 1. Delirium care pathway.

of delirium is tapering or discontinuing medications that increase its risk or have a change in pharmacokinetics due to illness. Benzodiazepines should be avoided unless delirium is due to alcohol or sedative withdrawal. A recent Cochrane review of 9 trials demonstrated no reduction in delirium severity or duration in patients receiving antipsychotics of different classes compared with those who did not receive antipsychotics.[58] At this time, antipsychotics should be reserved for patients who are a danger to themselves or to staff. When used, the lowest dose should be used, and cardiac complications (eg, prolonged QT) should be monitored.[59] Use of antipsychotics should be reserved for extenuating circumstances because of both lack of effectiveness and risk of harm, as demonstrated in US Food and Drug Administration warnings of increased mortality in older adults with their use.[60]

There is increasing interest in other pharmacologic interventions, although current evidence does not support the use of any medication explicitly for delirium prevention or treatment. One Cochrane review of 14 trials of pharmacologic interventions (encompassing 6 drug classes) in critically ill patients found no difference between placebo and any drug with regard to delirium-free and coma-free days, or length of stay, although it did find that dexmedetomidine may shorten delirium duration.[61] In recently published sweeping practice guidelines for clinical management of ICU patients, no pharmacologic agent was recommended for delirium prevention or treatment, except for dexmedetomidine for when agitation from delirium may be precluding extubation.[62] Given mixed results, further research regarding the use of dexmedetomidine for delirium treatment is warranted. Although alterations in sleep-wake cycle are implicated in the development of delirium, administration of melatonin, or melatonin receptor agonist ramelteon, has been associated with delirium reduction in some, but not all, randomized controlled trials.[63–66] Melatonin is commonly used as the one pharmacologic intervention in multidisciplinary delirium care pathways given potential benefit and benign side-effect profile.

SUMMARY

Altered mental status is common in people presenting to the hospital, especially in older adults and those with cognitive impairment. Altered mental status is a helpful description that should result in a rapid search for the underlying diagnosis, which includes broad differential of life-threatening and reversible precipitants, to provide a targeted treatment plan.

CLINICS CARE POINTS

- Acute altered mental status should be evaluated as quickly as possible in order to identify and treat reversible causes.
- Altered mental status may be caused by neurologic and non-neurologic etiologies and so a broad work-up is warranted.
- Pharmacology has largely been unhelpful, and at times harmful, when applied to delirium management. Antipsychotics should only be reserved for patients who are a danger to themselves or to staff.

DISCLOSURE

Dr LaHue has nothing to disclose. Funding for Dr Douglas: Sara & Evan Williams Foundation Endowed Neurohospitalist Chair.

REFERENCES

1. Smith AT, Han JH. Altered mental status in the emergency department. Semin Neurol 2019;39(1):5–19.
2. Wijdicks EFM. Metabolic encephalopathy: behind the name. Neurocrit Care 2018;29(3):385–7.
3. American Psychiatric Association. Desk reference to the diagnostic criteria from DSM-5. Arlington, Va: American Psychiatric Association; 2013.
4. Wofford JL, Loehr LR, Schwartz E. Acute cognitive impairment in elderly ED patients: etiologies and outcomes. Am J Emerg Med 1996;14(7):649–53.
5. Hustey FM, Meldon SW. The prevalence and documentation of impaired mental status in elderly emergency department patients. Ann Emerg Med 2002;39(3):248–53.
6. Kanich W, Brady WJ, Huff JS, et al. Altered mental status: evaluation and etiology in the ED. Am J Emerg Med 2002;20(7):613–7.
7. Marcantonio ER. Delirium in hospitalized older adults. N Engl J Med 2017; 377(15):1456–66.
8. American Geriatrics Society Expert Panel on Postoperative Delirium in OlderAdults. Postoperative delirium in older adults: best practice statement from the American Geriatrics Society. J Am Coll Surg 2015;220(2):136–148 e131.
9. Inouye SK, Westendorp RG, Saczynski JS. Delirium in elderly people. Lancet 2014;383(9920):911–22.
10. McNicoll L, Pisani MA, Zhang Y, et al. Delirium in the intensive care unit: occurrence and clinical course in older patients. J Am Geriatr Soc 2003;51(5):591–8.

11. Gibb K, Seeley A, Quinn T, et al. The consistent burden in published estimates of delirium occurrence in medical inpatients over four decades: a systematic review and meta-analysis study. Age Ageing 2020;49(3):352–60.

12. Francis J, Martin D, Kapoor WN. A prospective study of delirium in hospitalized elderly. JAMA 1990;263(8):1097–101.

13. Salluh JI, Soares M, Teles JM, et al. Delirium epidemiology in critical care (DECCA): an international study. Crit Care 2010;14(6):R210.

14. Ely EW, Shintani A, Truman B, et al. Delirium as a predictor of mortality in mechanically ventilated patients in the intensive care unit. JAMA 2004;291(14):1753–62.

15. McCusker J, Cole MG, Dendukuri N, et al. Does delirium increase hospital stay? J Am Geriatr Soc 2003;51(11):1539–46.

16. Inouye SK, Rushing JT, Foreman MD, et al. Does delirium contribute to poor hospital outcomes? A three-site epidemiologic study. J Gen Intern Med 1998;13(4):234–42.

17. Siddiqi N, House AO, Holmes JD. Occurrence and outcome of delirium in medical in-patients: a systematic literature review. Age Ageing 2006;35(4):350–64.

18. LaHue SC, Douglas VC, Kuo T, et al. Association between inpatient delirium and hospital readmission in patients >/= 65 years of age: a retrospective cohort study. J Hosp Med 2019;14(4):201–6.

19. Leslie DL, Marcantonio ER, Zhang Y, et al. One-year health care costs associated with delirium in the elderly population. Arch Intern Med 2008;168(1):27–32.

20. Gustafson Y, Brannstrom B, Norberg A, et al. Underdiagnosis and poor documentation of acute confusional states in elderly hip fracture patients. J Am Geriatr Soc 1991;39(8):760–5.

21. Inouye SK, Foreman MD, Mion LC, et al. Nurses' recognition of delirium and its symptoms: comparison of nurse and researcher ratings. Arch Intern Med 2001;161(20):2467–73.

22. Inouye SK. Delirium in older persons. N Engl J Med 2006;354(11):1157–65.

23. Shaw RC, Walker G, Elliott E, et al. Occurrence rate of delirium in acute stroke settings: systematic review and meta-analysis. Stroke 2019;50(11):3028–36.

24. American Psychiatric Association., American psychiatric association. DSM-5 task force. Diagnostic and statistical manual of mental disorders : DSM-5. 5th edition. Arlington, VA Washington, D.C.: American Psychiatric Association; 2013.

25. Inouye SK, van Dyck CH, Alessi CA, et al. Clarifying confusion: the confusion assessment method. A new method for detection of delirium. Ann Intern Med 1990;113(12):941–8.

26. Gaudreau JD, Gagnon P, Harel F, et al. Fast, systematic, and continuous delirium assessment in hospitalized patients: the nursing delirium screening scale. J Pain Symptom Manage 2005;29(4):368–75.

27. Helfand BKI, D'Aquila ML, Tabloski P, et al. Detecting delirium: a systematic review of identification instruments for non-ICU settings. J Am Geriatr Soc 2021;69(2):547–55.

28. De J, Wand AP. Delirium screening: a systematic review of delirium screening tools in hospitalized patients. Gerontologist 2015;55(6):1079–99.

29. Bellelli G, Morandi A, Davis DH, et al. Validation of the 4AT, a new instrument for rapid delirium screening: a study in 234 hospitalised older people. Age Ageing 2014;43(4):496–502.

30. Brown EG, Douglas VC. Moving beyond metabolic encephalopathy: an update on delirium prevention, workup, and management. Semin Neurol 2015;35(6):646–55.

31. Hasbun R, Abrahams J, Jekel J, et al. Computed tomography of the head before lumbar puncture in adults with suspected meningitis. N Engl J Med 2001;345(24):1727–33.
32. Metersky ML, Williams A, Rafanan AL. Retrospective analysis: are fever and altered mental status indications for lumbar puncture in a hospitalized patient who has not undergone neurosurgery? Clin Infect Dis 1997;25(2):285–8.
33. Onorato IM, Wormser GP, Nicholas P. 'Normal' CSF in bacterial meningitis. JAMA 1980;244(13):1469–71.
34. Koskiniemi M, Vaheri A, Taskinen E. Cerebrospinal fluid alterations in herpes simplex virus encephalitis. Rev Infect Dis 1984;6(5):608–18.
35. Dubey D, Pittock SJ, Kelly CR, et al. Autoimmune encephalitis epidemiology and a comparison to infectious encephalitis. Ann Neurol 2018;83(1):166–77.
36. Clarke JL, Perez HR, Jacks LM, et al. Leptomeningeal metastases in the MRI era. Neurology 2010;74(18):1449–54.
37. Scott BJ, Douglas VC, Tihan T, et al. A systematic approach to the diagnosis of suspected central nervous system lymphoma. JAMA Neurol 2013;70(3):311–9.
38. Brahmer JR, Lacchetti C, Thompson JA. Management of immune-related adverse events in patients treated with immune checkpoint inhibitor therapy: american society of clinical oncology clinical practice guideline summary. J Oncol Pract 2018;14(4):247–9.
39. Gust J, Ponce R, Liles WC, et al. Cytokines in CAR T cell-associated neurotoxicity. Front Immunol 2020;11:577027.
40. Betjemann JP, Nguyen I, Santos-Sanchez C, et al. Diagnostic yield of electroencephalography in a general inpatient population. Mayo Clin Proc 2013;88(4):326–31.
41. Douglas VC, Josephson SA. Altered mental status. Continuum (Minneap Minn) 2011;17(5 Neurologic Consultation in the Hospital):967–83.
42. Raskin NH, Price JB, Fishman RA. Portal-systemic encephalopathy due to congenital intrahepatic shunts. N Engl J Med 1964;270:225–9.
43. Inouye SK. Predisposing and precipitating factors for delirium in hospitalized older patients. Dement Geriatr Cogn Disord 1999;10(5):393–400.
44. Inouye SK, Zhang Y, Jones RN, et al. Risk factors for delirium at discharge: development and validation of a predictive model. Arch Intern Med 2007;167(13):1406–13.
45. LaHue SC, Liu VX. Loud and clear: sensory impairment, delirium, and functional recovery in critical illness. Am J Respir Crit Care Med 2016;194(3):252–3.
46. Ryan DJ, O'Regan NA, Caoimh RO, et al. Delirium in an adult acute hospital population: predictors, prevalence and detection. BMJ Open 2013;3(1):e001772.
47. LaHue SC, Douglas VC, Miller BL. The one-two punch of delirium and dementia during the COVID-19 pandemic and beyond. Front Neurol 2020;11:596218.
48. LaHue SC, James TC, Newman JC, et al. Collaborative delirium prevention in the age of COVID-19. J Am Geriatr Soc 2020;68(5):947–9.
49. Inouye SK, Charpentier PA. Precipitating factors for delirium in hospitalized elderly persons. Predictive model and interrelationship with baseline vulnerability. JAMA 1996;275(11):852–7.
50. Wang Y, Sands LP, Vaurio L, et al. The effects of postoperative pain and its management on postoperative cognitive dysfunction. Am J Geriatr Psychiatry 2007;15(1):50–9.
51. Young J, Murthy L, Westby M, et al. Diagnosis, prevention, and management of delirium: summary of NICE guidance. BMJ 2010;341:c3704.

52. Hshieh TT, Yue J, Oh E, et al. Effectiveness of multicomponent nonpharmacological delirium interventions: a meta-analysis. JAMA Intern Med 2015;175(4): 512–20.
53. Inouye SK, Bogardus ST Jr, Charpentier PA, et al. A multicomponent intervention to prevent delirium in hospitalized older patients. N Engl J Med 1999;340(9): 669–76.
54. Strijbos MJ, Steunenberg B, van der Mast RC, et al. Design and methods of the Hospital Elder Life Program (HELP), a multicomponent targeted intervention to prevent delirium in hospitalized older patients: efficacy and cost-effectiveness in Dutch health care. BMC Geriatr 2013;13:78.
55. LaHue SC, Maselli J, Rogers S. Outcomes following implementation of a hospital-wide multicomponent delirium care pathway. J Hosp Med 2021;16(7):397–403.
56. Siddiqi N, Harrison JK, Clegg A, et al. Interventions for preventing delirium in hospitalised non-ICU patients. Cochrane Database Syst Rev 2016;3:CD005563.
57. Douglas VC, Hessler CS, Dhaliwal G, et al. The AWOL tool: derivation and validation of a delirium prediction rule. J Hosp Med 2013;8(9):493–9.
58. Burry L, Mehta S, Perreault MM, et al. Antipsychotics for treatment of delirium in hospitalised non-ICU patients. Cochrane Database Syst Rev 2018;6:CD005594.
59. Nikooie R, Neufeld KJ, Oh ES, et al. Antipsychotics for treating delirium in hospitalized adults: a systematic review. Ann Intern Med 2019;171(7):485–95.
60. Kuehn BM. FDA warns antipsychotic drugs may be risky for elderly. JAMA 2005; 293(20):2462.
61. Burry L, Hutton B, Williamson DR, et al. Pharmacological interventions for the treatment of delirium in critically ill adults. Cochrane Database Syst Rev 2019; 9:CD011749.
62. Devlin JW, Skrobik Y, Gelinas C, et al. Executive summary: clinical practice guidelines for the prevention and management of pain, agitation/sedation, delirium, immobility, and sleep disruption in adult patients in the ICU. Crit Care Med 2018;46(9):1532–48.
63. Hatta K, Kishi Y, Wada K, et al. Preventive effects of ramelteon on delirium: a randomized placebo-controlled trial. JAMA Psychiatry 2014;71(4):397–403.
64. Al-Aama T, Brymer C, Gutmanis I, et al. Melatonin decreases delirium in elderly patients: a randomized, placebo-controlled trial. Int J Geriatr Psychiatry 2011; 26(7):687–94.
65. de Jonghe A, van Munster BC, Goslings JC, et al. Effect of melatonin on incidence of delirium among patients with hip fracture: a multicentre, double-blind randomized controlled trial. CMAJ 2014;186(14):E547–56.
66. Nishikimi M, Numaguchi A, Takahashi K, et al. Effect of administration of ramelteon, a melatonin receptor agonist, on the duration of stay in the ICU: a single-center randomized placebo-controlled trial. Crit Care Med 2018;46(7):1099–105.

Prognostication, Ethical Issues, and Palliative Care in Disorders of Consciousness

Adeline L. Goss, MD[a],*, Claire J. Creutzfeldt, MD[b]

KEYWORDS

- Consciousness • Palliative care • Ethics • Traumatic brain injury • Neurocritical care

KEY POINTS

- A subset of patients with disorders of consciousness who are behaviorally unresponsive may have awareness detected only by neuroimaging or electrophysiology.
- These and other recent research advances in disorders of consciousness raise ethical questions that have important implications for acute and postacute care of these patients.
- A palliative care framework can help providers deliver ethical, compassionate care to these patients and their loved ones.

INTRODUCTION

Advances in the care of severe acute brain injury (SABI) have enabled the survival of patients in states of diminished consciousness. Recent research has offered an increasingly complex picture of the possible inner lives of these patients and their potential for recovery. This shift opens new ethical questions and intensifies the challenges facing patients' surrogate decision-makers, who in the acute period of SABI are tasked with making life-or-death decisions in the face of profound uncertainty. In this article, we define disorders of consciousness (DoC), describe newer findings around DoC diagnosis and prognosis, and discuss ethical questions surrounding the clinical management of patients with DoC. We conclude by illustrating a palliative care approach to some of the more difficult aspects of providing care to these patients and their loved ones.

DEFINITIONS OF DISORDERS OF CONSCIOUSNESS

Consciousness is often separated into 2 components: wakefulness (or arousal, the so-called "level of consciousness") and awareness (the contents of consciousness). Disorders of consciousness are currently classified in terms of clinically observed

Disclosure: The authors have nothing to disclose.
[a] Department of Neurology, University of California San Francisco, 505 Parnassus Avenue, Box 0114, San Francisco, CA 94143, USA; [b] Department of Neurology, University of Washington, 325 Ninth Avenue, Seattle, WA 98104, USA
* Corresponding author.
E-mail address: adeline.goss@ucsf.edu

Neurol Clin 40 (2022) 59–75
https://doi.org/10.1016/j.ncl.2021.08.005
0733-8619/22/© 2021 Elsevier Inc. All rights reserved.

behavior and include coma, vegetative state, minimally conscious, and the emergence from minimally conscious state (MCS) (**Table 1**).

In coma, the patient is unaware and cannot be aroused; eyes are closed, and noxious stimulation elicits posturing or no response. Progression to vegetative state (VS) is characterized by spontaneous eye opening, giving the appearance of wakefulness, but patients show only reflexive behavior.

Some patients with VS emerge to a MCS. In MCS, patients show inconsistent but reproducible behavioral evidence of consciousness, such as command-following, gesturing yes/no to questions, appropriate smiling or crying, reaching for objects, visual pursuit, or intelligible speech.[1] Visual pursuit is the most common initial sign of MCS, followed by command following and automatic movements.[2] Some divide MCS into 'MCS+' and 'MCS−' according to the presence (+) or absence (−) of behavioral evidence of language comprehension or expression.[3,4] The transition from VS to MCS has prognostic importance.

DoC syndromes can further be classified according to chronicity. Acute DoC describes the first 28 days after brain injury, whereas prolonged DoC describes the period after 28 days. The term 'permanent VS' is no longer felt to be justified given evidence that some patients can emerge from VS months or years after injury. Instead, the term 'chronic VS' has been suggested to describe patients who have reached stability in the VS state.[5]

Emergence from MCS (eMCS) is characterized by demonstration of functional object use or reliable communication (whether through speech, writing, yes/no signals, or communication devices).[1] Patients with eMCS typically are disoriented, cognitively impaired, inattentive, and unaware of their health state.[6,7] They may have sleep disturbance and restlessness or agitation.[6]

The categories of DoC discussed so far all rely on skilled and repeated neurobehavioral assessment, and misdiagnosis is common.[8] In addition, this taxonomy has recently been challenged by experiments demonstrating that a minority of patients with VS—showing no detectible behavior at bedside—can follow simple commands detected only by neuroimaging or electrophysiology.[9,10] This state has been called "cognitive-motor disassociation" (CMD) and is described further below.[11]

CLINICAL EXAMINATION IN DISORDERS OF CONSCIOUSNESS

The range of physical and cognitive impairments in DoC, including aphasia, motor, and sensory deficits, make it difficult to distinguish behaviors that indicate awareness from those that are nonpurposeful.[5] Diagnosis is further complicated by fluctuations in arousal and the time required for thorough examination.[5,12] Overcoming these challenges to establish an accurate diagnosis in DoC is important to educate family members about a patient's current state, inform prognosis, and guide treatment decisions including around the continuation of life-sustaining therapy (LST).

The traditional method of diagnosis in DoC is by qualitative bedside examination for reproducible responses to visual, auditory, and/or noxious stimuli, command-following, and communication. However, studies have shown that about 40% of patients with MCS are misclassified as VS using this approach.[8,13,14] Sources of error in the examination include incomplete, ill-timed, or infrequent examinations.[5,12,15,16]

Diagnosis can be improved through the use of standardized neurobehavioral assessments.[5] The most sensitive is the Coma Recovery Scale-Revised (CRS-R),[12,17] which is composed of 6 subscales and incorporates the existing diagnostic criteria for VS, MCS, and eMCS.[18] Diagnosis in DoC may further be improved using relevant stimuli, such as a mirror (so patients can follow their own eyes)[19]; involving patients' caregivers in the examination[20]; reducing sedating medications; and following

Table 1
Clinical features of disorders of consciousness

	Coma	VS	MCS	eMCS	CMD
Eye opening	None	Spontaneous	Spontaneous	Spontaneous	Spontaneous
Movement	None	Reflexive; nonpurposeful	Automatic; object manipulation	Functional object use	Reflexive; patterned
Response to noxious stimuli	Reflexive; posturing; none	Posturing; withdrawal	Localization	N/A	Posturing; withdrawal
Visual response	None	Startle; none	Sustained pursuit and/or fixation, may reach for objects (MCS-) or recognize objects (MCS+)	Recognizes objects	Startle or none
Affective response	None	Random	Congruent with stimulus	Congruent with stimulus	Random
Response to command	None	None	Inconsistent, reproducible	Consistent, reproducible	Consistent, reproducible (as detected by neuroimaging or electrophysiology)
Vocalization	None	None	Inconsistent, random vocalization or none (MCS-); inconsistent, intelligible words (MCS+)	Intelligible words	None
Communication	None	None	Unreliable	Reliable	In rare individuals, detected by neuroimaging or electrophysiology

Abbreviations: CMD, cognitive-motor dissociation; eMCS, emergence from minimally conscious state; MCS, minimally conscious state; VS, vegetative state.

protocols to enhance arousal (eg, CRS-R Arousal Facilitation Protocol).[18] If possible, examinations should be conducted in the morning, when behaviors suggestive of MCS are more likely to be detected.[16] Performing an assessment more than once may improve diagnostic accuracy.[15]

MULTIMODAL DIAGNOSIS IN DISORDERS OF CONSCIOUSNESS

Even rigorous bedside assessment may fail to detect the presence of covert awareness. Investigational techniques to detect covert awareness have been developed for functional MRI (fMRI), fluorodeoxyglucose (FDG)-PET, single-photon emission computerized tomography (SPECT), and electroencephalography (EEG). These techniques offer more robust evaluation of consciousness than the bedside examination[12,21] and demonstrate differences between patients with VS and MCS at the group level. However, they have not been rigorously evaluated for diagnosing DoC in individual patients. Practical issues like interrater reliability and technical challenges like motion/muscle artifact may limit their utility, there is no consensus about when to use them or how to interpret them. With that said, these techniques hold promise for advancing diagnosis and prognosis for individuals with DoC.

These techniques can be classified in terms of resting state, passive, and active paradigms. Resting-state paradigms measure the presence of intact resting-state neuronal networks that are believed to be closely associated with a conscious state. One approach uses FDG-PET to measure differences in metabolic rates in the frontoparietal associative cortices. Using CRS-R as the reference, this technique has high sensitivity and specificity to differentiate between VS and MCS.[12,21,22] In research settings, visual analysis of standard resting EEG in the postacute setting (after hospital discharge) for background organization and presence of sleep architecture also has high specificity but low sensitivity for detecting signs of MCS.[12] These resting-state paradigms rely on assumptions about the relationship between these networks and awareness; they measure the integrity of what is believed to be the substrate of consciousness.

Passive paradigms examine preserved large-scale functional cortical connectivity following an external stimulus. These techniques detect brain activity that is believed to be closely associated with a conscious state, for example, the activation of "higher-order" associative cortical networks for auditory, somatosensory, or visual sensation, in contrast to "lower-level" primary sensory cortices. An estimated 55% of MCS and 26% of patients with VS show preserved functional cortical connectivity in passive paradigms.[23] Like resting-state paradigms, these approaches have not been rigorously evaluated in the real-world setting and rely on assumptions about the relationship between measurable brain activity and awareness.[21]

Active paradigms measure brain activity as patients are instructed to engage in mental tasks. For example, in a 2006 study by Owen and colleagues, a patient with a clinical diagnosis of VS from traumatic brain injury (TBI) was instructed to imagine playing tennis or imagine moving from room to room in her house while undergoing fMRI; in response, there was reliable activation in her supplementary motor area (SMA) and parahippocampal gyrus (PPA), respectively. These responses were sustained for about 30 seconds, until she was presented with another instruction, a pattern indistinguishable from that observed in healthy volunteers.[24] A meta-analysis of 6 such studies using fMRI or EEG active paradigms suggested that 14.4% of patients with clinically confirmed VS could modulate their brain activity to command.[23] Twice as many patients with MCS could do so. Command following through active paradigms was more common in patients with DoC after TBI than after nontraumatic injury.[23]

The absence of a gold standard for detecting consciousness complicates our ability to calculate sensitivity and specificity for active paradigms. The fact that most patients with MCS are unable to follow commands using these protocols—despite, by definition, being able to demonstrate intentional behavior at the bedside[25]—suggests low sensitivity. In fact, a substantial number of healthy controls cannot cooperate with active paradigms.[23,26] Recent guidelines from the European Academy of Neurology concluded that active paradigms have high specificity but low sensitivity in identifying patients with VS who can follow commands despite appearing unresponsive.[12]

THE PROBLEM OF OTHER MINDS

In active paradigm studies, the ability to follow commands is interpreted as agency—a marker of consciousness. Some have argued, however, that a person in possession of motivational and cognitive states and capacities, such as the ability to visualize playing tennis, is not necessarily "conscious" in the sense that we typically think of the term—that is, that person does not necessarily have a qualitative, inner experience of being aware.[27] This latter concept is known as *phenomenal consciousness:* there is something "it is like" to be that person.[28] The philosophic barrier here is known as the "problem of other minds." It is impossible for one person to directly assess the conscious experience of another person[29]; we can only infer it by assessing their behaviors and responses to stimuli.[10] We are particularly reassured that another person is having a conscious experience when they can tell us about it.

A small handful of studies have attempted to teach behaviorally unresponsive individuals to use mental imagery to communicate. In 2010, Monti and colleagues again asked patients with VS and MCS to imagine hitting a tennis ball back and forth with an instructor (SMA) or imagine navigating a familiar place (PPA). Five of 54 patients had measurable brain activity in the SMA or PPA to these commands. One patient with VS 5 years after TBI, with no behavioral evidence of awareness on repeated examinations, was then asked to use one type of imagery (either tennis or spatial imagery) for yes, and the other for no. He answered 5 of 6 biographic questions correctly.[30] This finding was replicated in 2013 in a man with VS due to TBI 12 years prior, who over many sessions in the fMRI scanner demonstrated accurate answers to biographic questions, although he did not respond on every occasion he was scanned.[31] Several other studies attempting to replicate communication using mental imagery with patients with DoC have had negative results. In one, 6 patients with MCS were unable to use mental imagery to communicate, 2 of whom demonstrated ability to communicate at the bedside.[25] It may be that the cognitive demand of communication tasks is too high for most patients with VS/MCS.[11]

There are several important limitations to these data. Most of these studies were single-center convenience samples, often lacking a clear statement about the number of excluded patients and why they were excluded. Patient numbers were generally low.[23] The reference standard of clinical examination is subject to error; in the study by Monti and colleagues discussed earlier, 2 patients with "VS" who performed the command-following task were re-examined and found to have behavior consistent with MCS.[30] Furthermore, the low sensitivity of these tests and lack of a gold standard for consciousness creates ambiguity around the meaning of a negative result.

PROGNOSIS IN DISORDERS OF CONSCIOUSNESS

Estimating prognosis for individual patients with DoC remains challenging, in part due to methodological issues with the longitudinal studies of these patients. Most available long-term studies have examined patients after admission to inpatient rehabilitation centers[32,33] and are therefore likely to overestimate the proportion of patients with good outcome, as patients are typically preselected for a rehabilitation stay if they are considered to have a good chance of recovery.[34] Studies also often pool patients with VS and MCS.[33,35,36] Separating these groups is important because patients admitted to acute rehabilitation with MCS have significantly better survival and functional prognosis than those with VS,[5,37,38] particularly patients with preserved language function (MCS+).[38,39] Studies that have pooled patients with VS/MCS have suggested that approximately 20% recover to a level where they are judged to be eventually capable of returning to employment.[32,33] The available data for patients with VS are less optimistic. Among those admitted to acute rehabilitation with VS, about 17% will reach MCS by 6 months after injury.[5] In one French study that tracked 33 patients with VS for up to 2.5 years, 28 (84.8%) had died by the end of the study period, 3 (9.1%) were in a state of severe disability [Glasgow Coma Outcome - Extended (GOSE) score of 3], and only one (3.0%), a 24-year-old man with VS due to intoxication, reached moderate disability (GOSE 5). This study was limited in that most patients had nontraumatic etiologies of VS, such as anoxic injury and intracerebral hemorrhage,[37] which are associated with worse outcomes.[33]

One important realization in recent years is that late emergence from VS to MCS is possible. In 1994, the AAN Multi-Society Task Force defined VS as "persistent" 3 months after non-TBI and 12 months after TBI, concluding that unexpected "recovery of consciousness" (ie, evidence of voluntary behavior or awareness of self/environment, both now considered criteria for MCS) after 3 months occurred in 2.4% of patients with nontraumatic injury and after 12 months in only 1.6% of patients with TBI.[40] However, a 1996 reanalysis of the Task Force data found that the study had suffered from inconsistent follow-up; of 434 patients with VS due to TBI, only 25 were followed up after 12 months and 6 had "recovery of consciousness" by 3 years after injury, putting the rate of late recovery at 14% or higher.[41] More recent studies suggest that late transition from VS to MCS may occur in as many as 20% of patients who met "permanent VS" criteria,[5] albeit with continued severe disability.[42] This realization has led to replacing the term "permanent VS" with the term "chronic VS."[5]

Newer multimodal strategies incorporating specialized functional imaging or electrophysiologic studies may improve prognostication. In VS due to TBI, several techniques have been proposed to improve estimates of the likelihood of reaching MCS at 12 months, including MRI at 6 to 8 weeks after injury, SPECT at 1 to 2 months after injury, and the presence of P300 or EEG reactivity at 2 to 3 months after injury. In VS due to non-traumatic etiologies, the CRS-R and somatosensory evoked potentials may assist in prognostication regarding reaching MCS at 24 months.[5]

ACUTE DISORDERS OF CONSCIOUSNESS

Research into covert awareness in DoC has focused on the postacute stage (after hospital discharge). The great majority of patients who have shown covert awareness on functional neuroimaging or electrophysiology have been months or years after injury. At this stage, end-of-life decisions tend not to be pressing. The highest-stakes time for patients with DoC is much earlier, in the first hours to weeks, when uncertainty is greatest and treatment decisions are first made around respiratory support, artificial nutrition, and hydration.

In the acute setting, prognostication relies on clinical, electrodiagnostic, and imaging findings seen within the first week as well as age and presence of other comorbidities. Different criteria are used for different etiologies of SABI, including stroke, TBI, and cardiac arrest.[43–45] Recent studies are looking at using multimodal imaging or artificial intelligence[46] to improve prognostication in the acute phase of SABI.

Despite these tools, uncertainty characterizes the early period of SABI. This uncertainty may lead providers to offer vague, inaccurate, and/or falsely confident prognoses to surrogate decision-makers.[47] Overly optimistic prognoses may lead to overtreatment, whereas overly pessimistic prognoses may lead to self-fulfilling prophecies through withdrawal of LST.[47–49] In one multicenter retrospective cohort study of 720 patients with TBI in Canada, withdrawal of LST accounted for 70% of in-hospital deaths and was more closely associated with the facility where care was provided than with patient characteristics. About half of withdrawal of LST decisions occurred during the first 72 hours of injury.[50]

ETHICAL CONSIDERATIONS IN THE CARE OF PATIENTS WITH DISORDERS OF CONSCIOUSNESS

The discovery 15 years ago of covert command following among a minority of patients with VS raised important ethical issues. Some are unique to DoC, whereas others reflect ethical challenges in the care of many patients with SABI.

Quality of Life

The presence of CMD among some patients with VS has led to concern about the quality of life (QoL) of these individuals. In traditional conceptions of VS, the absence of behavior was assumed to mean the absence of consciousness, and therefore the absence of suffering. With knowledge of CMD comes concern that some behaviorally unresponsive patients may experience suffering but may be unable to communicate their wishes or needs at the bedside. Savulescu and Kahane have characterized the situation as "far worse than someone in the worst form of solitary confinement" and have argued that "terminating these patients' lives might be morally required, not merely permissible."[27]

Many clinicians and members of the general public share this attitude. A study of European physicians found that even after education about the rate of diagnostic error in VS and evidence of residual cognition in VS, 82% would prefer not to be kept alive in a chronic VS.[51] Avoidance of suffering is a common justification for LST withdrawal in many patients with VS.[52] Yet the concepts of suffering and QoL are speculative in noncommunicating patients[53] and needs to be regarded in the context of the disability paradox, wherein people with a disability rate their QoL higher than nondisabled people imagining life with disability.[54]

In individuals with DoC who cannot self-report, there have been attempts to consider objective factors thought to be important to QoL. Three generally accepted domains of QoL include having pleasant experiences, personal achievements, and desirability of health status according to the values of a population.[53,55] It has been argued that aware patients with DoC can enjoy well-being in the first domain only, and that this results in a low QoL.[27] Yet this argument does not account for response shifts, in which individuals with severe chronic illness or disability experience a reprioritization of the factors that contribute to QoL.[21,56–58] In DoC, QoL may depend more on perceived social support and "hedonic experiences" both negative (pain, depression, and boredom) and positive (physical contact, companionship, and mental stimulation).[55,57,59]

More research is needed to attempt to assess the subjective well-being of aware patients with DoC. Without such tools, medical decision-making is subject to the inference, suppositions, and preconceptions of medical providers and surrogate decision-makers, an issue discussed further below.[53,55]

Medical Decision-Making

Patients with VS or MCS need various degrees of support to remain alive, most commonly artificial nutrition and hydration provided through a gastrostomy tube and ventilatory support using a tracheostomy. They also lack the capacity to make and communicate treatment decisions. How treatment decisions are made in such scenarios varies by nation.

In the United States, patients enjoy a constitutionally protected right to refuse both the initiation and the continuation of LST. When a brain-injured patient cannot make treatment decisions, that right is transferred to a lawful surrogate decision-maker. The legality of discontinuing artificial nutrition and hydration in accordance with a patient's previously stated wishes was upheld in 1990 surrounding the case of Nancy Beth Cruzan, a young woman with VS.[60] All subsequent legal decisions on withdrawing of LST have cited Cruzan as the precedent, including the heavily publicized 2005 case of Theresa Schiavo.[61,62]

Surrogate decision-making is founded in patient autonomy. Surrogates make decisions for patients using established standards. If a patient has relevant, previously expressed wishes, they should be followed. If not, the surrogate should use substituted judgment and attempt to reproduce the decision the patient would have made by applying the patient's values and preferences to the clinical circumstance. When that is not possible, surrogates should attempt to determine what is in the best interest of the patient.[61–64]

There are real-life limitations to this established system of surrogate decision-making. First, there is only moderate concordance between surrogates and patients around treatment preferences; one meta-analysis of 16 studies showed that surrogates predicted patients' treatment preferences (including around a VS scenario) with 68% accuracy, a rate that did not improve among patients who had previously discussed treatment preferences with their surrogates.[65] Moreover, some surrogates for patients with DoC choose to continue LST despite the patient's clearly stated wishes not to receive it. In one qualitative study, caregivers for patients with chronic VS described overruling the patient's wishes for several reasons, including expectation of recovery and a perception that artificial nutrition and hydration do not constitute LST. Other surrogate decision-makers may make decisions incrementally in the acute setting, not realizing that there is often a "window of opportunity" for death in SABI, after which the dependence on LST decreases, with the last LST usually being artificial nutrition and hydration.[66] Surrogate decision-makers develop their understanding of diagnosis and prognosis using personal observations and beliefs, not just the information communicated by clinicians.[67] One study found that 90% of caregivers of patients in VS regarded the patient as conscious.[68] These observations highlight the importance of sensitive, empathetic communication with surrogate decision-makers.

There has been recent debate around whether clinicians are obligated to disclose to families of patients with VS the fact that some patients with VS may demonstrate covert awareness by investigational neuroimaging.[21] On the one hand, the withholding of medical information from patients/surrogates without their consent represents a violation of the principle of autonomy. On the other hand, at present, few patients can access testing to detect covert awareness, and disclosing the presence of CMD in some patients without being able to test for it in an individual patient could lead to false hope and overtreatment. Disclosures ought to include caveats that multimodal evaluations return negative findings in most of the patients with VS/MCS, and that the link between positive findings and phenomenal consciousness remains unclear.[21]

Therapeutic Nihilism

The traditional understanding of VS as a permanent state of unresponsiveness may lead to perceptions that prolonging life for such patients is potentially inappropriate or medically futile.[69] Medical futility is invoked when a therapy that is hoped to benefit a patient's medical condition is expected not to do so based on the best available evidence.[70] Declarations of medical futility in DoC need to take into account evolving understanding of diagnosis and prognosis in DoC. The AAN now recommends that clinicians discussing prognosis with caregivers of patients with acute DoC (during the first 28 days after injury) should avoid statements that suggest these patients have a universally poor prognosis,[5] to avoid self-fulfilling prophecies.[71]

Systems of Care

Evidence of covert awareness among patients with VS, frequent misdiagnosis of VS/MCS, and the possibility of late recovery from both conditions raise ethical concerns about the systems of care in place for these patients. Erp and colleagues have described a "vicious circle" of epidemiology, organization of care, and end-of-life decisions for patients with VS: this group of patients is small and recovery is rarely witnessed by those providing acute care; because of this, care is organized ad-hoc, resulting in misdiagnosis and lack of specialized rehabilitation; and decisions about whether to continue life-supporting treatment are made without an accurate diagnosis or evidence-based prognostication.[72] At the same time, the aggressive care of patients with limited or no awareness raises questions of distributive justice and allocation of resources.[73] Research is needed to develop evidence-based systems of care for patients with VS/MCS and better identify those who are likely to benefit from early intensive neurorehabilitation.

INPATIENT CARE FOR PATIENTS WITH DISORDERS OF CONSCIOUSNESS: A NEUROPALLIATIVE CARE APPROACH

The changing medical and scientific understanding of DoC and the ethical issues described earlier add to the complexity of caring for patients with DoC and supporting their loved ones, surrogate decision-makers, and/or family members. We recommend a palliative care approach to dealing with these complex issues. Palliative care aims at preventing and relieving physical, social, psychological, and spiritual suffering; it encompasses symptom management as well as communication around diagnosis, prognosis, treatment options, goals of care, shared decision-making, and advance care planning.[74] "Primary" palliative care is provided by a patient's primary team and is based on the idea that all health care providers should possess certain palliative care skills, with the support of specialists as needed. **Table 2** summarizes a list of proposed palliative care skills for the neurohospitalist caring for patients with DoC.

SYMPTOM MANAGEMENT

Symptom management in DoC remains difficult because of patients' limited ability or inability to communicate. The very concept of a "symptom" is ambiguous in this population because it implies phenomenal consciousness, the presence of which is uncertain. Experiencing pain requires nociception, sensory/discriminative dimensions of pain (which may produce autonomic responses and patterned behavior like grimacing), and the affective/motivational dimensions of pain (which are thought to generate the feeling of pain and may produce an urge to avoid the stimulus).[53,55,75] In PET studies, patients with VS exposed to pain consistently show activation of the midbrain,

Table 2
Primary palliative care skills for patients with disorders of consciousness

	Primary Palliative Care Skills
Symptom management	Recognize subtle signs of awareness and address all patients as if they are aware Recognize and treat reproducible signs of pain, agitation, and delirium Offer pleasant experiences and minimize uncomfortable experiences for all patients, including those whose subjective experience is unknown
Communication skills and goals of care	Communicate with patients and surrogates with empathy and compassion Effectively elicit the patient's goals, values, and treatment preferences Effectively communicate information to surrogate decision-makers in the language they understand Offer evidence-based prognostic estimates and avoid overly negative or positive prognostication Effectively communicate about uncertainty Avoid making assumptions about the quality of life for noncommunicative patients Provide anticipatory guidance regarding treatment trajectories Help decision-makers establish goals of care based on the patient's values, goals, and treatment preferences Incorporate ethical principles into communication and decision-making Develop consensus for difficult decisions Identify and manage moral distress among interdisciplinary team members
Psychosocial and spiritual support	Identify psychosocial and emotional needs among the patient's loved ones/caregivers Identify needs for spiritual or religious support and provide referrals Access resources to support the patient's loved ones/caregivers Practice cultural humility
Systems of care	Establish a follow-up plan in which the patient's/caregivers' palliative care needs will continue to be addressed
End of life care	Emphasize nonabandonment and provide continued emotional support through the dying process Provide anticipatory guidance regarding the dying process Facilitate bereavement support

Adapted from Creutzfeldt CJ, Holloway RG, Curtis JR. Palliative Care: A Core Competency for Stroke Neurologists. *Stroke.* 2015;46(9):2714-2719; with permission.

contralateral thalamus, and S1 areas,[76,77] suggesting relatively preserved nociception and at least partial sensory-discriminative pain processing.[55] Higher-order associative areas such as S2, insula, and anterior cingulate cortexes also tend to activate in response to pain in patients with VS, but appear functionally disconnected from each other.[76,78,79] These connections are typically preserved in patients with MCS,[78] which may suggest that patients with MCS can experience pain as noxious, whereas patients with VS cannot. However, there is no way to confirm this hypothesis in patients who are unable to self-report.

Given ongoing ambiguity on the extent to which patients with DoC can experience discomfort, attempts should be made to try to minimize it[55] and offer pleasurable experiences when possible, like pleasant tastes, smells, and music. Sources of discomfort may include immobility, spasticity, pressure ulcers, infections, paroxysmal sympathetic hyperactivity, and invasive procedures, and confusion or agitation. Providers should attempt to minimize discomfort and generally keep in mind the possibility of covert awareness while examining and speaking to these patients.[80]

COMMUNICATING UNCERTAINTY

Outcomes from SABI can range from lifelong unresponsiveness to functional independence. Markers for very poor prognosis have been identified in certain types of SABI, but we are only beginning to develop tools to estimate prognosis for most of the individual patients. One of the central challenges in caring for patients with DoC is communicating this uncertainty.

Two principles of managing uncertainty in SABI are to remove uncertainty when possible, and to be transparent about the uncertainty that remains. Clinicians should minimize misdiagnosis using evidence-based behavioral assessments, strategies to enhance arousal, and multimodal evaluation where applicable and available.

Most surrogates appreciate receiving prognostic information early in the course of critical illness, even if that prognosis is uncertain.[81,82] Several strategies exist to help clinicians communicate uncertainty.[83] First, clinicians need to be able to acknowledge their own uncertainty, because suppressing this knowledge can lead to premature closure, the single most common phenomenon in misdiagnosis.[83,84] Clinicians should disclose prognostic uncertainty to surrogate decision-makers while bracketing estimates with ranges where possible (eg, sharing the best-case and worst-case scenario).[85] Misleading language ("no hope") or ambiguous language ("meaningful recovery")[86] should be avoided. Clinicians should acknowledge the difficult emotions evoked by uncertainty and show their commitment to ongoing engagement with the patient and family going forward ("I don't know right now, but I will continue to be honest with you as we learn more").[83] Finally, anticipatory guidance can help families know what to expect in terms of a time course of treatment and possible future complications.[5] If a decision is made to pursue LST including artificial nutrition and hydration, clinicians might suggest a time-limited trial, with a plan to revisit goals of care in a predetermined number of weeks or months pending the patient's clinical course.[87,88]

CAREGIVER SUPPORT

In SABI, patients' loved ones assume the role of caregiver suddenly. From the first moment in the emergency department or ICU, they must simultaneously learn new medical information, navigate new systems of care, and confront financial and logistical barriers, all while grieving.

Caregivers for patients with chronic DoC have been shown to experience a prolonged grief reaction.[89,90] The patient's ongoing physical presence but absent or limited behavioral presence creates ambiguity around the nature of the loss. Whereas grieving for death typically recedes over time, caregivers for patients with DoC may find the patient's "concurrent presence-absence" challenging and may struggle to find a strategy for mourning.[90,91] Meanwhile, they may serve simultaneously as the patient's caregiver, care coordinator, advocate, and financial provider. The responsibility of caregiving affects how they can contribute to other relationships and roles in their lives.[90]

Greater access to resources and stronger social networks may decrease caregiver burden.[90,92] Inpatient providers can begin this process by connecting caregivers to existing services and establishing a robust follow-up plan.

SUMMARY

Advances in the understanding of diagnosis and prognosis in DoC raise important ethical questions and underline the need to provide a palliative care approach to these patients and their caregivers. As described earlier, many gaps in knowledge remain. There is an urgent need for improved prognostic tools in the acute setting, when stakes are high and uncertainty is greatest. More research is needed to facilitate communication with capable individuals with DoC, both for therapeutic purposes and to directly involve these individuals in medical decision-making. Despite ongoing advances in DoC research, uncertainty continues to characterize these patients' diagnosis, prognosis, and QoL. Clinicians should clearly communicate this uncertainty, provide support to patients' loved ones, and facilitate difficult decision-making in the face of the unknown.

Clinics care points

- About 40% of patients with minimally conscious state are erroneously classified with vegetative state using bedside examination.
- Bedside diagnosis of disorders of consciousness can be improved through the use of standardized neurobehavioral assessments and through simple practices like evaluating visual pursuit using a mirror, involving caregivers in the examination, and performing serial examinations.
- About 14% of patients diagnosed with vegetative state on neurobehavioral assessments can follow commands as detected by neuroimaging and electrophysiology techniques. A handful of these patients have used these technologies to communicate.
- The discovery of covert awareness among some patients with VS raises ethical questions around quality of life and medical decision-making.

ACKNOWLEDGEMENT

Dr Creutzfeldt is funded through a NINDS career development award (K23 NS099421-01A1).

REFERENCES

1. Giacino JT, Ashwal S, Childs N, et al. The minimally conscious state: definition and diagnostic criteria. Neurology 2002;58(3):349–53.
2. Martens G, Bodien Y, Sheau K, et al. Which behaviours are first to emerge during recovery of consciousness after severe brain injury? Ann Phys Rehabil Med 2020; 63(4):263–9.
3. Aubinet C, Cassol H, Gosseries O, et al. Brain Metabolism but Not Gray Matter Volume Underlies the Presence of Language Function in the Minimally Conscious State (MCS): MCS+ Versus MCS− Neuroimaging Differences. Neurorehabil Neural Repair 2020;34(2):172–84.
4. Thibaut A, Bodien YG, Laureys S, et al. Minimally conscious state "plus": diagnostic criteria and relation to functional recovery. J Neurol 2020;267(5):1245–54.
5. Giacino JT, Katz DI, Schiff ND, et al. Practice Guideline Update Recommendations Summary: Disorders of Consciousness. Arch Phys Med Rehabil 2018; 99(9):1699–709.
6. Bodien YG, Martens G, Ostrow J, et al. Cognitive impairment, clinical symptoms and functional disability in patients emerging from the minimally conscious state. NeuroRehabilitation 2020;46(1):65–74.

7. Nakase-Richardson R, Yablon SA, Sherer M, et al. Emergence from minimally conscious state: insights from evaluation of posttraumatic confusion. Neurology 2009;73(14):1120–6.

8. Schnakers C, Vanhaudenhuyse A, Giacino J, et al. Diagnostic accuracy of the vegetative and minimally conscious state: Clinical consensus versus standardized neurobehavioral assessment. BMC Neurol 2009;9(1):1–5.

9. Bayne T, Hohwy J, Owen AM. Reforming the taxonomy in disorders of consciousness. Ann Neurol 2017;82(6):866–72.

10. Bernat JL. Nosologic considerations in disorders of consciousness. Ann Neurol 2017;82(6):863–5.

11. Schiff ND. Cognitive Motor Dissociation Following Severe Brain Injuries. JAMA Neurol 2015;72(12):1413.

12. Kondziella D, Bender A, Diserens K, et al. European Academy of Neurology guideline on the diagnosis of coma and other disorders of consciousness. Eur J Neurol 2020;27(5):741–56.

13. Andrews K, Murphy L, Munday R, et al. Misdiagnosis of the vegetative state: retrospective study in a rehabilitation unit. BMJ 1996;313(7048):13–6.

14. Wade DT. How often is the diagnosis of the permanent vegetative state incorrect? A review of the evidence. Eur J Neurol 2018;25(4):619–25.

15. Wannez S, Heine L, Thonnard M, et al. The repetition of behavioral assessments in diagnosis of disorders of consciousness. Ann Neurol 2017;81(6):883–9.

16. Cortese Md, Riganello F, Arcuri F, et al. Coma recovery scale-r: variability in the disorder of consciousness. BMC Neurol 2015;15(1):186.

17. Seel RT, Sherer M, Whyte J, et al. Assessment Scales for Disorders of Consciousness: Evidence-Based Recommendations for Clinical Practice and Research. Arch Phys Med Rehabil 2010;91(12):1795–813.

18. Giacino JT, Kalmar K, Whyte J. The JFK Coma Recovery Scale-Revised: Measurement characteristics and diagnostic utility1. Arch Phys Med Rehabil 2004; 85(12):2020–9.

19. Sun Y, Wang J, Heine L, et al. Personalized objects can optimize the diagnosis of EMCS in the assessment of functional object use in the CRS-R: a double blind, randomized clinical trial. BMC Neurol 2018;18:38. Available at: https://www.ncbi.nlm.nih.gov/pmc/articles/PMC5897931/. Accessed April 7, 2021.

20. Formisano R, Contrada M, Iosa M, et al. Coma Recovery Scale-Revised With and Without the Emotional Stimulation of Caregivers. Can J Neurol Sci 2019;46(5): 607–9.

21. Peterson A, Owen AM, Karlawish J. Alive inside. Bioethics 2020;34(3):295–305.

22. Stender J, Kupers R, Rodell A, et al. Quantitative rates of brain glucose metabolism distinguish minimally conscious from vegetative state patients. J Cereb Blood Flow Metab 2015;35(1):58–65.

23. Kondziella D, Friberg CK, Frokjaer VG, et al. Preserved consciousness in vegetative and minimal conscious states: systematic review and meta-analysis. J Neurol Neurosurg Psychiatry 2016;87(5):485–92.

24. Owen AM, Coleman MR, Boly M, et al. Detecting awareness in the vegetative state. Science 2006;313(5792):1402.

25. Bardin JC, Fins JJ, Katz DI, et al. Dissociations between behavioural and functional magnetic resonance imaging-based evaluations of cognitive function after brain injury. Brain 2011;134(3):769–82.

26. Cruse D, Chennu S, Chatelle C, et al. Bedside detection of awareness in the vegetative state: a cohort study. Lancet 2011;378(9809):2088–94.

27. Savulescu J, kahane G. Brain damage and the moral significance of consciousness. J Med Philos 2009;34(1):6–26.
28. Nagel T. What is it like to be a bat? Philosophical Rev 1974;83(4):435–50.
29. Farah MJ. Neuroethics and the problem of other minds: implications of neuroscience for the moral status of brain-damaged patients and nonhuman animals. Neuroethics 2008;1(1):9–18.
30. Monti MM, Vanhaudenhuyse A, Coleman MR, et al. Willful modulation of brain activity in disorders of consciousness. N Engl J Med 2010;362(7):579–89.
31. Fernández-Espejo D, Owen AM. Detecting awareness after severe brain injury. Nat Rev Neurosci 2013;14(11):801–9.
32. Nakase-Richardson R, Whyte J, Giacino JT, et al. Longitudinal Outcome of Patients with Disordered Consciousness in the NIDRR TBI Model Systems Programs. J Neurotrauma 2011;29(1):59–65.
33. Katz DI, Polyak M, Coughlan D, et al. Natural history of recovery from brain injury after prolonged disorders of consciousness: outcome of patients admitted to inpatient rehabilitation with 1-4 year follow-up. Progress in Brain Research 2009;177:73–88.
34. Kowalski RG, Hammond FM, Weintraub AH, et al. Recovery of Consciousness and Functional Outcome in Moderate and Severe Traumatic Brain Injury. JAMA Neurol 2021;78(5):548–57. Available at: https://jamanetwork.com/journals/jamaneurology/fullarticle/2776794. Accessed May 1, 2021.
35. deGuise E, LeBlanc J, Feyz M, et al. Long-Term Outcome After Severe Traumatic Brain Injury: The McGill Interdisciplinary Prospective Study. J Head Trauma Rehabil 2008;23(5):294–303.
36. Whyte J, Nakase-Richardson R, Hammond FM, et al. Functional outcomes in traumatic disorders of consciousness: 5-year outcomes from the National Institute on Disability and Rehabilitation Research Traumatic Brain Injury Model Systems. Arch Phys Med Rehabil 2013;94(10):1855–60.
37. Faugeras F, Rohaut B, Valente M, et al. Survival and consciousness recovery are better in the minimally conscious state than in the vegetative state. Brain Inj 2018; 32(1):72–7.
38. Giacino JT, Sherer M, Christoforou A, et al. Behavioral Recovery and Early Decision Making in Patients with Prolonged Disturbance in Consciousness after Traumatic Brain Injury. J Neurotrauma 2020;37(2):357–65.
39. Aubinet C, Larroque SK, Heine L, et al. Clinical subcategorization of minimally conscious state according to resting functional connectivity. Hum Brain Mapp 2018;39(11):4519–32.
40. Multi-Society Task Force on PVS. Medical aspects of the persistent vegetative state (1). N Engl J Med 1994;330(21):1499–508.
41. Childs NL, Mercer WN. Late Improvement in Consciousness after Post-Traumatic Vegetative State. N Engl J Med 1996;334(1):24–5.
42. Estraneo A, Moretta P, Loreto V, et al. Late recovery after traumatic, anoxic, or hemorrhagic long-lasting vegetative state. Neurology 2010;75(3):239–45.
43. Rossetti AO, Rabinstein AA, Oddo M. Neurological prognostication of outcome in patients in coma after cardiac arrest. Lancet Neurol 2016;15(6):597–609.
44. Azabou E, Navarro V, Kubis N, et al. Value and mechanisms of EEG reactivity in the prognosis of patients with impaired consciousness: a systematic review. Crit Care 2018;22(1):184.
45. Wijdicks EFM, Hijdra A, Young GB, et al. Quality Standards Subcommittee of the American Academy of Neurology. Practice parameter: prediction of outcome in comatose survivors after cardiopulmonary resuscitation (an evidence-based

review): report of the Quality Standards Subcommittee of the American Academy of Neurology. Neurology 2006;67(2):203-10.

46. Smith LGF, Milliron E, Ho M-L, et al. Advanced neuroimaging in traumatic brain injury: an overview. Neurosurg Focus 2019;47(6):E17.

47. Hemphill JC, White DB. Clinical Nihilism in Neuroemergencies. Emerg Med Clin North Am 2009;27(1):27-37.

48. Zurasky JA, Aiyagari V, Zazulia AR, et al. Early mortality following spontaneous intracerebral hemorrhage. Neurology 2005;64(4):725-7.

49. Zahuranec DB, Brown DL, Lisabeth LD, et al. Early care limitations independently predict mortality after intracerebral hemorrhage. Neurology 2007;68(20):1651-7.

50. Turgeon AF, Lauzier F, Simard J-F, et al. Mortality associated with withdrawal of life-sustaining therapy for patients with severe traumatic brain injury: a Canadian multicentre cohort study. CMAJ 2011;183(14):1581-8.

51. Demertzi A, Ledoux D, Bruno M-A, et al. Attitudes towards end-of-life issues in disorders of consciousness: a European survey. J Neurol 2011;258(6):1058-65.

52. Gipson J, Kahane G, Savulescu J. Attitudes of Lay People to Withdrawal of Treatment in Brain Damaged Patients. Neuroethics 2014;7(1):1-9.

53. Johnson LSM. Can they suffer? The ethical priority of quality of life research in disorders of consciousness 2013;6(4):8.

54. Albrecht GL, Devlieger PJ. The disability paradox: high quality of life against all odds. Soc Sci Med 1999;48(8):977-88.

55. Graham M, Weijer C, Cruse D, et al. An Ethics of Welfare for Patients Diagnosed as Vegetative With Covert Awareness. AJOB Neurosci 2015;6(2):31-41.

56. Dijkers MP. Quality of life after traumatic brain injury: a review of research approaches and findings. Arch Phys Med Rehabil 2004;85(4 Suppl 2):S21-35.

57. Graham M. Domains of Well-Being in Minimally Conscious Patients: Illuminating a Persistent Problem. AJOB Neurosci 2018;9(2):128-30.

58. Schwartz CE, Bode R, Repucci N, et al. The clinical significance of adaptation to changing health: a meta-analysis of response shift. Qual Life Res 2006;15(9):1533-50.

59. Tung J, Speechley KN, Gofton T, et al. Towards the assessment of quality of life in patients with disorders of consciousness. Qual Life Res 2020;29(5):1217-27.

60. Annas GJ. Nancy Cruzan and the Right to Die. N Engl J Med 1990;323(10):670-3.

61. Racine E, Rodrigue C, Bernat JL, et al. Observations on the Ethical and Social Aspects of Disorders of Consciousness. Can J Neurol Sci 2010;37(6):758-68.

62. Bernat JL. Clinical Decision-Making for Patients with Disorders of Consciousness. Ann Neurol 2020;87(1):19-21.

63. Bernat JL. Ethical Issues in the Treatment of Severe Brain Injury. Ann N Y Acad Sci 2009;1157(1):117-30.

64. Graham M. Precedent Autonomy and Surrogate Decisionmaking After Severe Brain Injury. Camb Q Healthc Ethics 2020;29(4):511-26.

65. Shalowitz DI, Garrett-Mayer E, Wendler D. The Accuracy of Surrogate Decision Makers: A Systematic Review. Arch Intern Med 2006;166(5):493-7.

66. Kitzinger J, Kitzinger C. The "window of opportunity" for death after severe brain injury: family experiences. Sociol Health Illn 2013;35(7):1095-112.

67. Boyd E, Lo B, Evans L, et al. "It's not just what the doctor tells me:" Factors that influence surrogate decision-makers' perceptions of prognosis*. Crit Care Med 2010;38(5):1270-5.

68. Tresch DD, Sims FH, Duthie EH, et al. Patients in a persistent vegetative state: Attitudes and reactions of family members. J Am Geriatr Soc 1991;39(1):17-21.

69. Bosslet GT, Pope TM, Rubenfeld GD, et al. An Official ATS/AACN/ACCP/ESICM/SCCM Policy Statement: Responding to Requests for Potentially Inappropriate Treatments in Intensive Care Units. Am J Respir Crit Care Med 2015;191(11):1318–30.

70. Laureys S. Science and society: death, unconsciousness and the brain. Nat Rev Neurosci 2005;6(11):899–909.

71. Becker KJ, Baxter AB, Cohen WA, et al. Withdrawal of support in intracerebral hemorrhage may lead to self-fulfilling prophecies. Neurology 2001;56(6):766–72.

72. Erp WS van, Lavrijsen JCM, Vos PE, et al. Unresponsive wakefulness syndrome: Outcomes from a vicious circle. Ann Neurol 2020;87(1):12–8.

73. Rubin EB, Bernat JL. Ethical aspects of disordered states of consciousness. Neurol Clin 2011;29(4):1055–71.

74. Tran LN, Back AL, Creutzfeldt CJ. Palliative Care Consultations in the Neuro-ICU: A Qualitative Study. Neurocrit Care 2016;25(2):266–72.

75. Graham M. Can they feel? the capacity for pain and pleasure in patients with cognitive motor dissociation. Neuroethics 2019;12(2):153–69.

76. Boly M, Faymonville M-E, Peigneux P, et al. Cerebral processing of auditory and noxious stimuli in severely brain injured patients: differences between VS and MCS. Neuropsychol Rehabil 2005;15(3–4):283–9.

77. Laureys S, Faymonville ME, Peigneux P, et al. Cortical processing of noxious somatosensory stimuli in the persistent vegetative state. Neuroimage 2002;17(2):732–41.

78. Kassubek J, Juengling FD, Els T, et al. Activation of a residual cortical network during painful stimulation in long-term postanoxic vegetative state: a 15O-H2O PET study. J Neurol Sci 2003;212(1–2):85–91.

79. Lutkenhoff E, Mcarthur D, Hua X, et al. Thalamic atrophy in antero-medial and dorsal nuclei correlates with six-month outcome after severe brain injury. NeuroImage Clin 2013;3:396–404.

80. Graham M. A Fate Worse Than Death? The Well-Being of Patients Diagnosed as Vegetative With Covert Awareness. Ethic Theor Moral Prac 2017;20(5):1005–20.

81. LeClaire MM, Oakes JM, Weinert CR. Communication of prognostic information for critically ill patients. Chest 2005;128(3):1728–35.

82. Anderson WG, Cimino JW, Ernecoff NC, et al. A Multicenter Study of Key Stakeholders' Perspectives on Communicating with Surrogates about Prognosis in Intensive Care Units. Ann ATS 2014;12(2):142–52.

83. Simpkin AL, Armstrong KA. Communicating Uncertainty: a Narrative Review and Framework for Future Research. J Gen Intern Med 2019;34(11):2586–91.

84. Graber ML, Franklin N, Gordon R. Diagnostic Error in Internal Medicine. Arch Intern Med 2005;165(13):1493.

85. Wittenberg E, Ferrell BR, Smith T, et al. Textbook of palliative care communication. Oxford: Oxford University Press; 2015.

86. Fins JJ. Disorders of Consciousness and Disordered Care: Families, Caregivers, and Narratives of Necessity. Arch Phys Med Rehabil 2013;94(10):1934–9.

87. Quill TE, Holloway R. Time-Limited Trials Near the End of Life. JAMA 2011;306(13):1483–4.

88. Holloway RG, Arnold RM, Creutzfeldt CJ, et al. Palliative and end-of-life care in stroke: a statement for healthcare professionals from the American Heart Association/American Stroke Association. Stroke 2014;45(6):1887–916.

89. de la Morena MJE, Cruzado JA. Caregivers of patients with disorders of consciousness: coping and prolonged grief. Acta Neurol Scand 2013;127(6):413–8.

90. Gonzalez-Lara LE, Munce S, Christian J, et al. The multiplicity of caregiving burden: a qualitative analysis of families with prolonged disorders of consciousness. Brain Inj 2021;35(2):200–8.
91. Zaksh Y, Yehene E, Elyashiv M, et al. Partially dead, partially separated: establishing the mechanism between ambiguous loss and grief reaction among caregivers of patients with prolonged disorders of consciousness. Clin Rehabil 2019; 33(2):345–56.
92. Manskow US, Sigurdardottir S, Røe C, et al. Factors Affecting Caregiver Burden 1 Year After Severe Traumatic Brain Injury: A Prospective Nationwide Multicenter Study. J Head Trauma Rehabil 2015;30(6):411–23.

Infectious Meningitis and Encephalitis

Rachel J. Bystritsky, MD[a],*, Felicia C. Chow, MD, MAS[b,c]

KEYWORDS

- Meningitis • Encephalitis • CNS infection

KEY POINTS

- Acute bacterial meningitis is a medical emergency that requires prompt recognition and therapy
- Chronic meningitis is defined as inflammation of the meninges associated with a duration of symptoms of at least 4 weeks
- Viruses are the most common etiologic agents of encephalitis, although in many cases, a specific pathogen is never identified
- Lumbar puncture for cerebrospinal fluid analysis is an essential component of evaluation for meningitis and encephalitis

INTRODUCTION

Meningitis and encephalitis are inflammatory conditions of the central nervous system (CNS) that can lead to high rates of mortality and disability. Although there is considerable overlap between the presentation, diagnostic evaluation, and etiologies of meningitis and encephalitis, defining the specific syndromes can be useful in developing an overall clinical approach. Meningitis, defined as inflammation of the meninges surrounding the brain and spinal cord, is typically characterized by headache, neck stiffness, and cerebrospinal fluid (CSF) pleocytosis. Encephalitis, however, involves inflammation of the brain parenchyma, the hallmark of which is encephalopathy, or diffuse alteration of brain function and altered mental status. Patients may have evidence of both meningeal and parenchymal inflammation, known as meningoencephalitis, or involvement of the meninges and/or brain parenchyma in combination with inflammation anywhere along the neuroaxis, including the spinal cord (encephalomyelitis) or nerve roots (encephalomyeloradiculitis or meningoradiculitis). Meningitis and

[a] Department of Medicine, University of California San Francisco, 513 Parnassus Avenue, Room S-280, San Francisco, CA 94143, USA; [b] Department of Neurology, University of California, San Francisco, 1001 Potrero Avenue, Building 1, Room 101, San Francisco, CA 94110, USA; [c] Department of Medicine, University of California, San Francisco, 1001 Potrero Avenue, Building 1, Room 101, San Francisco, CA 94110, USA
* Corresponding author.
E-mail address: rachel.bystritsky@ucsf.edu

Neurol Clin 40 (2022) 77–91
https://doi.org/10.1016/j.ncl.2021.08.006
0733-8619/22/© 2021 Elsevier Inc. All rights reserved.
neurologic.theclinics.com

encephalitis have various causes, both infectious and noninfectious. This review will focus on infectious meningitis and encephalitis.

EPIDEMIOLOGY
Bacterial Meningitis

Meningitis is a significant cause of mortality and morbidity worldwide. Despite the availability of highly active antibacterial agents, poor outcomes associated with bacterial meningitis remain high, with a case fatality rate of approximately 15%.[1] Before the advent of antimicrobial therapy, bacterial meningitis was almost uniformly fatal. Furthermore, among survivors of meningitis, neurologic disability and persistent sequelae that impact day-to-day function are prevalent, ranging from hearing loss and other focal neurologic deficits to seizures and cognitive impairment.[2]

The incidence of bacterial meningitis varies by geographic region. In the United States, the annual incidence of bacterial meningitis as of 2006 to 2007 surveillance data was 1.38 cases per 100,000.[1] Among cases of bacterial meningitis across age groups, the predominant causal organisms in the United States are Streptococcus pneumoniae (58.0%), group B Streptococcus (18.1%), Neisseria meningitidis (13.9%), Haemophilus influenzae (6.7%), and Listeria monocytogenes (3.4%).[1] Worldwide, the highest rates of bacterial meningitis occur in the "meningitis belt" of sub-Saharan Africa stretching from Senegal to Ethiopia, where meningococcal disease is hyperendemic, although the introduction of conjugated meningococcal vaccines has decreased the incidence significantly.[3] The relative frequency of different pathogens varies with age, with group B Streptococcus being the most common etiology of meningitis in neonates[4] and L monocytogenes primarily affecting infants and persons over the age of 50 years (**Table 1**). Gram-negative bacillary meningitis is exceedingly rare in immunocompetent adults in the absence of CNS instrumentation (ie, preceding neurosurgery or indwelling devices).

Viral Meningitis

Although bacterial meningitis is a "can't miss" diagnosis, viral meningitis is actually the most common type of infectious meningitis.[4] The proportion of meningitis cases attributed to viruses is growing as the incidence of bacterial meningitis falls and as molecular diagnostic techniques to identify viral infections become more widely available. The term "aseptic meningitis," which is often misused interchangeably with viral meningitis, refers to meningitis in which no infectious agent is identified after an initial

Table 1 Common etiologic agents of bacterial meningitis	
Predisposing Factor	**Bacterial Pathogens**
Age[1]	
<2 mo	Group B strep, S pneumoniae, Listeria monocytogenes, E coli
2–23 mo	S pneumoniae, N meningitidis, H influenza type B (Hib), group B strep
2–50 y	N meningitidis, S pneumoniae
>50	S pneumoniae, N meningitidis, Hib, group B Strep, L monocytogenes
Health care associated	S aureus, gram negative bacilli, coagulase negative staphylococci
Basilar skull fracture[5,6]	S pneumoniae, beta-hemolytic strep

evaluation for bacterial etiologies. Among cases of aseptic meningitis in high-income countries in which a cause is identified, nonpolio enteroviruses and herpesviruses are the most frequently detected pathogens, although their relative distributions are variable.[7,8] In a study of adult immunocompetent patients in Finland presenting with aseptic meningitis, enteroviruses were the causative agent in 26% of cases, herpes simplex virus-2 (HSV-2) in 17%, and varicella-zoster virus (VZV) in 8%.[8] In another study from Spain that included both adults and children with aseptic meningitis, enteroviruses accounted for 44% of cases compared with only 6% attributed to HSV-2 and VZV.[7] Other viral etiologies of meningitis include mumps and measles viruses, arboviruses, and lymphocytic choriomeningitis virus (LCMV). In a large proportion of patients with aseptic meningitis, ranging from 33% to nearly 50% of cases, no etiology may be identified.[4,7,8] Although viral infection is often viewed as a benign form of meningitis, viral meningitis can lead to substantial morbidity and decrease in quality of life.[5]

Recurrent and Chronic Meningitis

Recurrent meningitis is rare. Recurrent benign lymphocytic meningitis (also known as Mollaret's) is thought to be predominantly caused by HSV-2 infection.[9] Recurrent bacterial meningitis is often associated with an underlying anatomic (59%) or immunologic (36%) defect.[10]

Chronic meningitis is distinguished from acute meningitis by the presence of symptoms and evidence of meningeal inflammation for at least 4 weeks. Chronic meningitis is less common than acute meningitis and is frequently caused by tuberculosis and fungal infections. The epidemiology of chronic meningitis varies widely by geographic location. *Mycobacterium tuberculosis* is believed to be the most common cause of chronic meningitis worldwide and occurs in 1% to 2% of cases of active tuberculosis.[11] *Cryptococcus neoformans* is the most common etiologic agent of fungal meningitis and primarily occurs in immunocompromised hosts, particularly those with advanced HIV and in recipients of solid organ transplants. *Cryptococcus gattii* is an emerging fungal pathogen and, in contrast to *C neoformans*, has a greater propensity for causing CNS infection in immunocompetent hosts.[12] Dimorphic fungi including *Coccidioides*, *Histoplasma*, and *Blastomyces*, which are endemic to particular geographic regions, and *Sporothrix schenckii* can also cause chronic meningitis.

Other Causes of Meningitis

The spirochetes *Treponema pallidum* (syphilis), *Borrelia* species, and *Leptospira* are other potential causes of meningitis, which can present relatively acutely but also in a more subacute to chronic fashion. Cranial neuropathies and peripheral radiculoneuropathies may occur with CNS infections caused by spirochete organisms.[13] Several zoonotic infections, including *Brucella* spp. and *Coxiella burnetii*, can present as meningitis. Parasitic causes of meningitis in the United States are rare, but more common in endemic regions of the world, and often associated with the detection of eosinophils in the CSF. Etiologic agents include *Angiostrongylus*, *Baylisascaris*, *Taenia solium,* and *Gnathostoma.*[14]

Viral Encephalitis

The burden of disease associated with encephalitis is substantial, with an overall rate of hospitalization of 7.3 per 100,000 population and a mortality rate of 5.6% to 5.8%.[15,16] Encephalitis occurs in all age groups but is more common in infants and adults over the age of 65 years. Most cases of infectious encephalitis are caused by viruses. The most common etiologic agent of encephalitis is HSV, followed by enteroviruses, arboviruses, and VZV. In contrast to HSV meningitis, HSV encephalitis is most often caused by HSV-1 and is associated with a high rate of mortality and neurologic sequelae.[17] Other human herpesviruses such as VZV, cytomegalovirus (CMV), Epstein-Barr virus (EBV), and human herpesvirus 6 (HHV-6) can also cause encephalitis. Of these, VZV is the most common and can occur in immunocompetent hosts, whereas CMV, EBV, and HHV-6 encephalitis predominantly occur in immunocompromised hosts.

A wide variety of enterovirus serotypes cause neuroinvasive disease and follow a seasonal pattern with cases peaking during the summer to early fall in the United States.[18] Enterovirus 71 has been associated with outbreaks of severe neurologic disease in children.[19] Arboviruses are transmitted to humans by arthropods, predominantly mosquitos and ticks, and thus typically occur in a seasonal pattern corresponding to peak activity of their vectors. West Nile virus (WNV) is by far the leading cause of arboviral encephalitis in the United States, with La Crosse, Jamestown Canyon, Powassan, St. Louis encephalitis, and Equine encephalitis viruses causing smaller numbers of cases each year.[20] Outside the United States, Japanese encephalitis is the most important cause of epidemic viral encephalitis worldwide, causing 68,000 cases and 13,000 to 20,000 deaths yearly.[21] Rabies virus infection, although rare in the United States, causes approximately 59,000 human deaths annually worldwide.[22] Encephalitis resulting from neuroinvasive influenza infection is uncommon, but maybe more prevalent with certain subtypes, as observed during the 2009 H1N1 pandemic.[23]

Nonviral Encephalitis

Nonviral causes of encephalitis are significantly less common. Rare etiologic agents include atypical bacteria (*Rickettsia, Brucella, Ehrlichia, Anaplasma*), fungi, and protozoa (*Toxoplasma, Plasmodium falciparum*). Of the free-living ameba, *Acanthamoeba* and *Balamuthia* cause granulomatous amebic encephalitis and *Naegleria fowleri* causes a primary amebic meningoencephalitis.[24]

CLINICAL PRESENTATION
Meningitis

Acute bacterial meningitis in adults classically presents with a triad of fever, neck stiffness, and altered mental status and is characterized by sudden onset of symptoms. However, the complete triad may be present in less than half of patients presenting with community-acquired bacterial meningitis,[25] whereas at least 1 of the 3 symptoms is found in nearly 100% of patients.[25,26] Most adults with acute bacterial meningitis either present with fever or develop fever within 1 day of presentation. Altered mental status, which may suggest the presence of meningoencephalitis, is common with acute bacterial meningitis but more unusual with other types of acute meningitis. Headache is another common complaint at presentation (87%).[26] When considering headache with the classic triad, at least 2 of 4 symptoms are present in 95% of patients with acute bacterial meningitis.[27] Meningismus on examination is present in most patients; however, it may be subtle or absent in up to 35% of patients.[28] Kernig's and Brudzinski's signs have similarly poor sensitivity (11% and 9%, respectively).[29] The absence of these clinical findings cannot be used to exclude bacterial meningitis. The presence of a rapidly evolving petechial or purpuric rash may suggest *N meningitidis* as the etiologic agent, although patients with pneumococcal meningitis may also present with rash, though less frequently.[30] Although viral meningitis can be a more benign, self-limited illness, the presentation of viral meningitis is similar to that of bacterial meningitis, particularly early in the disease course, and the two cannot be distinguished reliably based on clinical findings.[28] Classic signs and symptoms of meningitis may be absent in very young, elderly, and immunocompromised hosts.

The clinical presentation of chronic meningitis, defined as evidence of meningeal inflammation, including persistent CSF pleocytosis and/or elevated protein, lasting at least 4 weeks, maybe subtle and highly variable. The development of symptoms is often insidious. Fever and meningismus may be absent. The diagnosis of chronic meningitis is challenging, and diagnostic delays are common. Symptoms may be progressive, static, or wax and wane. Cranial nerve and other focal neurologic deficits may be observed late in the course of disease, as a consequence of hydrocephalus or cerebral infarction.

Encephalitis

The key presenting feature of encephalitis is altered mental status. Headache is common,[31] and presence of fever, seizures, and focal neurologic deficits are considered minor criteria for the diagnosis of encephalitis.[32] Signs and symptoms of encephalitis may overlap with meningitis and other intracranial infections. Neck stiffness and photophobia are typically absent in pure encephalitis and when present suggest a meningoencephalitis with concomitant meningeal inflammation. The pattern of involvement of the nervous system may also offer clues to potential causative agents.[33] For example, enteroviruses and *Listeria* should be considered in patients presenting with rhombencephalitis. Extrapyramidal symptoms may be seen in WNV and other arboviral encephalitides, as well as CNS toxoplasmosis. Prominent limbic symptoms may point to HSV-1 or HHV-6 encephalitis. Acute flaccid paralysis is suggestive of WNV and enterovirus infection.

Although differences in clinical manifestations may be noted in observational studies, no initial clinical features reliably distinguish etiologies of acute encephalitis[34]; therefore, early empirical therapy for treatable causes of acute encephalitis (ie, HSV and VZV) is imperative. HSV-1 exhibits tropism for the temporal lobe, resulting in seizures in greater than 50% of patients with HSV encephalitis.[31] Herpetic skin lesions are seldom seen with HSV-1 encephalitis.[30] VZV encephalitis in adults is most commonly a manifestation of viral reactivation and may occur in the absence of or may precede skin lesions,[35] whereas in children, it is a complication of primary varicella infection. Arboviral encephalitis is often preceded by a viral prodrome, usually within days of a mosquito or tick bite.[36] Rash is reported in 15% to 57% of patients with WNV infection.[37]

EVALUATION

Diagnostic evaluation should be guided by the patient's clinical presentation, immune status, and potential exposures, including geographic location, travel history, vaccination status, occupational history, sexual history, and substance use. Lumbar puncture (LP) to obtain CSF for analysis is an essential component of the evaluation for any patient presenting with suspected meningitis or encephalitis. US guidelines[38] recommend neuroimaging with computed tomography (CT) for selected patients before performing an LP to exclude a mass lesion which could predispose the patient to cerebral herniation. These include patients who are immunocompromised or have a history of CNS disease (eg, mass lesion, stroke, focal infection), or are presenting with new-onset seizure, papilledema, abnormal level of consciousness, or focal neurologic deficit. For patients without these risk factors, CT before LP is of limited utility[39] and may lead to unnecessary delays in diagnosis and treatment. Controversy exists regarding whether the presence of altered mental status requires imaging before

LP. Swedish guidelines were revised in 2009 to remove this recommendation, which was associated with significantly earlier treatment and improved outcomes.[40]

CSF Analysis

CSF should be sent for cell count and differential, protein, glucose, gram stain, and bacterial culture for all patients with suspected CNS infection, with additional studies based on clinical suspicion for specific etiologies. CSF analysis can help differentiate between categories of infectious causes of meningitis (**Table 2**),[41–43] although significant overlap in the CSF profile among pathogens exists.[44] CSF lactate may be helpful as an adjunctive assay to identify bacterial meningitis when measured before treatment with antibiotics.[45] The presence of eosinophils provides a valuable clue to the diagnosis as a limited number of infectious agents are associated with eosinophilic meningitis (predominantly helminths and *Coccidioides*).[14]

An opening pressure should be measured when performing an LP. The opening pressure is often elevated in cases of bacterial, fungal, and tuberculous meningitis and may be slightly raised in cases of viral encephalitis.[41]

Microbiologic Investigations and Serologic Testing

The priority of investigations should be dictated by clinical suspicion combined with evaluation for "can't miss" infections (eg, acute bacterial meningitis, HSV-1 encephalitis), infections that are common (eg, HSV, VZV, syphilis, cryptococcus), or for which there are targeted treatments (eg, endemic fungal infections, tuberculosis). All patients with suspected meningitis or encephalitis should have serum HIV and syphilis testing and blood cultures, in addition to other selected serologic testing based on the clinical scenario, immune status of the host, exposure history, and time of year. In addition to blood and CSF, other biological specimens, including nasopharyngeal swabs, sputum, and stool samples, may also aid in making a diagnosis.

The sensitivity of CSF gram stain for the identification of bacterial meningitis varies from 40% to 90%[46,47] across case series. CSF bacterial cultures are positive in more than 80% of cases of acute bacterial meningitis when collected before the initiation of antimicrobial therapy.[48] The sensitivity of culture for the detection of bacterial meningitis is significantly reduced by pretreatment with antibiotics, although may remain as high as 73% if LP is performed within 4 hours.[49] As a result, it is imperative to ascertain whether an LP occurred before or after antibiotic therapy when interpreting the results of CSF bacterial cultures. Other CSF parameters, including glucose and protein, can also begin to normalize within 24 hours of initiation of antibiotics, whereas the CSF pleocytosis is less rapidly affected.[50] Blood cultures are valuable in detecting an etiologic agent in bacterial meningitis, particularly if LP is delayed.[25] Multiplex polymerase chain reaction (PCR) panels have been developed for the rapid diagnosis of meningitis and serve as a helpful adjunct to culture-based testing. These panels may include

Table 2					
CSF analysis in meningitis					
	Opening Pressure	**Cell Count (Cells/mm³)**	**Predominant Cell Type**	**Glucose**	**Protein**
Viral	Normal	<1000	Lymphocytes	Normal	Normal to high
Bacterial	Elevated	Often >1000	Neutrophils	Low	High
Fungal	Elevated	Variable	Lymphocytes	Normal to low	Normal to high
Tuberculosis	Normal or elevated	100–500	Lymphocytes	Low to very low	High to very high

testing for common causes of bacterial meningitis and viral meningitis and encephalitis, and for *Cryptococcus* species.

The diagnosis of viral meningitis and encephalitis relies on PCR-based testing for the detection of viral pathogens. Initial testing for immunocompetent adults presenting with suspected viral meningitis should include CSF PCR testing for HSV-1, HSV-2, and VZV. Enterovirus testing can be considered if a definitive diagnosis is desired or in the setting of an outbreak, although detection of these viruses does not change clinical management as no specific therapies are available. For patients presenting with acute encephalitis, first-pass testing should include CSF PCR for HSV-1, HSV-2, VZV, enteroviruses, and, in children, human parechovirus, as well as CSF serologies for VZV. During summer and fall, CSF and serum serologic testing for WNV should be performed.[51] Additional testing for immunocompromised patients includes PCR testing for CMV, HHV-6, HHV-7, JC virus, LCMV, and WNV as well as CSF serology for LCMV.[51] The sensitivity of CSF HSV PCR is excellent although varies with the timing of the assay and may be negative early in the course of illness or after exposure to antiviral therapy.[52] For patients with a negative CSF HSV PCR in whom the pretest probability for HSV-1 encephalitis is high, repeat LP and CSF HSV PCR testing should be obtained.

CSF culture is the gold standard for the diagnosis of cryptococcal meningitis but may take several days to grow and can be negative in a minority of cases.[53] CSF cryptococcal antigen testing is an important adjunct to CSF culture and was the first fungal antigen detection assay to be adopted for widespread clinical use.[54] More recently developed lateral flow assay cryptococcal antigen tests are highly accurate, inexpensive, and can be implemented in resource-limited settings.[55] Although the sensitivity of cryptococcal antigen testing is high, false negatives can occur in the presence of capsule-deficient *C neoformans*.[56] Other fungal etiologies of meningitis, including *Coccidioides* and *Histoplasma*, may be more difficult to diagnose as cultures are frequently negative and diagnosis often relies on serologic testing. CSF *Coccidioides* antigen testing has recently become available with a reported sensitivity as high as 93%.[57] Similarly, a combination of CSF antigen and antibody testing is the most sensitive approach for the diagnosis of *Histoplasma* meningitis.[58] The measurement of (1,3)-beta-D-glucan in CSF may be positive in meningitis because of a wide variety of fungal pathogens, although clinical studies are limited.[59]

The diagnosis of tuberculous meningitis is notoriously difficult, given poor sensitivity of CSF acid-fast bacilli (AFB) staining and culture. A minimum of 10 mL of CSF is recommended for AFB testing, as the yield of AFB smear and culture is improved with repeat high volume LP.[60] Sensitivity of culture is imperfect and varies from 70% to 86%.[60,61] Even when culture is positive, results take several weeks, limiting the utility of culture for the clinical management of patients with suspected tuberculous meningitis. Nucleic acid amplification tests (eg, GeneXpert, GeneXpert Ultra MTB/RIF assays) are an important clinical tool that allows for the rapid detection of *M tuberculosis* in CSF with high specificity (99%) and fair sensitivity of 68% to 82% depending on the reference standard used,[62] although this sensitivity is insufficient to rule out tuberculosis in those with a high pretest probability. Tuberculin skin testing and interferon-gamma release assay are of limited clinical value as they do not distinguish between active and latent disease and are frequently negative in patients with active tuberculosis, including specifically in CNS tuberculosis.[63]

For patients presenting with aseptic meningitis or encephalitis, in addition to considering fungal and mycobacterial causes, studies should be sent to evaluate for atypical causes, including syphilis (CSF VDRL[64] and treponemal testing), brucellosis (CSF antibody testing by agglutination), toxoplasmosis (serology and PCR), Lyme disease (simultaneous measurement of serum and CSF antibodies), and Rickettsial infection (serum antibodies) based on clinical presentation and epidemiologic risk. Despite thorough evaluation using traditional microbiological techniques, serologies and PCR-based testing, in many cases of meningoencephalitis and meningitis, the etiologic agent remains unknown.[65] Metagenomic next-generation sequencing is a promising new technology in the diagnosis of CNS infections and can detect a wide range of pathogens in a single assay.[66] Broad-range PCR (universal PCR) can detect bacterial, fungal, or mycobacterial pathogens missed on routine culture and may be positive in 30% of cases of culture-negative presumed bacterial meningitis.[67] In addition to factors such as the volume of CSF tested and whether CSF was collected before or after initiation of antimicrobial therapy, another critical consideration when interpreting CSF results is the compartment from which CSF was obtained. For example, in patients with basilar meningitis, the CSF profile and yield of microbiological and molecular testing from ventricular fluid may be starkly different from lumbar CSF. These potential differences should be taken into account when interpreting CSF test results for diagnostic purposes and monitoring treatment response.[68]

Imaging

Beyond excluding mass lesions before LP in selected patients, the utility of brain imaging in the diagnosis of acute meningitis, or in the identification of the infectious etiology, is limited. However, brain imaging is essential for evaluating potential complications of acute meningitis including cerebritis/abscess, subdural empyema, venous sinus thrombosis, stroke, ventriculitis, or hydrocephalus[28] and should be considered in patients with persistent fevers, focal neurologic findings, or seizures. MRI is the imaging modality of choice for detecting complications of acute bacterial meningitis.[56] When vascular involvement is suspected or confirmed with the presence of strokes, magnetic resonance or CT angiography is recommended. Contrast-enhanced brain MRI with diffusion-weighted and iron-sensitive sequences when feasible is useful in the diagnostic evaluation of chronic meningitis. Patterns of enhancement (ie, basilar meningitis and ventriculitis) may help narrow the differential diagnosis, as may the presence of focal lesions or strokes.

MRI of the brain should be performed in all patients with suspected encephalitis.[33] Diffusion-weighted imaging is more sensitive than conventional MRI in detecting early changes in viral encephalitis.[69] Characteristic patterns of involvement can be seen in encephalitis caused by specific infectious agents.[33] For example, abnormalities of the inferomedial region of one or both temporal lobes are seen in most patients with HSV encephalitis,[70] although atypical neuroimaging patterns can be seen in immunocompromised patients and neonates or younger children.[71] Progressive multifocal leukoencephalopathy caused by JC virus usually presents with single or multifocal T2/FLAIR hyperintense and T1 hypointense confluent lesions affecting the white matter[66] without associated mass effect or enhancement.[72]

Brain Biopsy

Brain biopsy is rarely used for the diagnosis of encephalitis in the modern era, given the availability of PCR-based testing and serologic assays, but retains a limited role for the evaluation of encephalitis of unknown etiology with progressive neurologic deterioration.[33] In one study of 29 patients with encephalitis of unknown etiology, brain biopsy and neuropathologic rereview of biopsy material did not yield a more specific diagnosis in over two-thirds of cases.[73] In the absence of an urgent clinical indication, empiric administration of corticosteroids should be deferred until after brain biopsy as they may decrease the yield of tissue sampling in certain conditions (eg, lymphoma).

TREATMENT
Acute Meningitis

Acute bacterial meningitis is a medical emergency that requires the prompt institution of therapy, preferably after CSF studies and blood cultures are obtained. If LP is delayed, either because preceding neuroimaging is required or due to technical issues, empirical therapy should be initiated immediately. Delay in the institution of antibiotic therapy is associated with increased mortality from acute bacterial meningitis.[74] Empirical therapy should be chosen to cover the most likely bacterial agents based on age, risk factors (see **Table 1**), and results of the CSF gram stain. Once an etiologic agent is identified, therapy should be tailored to the specific pathogen (**Table 3**). In practice, it may be difficult to distinguish bacterial meningitis from viral meningoencephalitis. As a result, depending on the clinical scenario, IV acyclovir may also be started empirically while awaiting CSF studies.

In addition to antibacterial therapy, adjunctive dexamethasone should be started with or before the first dose of antibiotics for adults and considered for pediatric patients aged 6 weeks or older presenting with community-acquired bacterial meningitis. In a randomized placebo-controlled trial that demonstrated a reduction in the risk of unfavorable outcomes including mortality with dexamethasone use in adults with bacterial meningitis, clinical benefit was only seen in patients with *S pneumoniae* meningitis.[75] Therefore, dexamethasone should be discontinued if diagnostic testing uncovers another pathogen. In children, adjunctive corticosteroids have been shown to reduce hearing loss in *H influenzae* type b meningitis.[76] The role of adjunctive corticosteroids for children with pneumococcal meningitis is uncertain.[28]

Table 3 Antibiotic therapy by organism	
Organism	**Recommended Therapy**
Streptococcus pneumoniae	
Penicillin MIC ≤0.06	Penicillin G or ampicillin
Penicillin MIC ≥0.12	
Ceftriaxone MIC ≤0.12	Ceftriaxone or cefotaxime
Ceftriaxone MIC >0.12	Vancomycin plus ceftriaxone or cefotaxime
Neisseria meningitidis	
Penicillin MIC 0.06	Penicillin or ampicillin
Penicillin MIC 0.12–1	Ceftriaxone or cefotaxime
Listeria monocytogenes	Ampicillin or penicillin G
Haemophilus influenzae	
Beta-lactamase negative	Ampicillin
Beta-lactamase positive	Third-generation cephalosporin
Group B streptococcus	Ampicillin or penicillin G
Staphylococcus aureus	
Methicillin susceptible	Nafcillin or oxacillin
Methicillin resistant	Vancomycin
Enterobacterales	Third-generation cephalosporin
Staphylococcus epidermidis	Vancomycin

Abbreviations: MIC, Minimum inhibitory concentration.
Data from Tunkel AR, Hartman BJ, Kaplan SL, et al. Practice guidelines for the management of bacterial meningitis. Clin Infect Dis 2004;39(9):1267-1284. doi:10.1086/425368.

Viral meningitis typically follows a more benign course, although viral meningitis is associated with worse patient-reported outcomes including quality of life. The necessity and efficacy of antiviral therapy for uncomplicated HSV meningitis in immunocompetent patients, including the duration and formulation of therapy, is uncertain and recovery without neurologic sequelae is the norm even in the absence of antiviral treatment.[77] However, in immunocompromised patients, neurologic outcomes are significantly improved with antiviral therapy.[77]

Chronic Meningitis

Therapy for chronic meningitis depends on the etiologic agent and the primary focus of initial management is establishing a specific diagnosis rather than empirical therapy given the varied causes and indolent nature of the disease. However, as the diagnosis of tuberculous meningitis is challenging and treatment delay is associated with poor outcomes, therapy for tuberculous meningitis should be started empirically when tuberculous meningitis is suspected and supported by CSF findings. Tuberculous meningitis is treated with adjunctive corticosteroids,[78] in addition to 4-drug combination therapy. The decision to start corticosteroids with empirical therapy should be made with caution as the anti-inflammatory effects may mask the progression of an unrecognized fungal or noninfectious cause of meningitis. Empirical therapy is often continued to complete a full treatment course (9–12 months) unless an alternative diagnosis is made.[79]

In the absence of compelling clinical or epidemiologic clues suggesting a specific fungal pathogen, empirical antifungal therapy is rarely warranted. In patients with clinical features highly suggestive of fungal meningitis who are not improving or are deteriorating, empirical therapy should be considered. The challenge, however, is that therapy for fungal meningitis varies by etiologic agent. Initial therapy for cryptococcal meningitis consists of amphotericin B plus flucytosine, followed by fluconazole for consolidation and maintenance therapy.[80] First-line therapy for coccidioidal meningitis, which requires lifelong therapy, is high dose fluconazole.[81] CNS histoplasmosis is initially treated with liposomal amphotericin B followed by itraconazole for at least 1 year.[82]

Encephalitis

Specific therapies are lacking for most causes of viral encephalitis apart from herpesviruses. The focus of initial management is on identifying treatable causes. Empirical therapy with high dose intravenous acyclovir should be initiated in all patients with suspected encephalitis while results of diagnostic testing are pending. If atypical bacterial infections are suspected, including with *Rickettsia*, *Ehrlichia*, *Anaplasma*, or *Brucella*, doxycycline should be started empirically.

For proven HSV encephalitis, intravenous acyclovir is continued for 14 to 21 days, as relapse has been reported with shorter treatment durations.[83] VZV encephalitis is treated with intravenous acyclovir for 10 to 14 days.[33] Adjunctive corticosteroids are used by some for the treatment of VZV encephalitis, particularly in the presence of associated VZV vasculopathy,[84] although robust clinical data are lacking. Optimal therapy for CMV encephalitis is unknown. Guidelines suggest the use of dual therapy with ganciclovir and foscarnet.[33] Therapeutic options for encephalitis due to enteroviral or arboviral infection are limited and treatment is primarily supportive. Intravenous immunoglobulin (IVIG) has been used for enteroviral and WNV encephalitis; however, the value of this therapy has not been established. One recent clinical trial of IVIG for WNV encephalitis demonstrated a lack of efficacy of both standard and high-titered immunoglobulin.[85]

SUMMARY

Infectious meningitis and encephalitis cause a high burden of mortality and morbidity worldwide. These syndromes comprise a heterogeneous group of diseases caused by a wide variety of pathogens. Prompt recognition and empirical therapy for treatable causes are imperative. LP for CSF analysis is an essential component of the evaluation. Therapeutic approaches differ by infecting pathogens.

CLINICS CARE POINTS

- Acute bacterial meningitis is a medical emergency requiring prompt recognition, lumbar puncture, and initiation of antimicrobial therapy.
- Significant overlap exists in the clinical presentation of infectious causes of meningitis. Clinical features, the immune status of the host, epidemiologic risk factors, and results of the cerebrospinal fluid analysis can aid in narrowing the differential diagnosis.
- Although there is no specific therapy for many causes of viral encephalitis, HSV-1 is a common treatable cause and high-dose acyclovir should be started empirically while awaiting the results of diagnostic testing.
- Tuberculosis is a common cause of chronic meningitis worldwide. Because diagnostic testing is insensitive and treatment delays result in poor outcomes, therapy is often started empirically.

DISCLOSURE

The authors have nothing to disclose.

REFERENCES

1. Thigpen MC, Messonnier NE, Hadler JL, et al. Bacterial meningitis in the United States, 1998–2007. N Engl J Med 2011;10.
2. Lucas MJ, Brouwer MC, van de Beek D. Neurological sequelae of bacterial meningitis. J Infect 2016;73(1):18–27.
3. Lingani C, Bergeron-Caron C, Stuart JM, et al. Meningococcal meningitis surveillance in the African Meningitis Belt, 2004–2013. Clin Infect Dis 2015;61(Suppl 5): S410.
4. McGill F, Griffiths MJ, Bonnett LJ, et al. Incidence, aetiology, and sequelae of viral meningitis in UK adults: a multicentre prospective observational cohort study. Lancet Infect Dis 2018;18(9):992–1003.
5. Leibu S, Rosenthal G, Shoshan Y, et al. Clinical significance of long-term follow-up of children with posttraumatic skull base fracture. World Neurosurg 2017;103: 315–21.
6. Dagi TF, Meyer FB, Poletti CA. The incidence and prevention of meningitis after basilar skull fracture. Am J Emerg Med 1983;1(3):295–8.
7. Ory F de, Avellón A, Echevarría JE, et al. Viral infections of the central nervous system in Spain: a prospective study. J Med Virol 2013;85(3):554–62.
8. Kupila L, Vuorinen T, Vainionpää R, et al. Etiology of aseptic meningitis and encephalitis in an adult population. Neurology 2006;66(1):75–80.
9. Tedder DG, Ashley R, Tyler KL, et al. Herpes simplex virus infection as a cause of benign recurrent lymphocytic meningitis. Ann Intern Med 1994;121(5):334–8.
10. Tebruegge M, Curtis N. Epidemiology, etiology, pathogenesis, and diagnosis of recurrent bacterial meningitis. Clin Microbiol Rev 2008;21(3):519–37.

11. Mezochow A, Thakur K, Vinnard C. Tuberculous meningitis in children and adults: new insights for an ancient foe. Curr Neurol Neurosci Rep 2017;17(11):85.

12. Baddley JW, Chen SC-A, Huisingh C, et al. MSG07: an international cohort study comparing epidemiology and outcomes of patients with cryptococcus neoformans or cryptococcus gattii infections. Clin Infect Dis 2021. https://doi.org/10.1093/cid/ciab268. ciab268.

13. Pachner AR, Steere AC. The triad of neurologic manifestations of Lyme disease: meningitis, cranial neuritis, and radiculoneuritis. Neurology 1985;35(1):47–53.

14. Re VL, Gluckman SJ. Eosinophilic meningitis. Am J Med 2003;114(3):217–23.

15. George BP, Schneider EB, Venkatesan A. Encephalitis hospitalization rates and inpatient mortality in the United States, 2000-2010. PLoS ONE 2014;9(9):e104169.

16. Vora NM, Holman RC, Mehal JM, et al. Burden of encephalitis-associated hospitalizations in the United States, 1998-2010. Neurology 2014;82(5):443–51.

17. Jørgensen LK, Dalgaard LS, Østergaard LJ, et al. Incidence and mortality of herpes simplex encephalitis in Denmark: a nationwide registry-based cohort study. J Infect 2017;74(1):42–9.

18. Fowlkes AL, Honarmand S, Glaser C, et al. Enterovirus-associated encephalitis in the california encephalitis project, 1998–2005. J Infect Dis 2008;198(11):1685–91.

19. Pérez-Vélez CM, Anderson MS, Robinson CC, et al. Outbreak of neurologic enterovirus type 71 disease: a diagnostic challenge. Clin Infect Dis 2007;45(8):950–7.

20. McDonald E. West nile virus and other domestic nationally notifiable arboviral diseases — United States, 2018. MMWR Morb Mortal Wkly Rep 2019;68:673–8.

21. Centers for Disease Control and Prevention (CDC). Expanding poliomyelitis and measles surveillance networks to establish surveillance for acute meningitis and encephalitis syndromes–Bangladesh, China, and India, 2006-2008. MMWR Morb Mortal Wkly Rep 2012;61(49):1008–11.

22. Hampson K, Coudeville L, Lembo T, et al. Estimating the global burden of endemic canine rabies. PLoS Negl Trop Dis 2015;9(4):e0003709.

23. Akins PT, Belko J, Uyeki TM, et al. H1N1 encephalitis with malignant edema and review of neurologic complications from influenza. Neurocrit Care 2010;13(3):396–406.

24. Ong TYY, Khan NA, Siddiqui R. Brain-eating amoebae: predilection sites in the brain and disease outcome. J Clin Microbiol 2017;55(7):1989–97.

25. Bijlsma MW, Brouwer MC, Kasanmoentalib ES, et al. Community-acquired bacterial meningitis in adults in the Netherlands, 2006–14: a prospective cohort study. Lancet Infect Dis 2016;16(3):339–47.

26. Durand ML, Calderwood SB, Weber DJ, et al. Acute bacterial meningitis in adults – a review of 493 episodes. N Engl J Med 1993;328(1):21–8.

27. van de Beek D, de Gans J, Spanjaard L, et al. Clinical features and prognostic factors in adults with bacterial meningitis. N Engl J Med. 351(18):1849-1859.

28. van de Beek D, Cabellos C, Dzupova O, et al. ESCMID guideline: diagnosis and treatment of acute bacterial meningitis. Clin Microbiol Infect 2016;22:S37–62.

29. Brouwer MC, Thwaites GE, Tunkel AR, et al. Dilemmas in the diagnosis of acute community-acquired bacterial meningitis. Lancet 2012;380(9854):1684–92.

30. Tsai J, Nagel MA, Gilden D. Skin rash in meningitis and meningoencephalitis. Neurology 2013;80(19):1808–11.

31. Granerod J, Ambrose HE, Davies NW, et al. Causes of encephalitis and differences in their clinical presentations in England: a multicentre, population-based prospective study. Lancet Infect Dis 2010;10(12):835–44.

32. Venkatesan A, Tunkel AR, Bloch KC, et al. Case definitions, diagnostic algorithms, and priorities in encephalitis: consensus statement of the international encephalitis consortium. Clin Infect Dis 2013;57(8):1114–28.

33. Tunkel AR, Glaser CA, Bloch KC, et al. The management of encephalitis: clinical practice guidelines by the infectious diseases society of America. Clin Infect Dis 2008;47(3):303–27.

34. Le Maréchal M, Mailles A, Seigneurin A, et al. A prospective cohort study to identify clinical, biological, and imaging features that predict the etiology of acute encephalitis. Clin Infect Dis 2020. https://doi.org/10.1093/cid/ciaa598. ciaa598.

35. Kennedy PGE, Gershon AA. Clinical features of varicella-zoster virus infection. Viruses 2018;10(11):609.

36. Rust RS. Human arboviral encephalitis. Semin Pediatr Neurol 2012;19(3):130–51.

37. Ferguson DD, Gershman K, LeBailly A, et al. Characteristics of the rash associated with west nile virus fever. Clin Infect Dis 2005;41(8):1204–7.

38. Tunkel AR, Hartman BJ, Kaplan SL, et al. Practice guidelines for the management of bacterial meningitis. Clin Infect Dis 2004;39(9):1267–84.

39. Salazar L, Hasbun R. Cranial imaging before lumbar puncture in adults with community-acquired meningitis: clinical utility and adherence to the infectious diseases Society of America guidelines. Clin Infect Dis 2017;64(12):1657–62.

40. Glimåker M, Johansson B, Grindborg Ö, et al. Adult bacterial meningitis: earlier treatment and improved outcome following guideline revision promoting prompt lumbar puncture. Clin Infect Dis 2015;60(8):1162–9.

41. Solomon T, Hart IJ, Beeching NJ. Viral encephalitis: a clinician's guide. Pract Neurol 2007;7(5):288–305.

42. Tamune H, Takeya H, Suzuki W, et al. Cerebrospinal fluid/blood glucose ratio as an indicator for bacterial meningitis. Am J Emerg Med 2014;32(3):263–6.

43. Dorsett M, Liang SY. Diagnosis and treatment of central nervous system infections in the emergency department. Emerg Med Clin North Am 2016;34(4):917–42.

44. Khatib U, van de Beek D, Lees JA, et al. Adults with suspected central nervous system infection: a prospective study of diagnostic accuracy. J Infect 2017;74(1):1–9.

45. Sakushima K, Hayashino Y, Kawaguchi T, et al. Diagnostic accuracy of cerebrospinal fluid lactate for differentiating bacterial meningitis from aseptic meningitis: a meta-analysis. J Infect 2011;62(4):255–62.

46. Taniguchi T, Tsuha S, Shiiki S, et al. Point-of-care cerebrospinal fluid Gram stain for the management of acute meningitis in adults: a retrospective observational study. Ann Clin Microbiol Antimicrob 2020;19:59.

47. Tissot F, Prod'hom G, Manuel O, et al. Impact of round-the-clock CSF Gram stain on empirical therapy for suspected central nervous system infections. Eur J Clin Microbiol Infect Dis 2015;34(9):1849–57.

48. Bohr V, Rasmussen N, Hansen B, et al. 875 cases of bacterial meningitis: diagnostic procedures and the impact of preadmission antibiotic therapy. Part III of a three-part series. J Infect 1983;7(3):193–202.

49. Michael B, Menezes BF, Cunniffe J, et al. Effect of delayed lumbar punctures on the diagnosis of acute bacterial meningitis in adults. Emerg Med J 2010;27(6):433–8.

50. Nigrovic LE, Malley R, Macias CG, et al. Effect of antibiotic pretreatment on cerebrospinal fluid profiles of children with bacterial meningitis. Pediatrics 2008; 122(4):726–30.

51. Tyler KL. Acute viral encephalitis. N Engl J Med 2018;379(6):557–66.

52. Weil AA, Glaser CA, Amad Z, et al. Patients with suspected herpes simplex encephalitis: rethinking an initial negative polymerase chain reaction result. Clin Infect Dis 2002;34(8):1154–7.

53. Dismukes WE, Cloud G, Gallis HA, et al. Treatment of cryptococcal meningitis with combination amphotericin B and flucytosine for four as compared with six weeks. N Engl J Med 317(6):334 341.

54. Nalintya E, Kiggundu R, Meya D. Evolution of cryptococcal antigen testing: what is new? Curr Fungal Infect Rep 2016;10(2):62–7.

55. Boulware DR, Rolfes MA, Rajasingham R, et al. Multisite validation of cryptococcal antigen lateral flow assay and quantification by laser thermal contrast. Emerg Infect Dis 2014;20(1):45–53.

56. Hughes DC, Raghavan A, Mordekar SR, et al. Role of imaging in the diagnosis of acute bacterial meningitis and its complications. Postgrad Med J 2010;86(1018): 478–85.

57. Kassis C, Zaidi S, Kuberski T, et al. Role of Coccidioides antigen testing in the cerebrospinal fluid for the diagnosis of coccidioidal meningitis. Clin Infect Dis 2015;61(10):1521–6.

58. Bloch KC, Myint T, Raymond-Guillen L, et al. Improvement in diagnosis of histoplasma meningitis by combined testing for histoplasma antigen and immunoglobulin G and Immunoglobulin M anti-histoplasma antibody in cerebrospinal fluid. Clin Infect Dis 2018;66(1):89–94.

59. Davis C, Wheat LJ, Myint T, et al. Efficacy of cerebrospinal fluid beta-d-glucan diagnostic testing for fungal meningitis: a systematic review. J Clin Microbiol 2020;58(4):e02094.

60. Thwaites GE, Chau TTH, Farrar JJ. Improving the bacteriological diagnosis of tuberculous meningitis. J Clin Microbiol 2004;42(1):378–9.

61. Bahr NC, Tugume L, Rajasingham R, et al. Improved diagnostic sensitivity for tuberculous meningitis with Xpert(®) MTB/RIF of centrifuged CSF. Int J Tuberc Lung Dis 2015;19(10):1209–15.

62. Pormohammad A, Nasiri MJ, McHugh TD, et al. A systematic review and meta-analysis of the diagnostic accuracy of nucleic acid amplification tests for tuberculous meningitis. J Clin Microbiol 2019;57(6):e01113.

63. Vidhate MR, Singh MK, Garg RK, et al. Diagnostic and prognostic value of Mycobacterium tuberculosis complex specific interferon gamma release assay in patients with tuberculous meningitis. J Infect 2011;62(5):400–3.

64. Davis LE, Schmitt JW. Clinical significance of cerebrospinal fluid tests for neurosyphilis. Ann Neurol 1989;25(1):50–5.

65. Khetsuriani N, Holman RC, Anderson LJ. Burden of encephalitis-associated hospitalizations in the United States, 1988–1997. Clin Infect Dis 2002;35(2):175–82.

66. Wilson MR, Sample HA, Zorn KC, et al. Clinical metagenomic sequencing for diagnosis of meningitis and encephalitis. N Engl J Med 2019;380(24):2327–40.

67. Srinivasan L, Pisapia JM, Shah SS, et al. Can broad-range 16s ribosomal ribonucleic acid gene polymerase chain reactions improve the diagnosis of bacterial meningitis? A systematic review and meta-analysis. Ann Emerg Med 2012; 60(5):609–20.e2.

68. Khan SF, Macauley T, Tong SYC, et al. When ventricular cerebrospinal fluid assessment misleads: basal meningitis and the importance of lumbar puncture sampling. Open Forum Infect Dis 2019;6(7):ofz324.
69. Maschke M, Kastrup O, Forsting M, et al. Update on neuroimaging in infectious central nervous system disease. Curr Opin Neurol 2004;17(4):475–80.
70. Domingues RB, Fink MCD, Tsanaclis AMC, et al. Diagnosis of herpes simplex encephalitis by magnetic resonance imaging and polymerase chain reaction assay of cerebrospinal fluid. J Neurol Sci 1998;157(2):148–53.
71. Tan IL, McArthur JC, Venkatesan A, et al. Atypical manifestations and poor outcome of herpes simplex encephalitis in the immunocompromised. Neurology 2012;79(21):2125–32.
72. Shah R, Bag AK, Chapman PR, et al. Imaging manifestations of progressive multifocal leukoencephalopathy. Clin Radiol 2010;65(6):431–9.
73. Gelfand JM, Genrich G, Green AJ, et al. Encephalitis of unclear origin diagnosed by brain biopsy: a diagnostic challenge. JAMA Neurol 2015;72(1):66.
74. Proulx N, Fréchette D, Toye B, et al. Delays in the administration of antibiotics are associated with mortality from adult acute bacterial meningitis. QJM 2005;98(4):291–8.
75. de Gans J, van de Beek D. Dexamethasone in adults with bacterial meningitis. N Engl J Med 347(20):1549-1556.
76. Brouwer MC, McIntyre P, Prasad K, et al. Corticosteroids for acute bacterial meningitis. Cochrane Database Syst Rev 2015;2015(9):CD004405.
77. Noska A, Kyrillos R, Hansen G, et al. The role of antiviral therapy in immunocompromised patients with herpes simplex virus meningitis. Clin Infect Dis 2015;60(2):237–42.
78. Thwaites GE, Bang ND, Dung NH, et al. Dexamethasone for the treatment of tuberculous meningitis in adolescents and adults. N Engl J Med 351(17):1741-1751
79. Thwaites G, Fisher M, Hemingway C, et al. British Infection Society guidelines for the diagnosis and treatment of tuberculosis of the central nervous system in adults and children. J Infect 2009;59(3):167–87.
80. Perfect JR, Dismukes WE, Dromer F, et al. Clinical practice guidelines for the management of cryptococcal disease: 2010 update by the infectious diseases Society of America. Clin Infect Dis 2010;50(3):291–322.
81. Galgiani JN, Ampel NM, Blair JE, et al. 2016 Infectious Diseases Society of America (IDSA) clinical practice guideline for the treatment of coccidioidomycosis. Clin Infect Dis 2016;63(6):e112–46.
82. Wheat LJ, Freifeld AG, Kleiman MB, et al. Clinical practice guidelines for the management of patients with histoplasmosis: 2007 update by the infectious diseases Society of America. Clin Infect Dis 2007;45(7):807–25.
83. Valencia I, Miles DK, Melvin J, et al. Relapse of herpes encephalitis after acyclovir therapy: report of two new cases and review of the literature. Neuropediatrics 2004;35(6):371–6.
84. Nagel MA, Niemeyer CS, Bubak AN. Central nervous system infections produced by varicella zoster virus. Curr Opin Infect Dis 2020;33(3):273–8.
85. Gnann JW, Agrawal A, Hart J, et al. Lack of efficacy of high-titered immunoglobulin in patients with west nile virus central nervous system disease. Emerg Infect Dis 2019;25(11):2064–73.

Autoimmune Meningitis and Encephalitis

Megan B. Richie, MD

KEYWORDS

- Autoimmune encephalitis • Autoimmune meningitis • Paraneoplastic disorder
- Limbic encephalitis

KEY POINTS

- Meningeal or parenchymal inflammation often indicates a treatable disorder, and clinicians should consider infectious, neoplastic, and autoimmune diseases in patients with undifferentiated meningitis or encephalitis. Suspicion for autoimmune meningitis or encephalitis is heightened in younger patients with subacute disease onset and/or a personal or family history of autoimmunity.
- Early evaluation of suspected autoimmune encephalitis should include assessment for specific neural autoantibodies, as the identification of a positive antibody often precludes the need for brain biopsy and allows therapeutics to commence.
- Numerous autoimmune processes without associated neural autoantibodies can cause meningitis, encephalitis, or both and may be categorized into histiocytic, fulminant demyelinating, vasculitic, amyloid-related, and systemic rheumatologic disorders. Many require tissue sampling to diagnose.
- Although clinicians should aggressively seek alternative systemic biopsy sites when available, brain biopsy is a high-yield and relatively low-morbidity procedure in the appropriate clinical setting.

INTRODUCTION

Evaluating undifferentiated meningitis or encephalitis is challenging due to their broad differential diagnoses with significant clinical and etiologic overlap. Meningitis denotes inflammation of the meningeal space and typically presents with headache, nuchal rigidity, cerebrospinal fluid (CSF) pleocytosis, or leptomeningeal enhancement on MRI. In contrast, encephalitis signifies inflammation of the brain parenchyma, resulting in focal or multifocal deficits, potentially with corresponding parenchymal imaging abnormalities. These syndromes commonly co-occur as meningoencephalitis and cause a combination of signs and symptoms.

Meningeal inflammation is demonstrated by CSF pleocytosis or intrathecal antibody production, including an elevated immunoglobulin G (IgG) index, independent CSF

Department of Neurology, University of California San Francisco, 505 Parnassus Avenue, Box 0114, San Francisco, CA 94143, USA
E-mail address: megan.richie@ucsf.edu

Neurol Clin 40 (2022) 93–112
https://doi.org/10.1016/j.ncl.2021.08.007
neurologic.theclinics.com

oligoclonal bands (OCBs), or identification of a specific neural autoantibody. Inflammation of brain parenchyma is demonstrated by tissue pathology or, more commonly, inferred based on the combination of meningeal inflammation and focal deficits, indicating concurrent parenchymal involvement. Importantly, although abnormally elevated CSF protein or parenchymal enhancement on MRI can suggest an inflammatory process, neither one is sufficient evidence in isolation.

Because the presence of inflammation usually indicates a treatable condition, etiologic diagnosis of meningitis and encephalitis becomes especially important and considerations include infections, neoplasms, and autoimmune disorders. Although all 3 categories should be considered in every patient, certain features increase the likelihood of an autoimmune cause. Autoimmune pathology is typically subacute in onset and more common in individuals with a personal or family history of autoimmunity.[1] Younger age, female sex, or postpartum status also raise suspicion.[2] Autoimmune meningitis or encephalitis requires a systematic workup, and this review provides one practical approach tailored to the risk factors, clinical presentation, and diagnostic features of the individual patient.

DIAGNOSTIC APPROACH

The presence of a specific neural autoantibody is a key early differentiating feature between causes of autoimmune meningitis and encephalitis because identifying such an antibody often allows treatment initiation without the need for invasive testing such as brain biopsy. In contrast, many autoimmune causes of meningitis or encephalitis without associated autoantibodies, such as neurosarcoidosis or primary angiitis of the central nervous system (PACNS), do require a tissue specimen for diagnosis and treatment.[3,4] Thus it becomes very useful for clinicians to predict when patients may have a specific autoantibody syndrome, in order to allow time for serologic results to return before pursuing biopsy. Certain autoantibody syndromes are also often associated with specific neoplasms, and identifying these paraneoplastic antibodies prompts a thorough search for associated malignancy. Finally, many antibody syndromes have established treatment practices and therapeutic decisions are frequently streamlined when an autoantibody is discovered.[5] In fact, identifying an autoantibody is so meaningful that within the medical literature, the phrase "autoimmune encephalitis" is often reserved for cases associated with a particular neural autoantibody.[6]

Autoantibody-Associated Encephalitis

All neural antibody-associated diseases of the CNS cause encephalitis or meningoencephalitis; none cause meningitis alone. These autoantibody-associated encephalitides are commonly divided based on whether the affected antigen is intracellular or extracellular (**Table 1**).[1,5] Syndromes related to antibodies against intracellular antigens are frequently associated with cancer and include the classic paraneoplastic disorders such as anti-Hu, anti-Ri, or anti-Yo. Neural injury is thought to occur via cytotoxic T cells, and identified antibodies are likely biomarkers rather than pathogenic because antibodies cannot enter live cells.[1,6] Prognosis for intracellular autoantibody syndromes is often poor, both because neuronal injury is usually irreversible and because the disorder is due to an associated malignancy. In contrast, antibodies targeting extracellular antigens, such as N-methyl-D-aspartic acid (NMDA), voltage-gated potassium channel (VGKC), or α-amino-3-hydroxy-5-methyl-4-isoxazolepropionic acid are thought to be directly pathogenic. These antibodies reversibly impair epitopes of cell surface or associated synaptic proteins and are variably associated with neoplasm. As a result, prognosis is more favorable.[5]

Table 1
General features associated with intracellular and extracellular autoantibody syndromes of the central nervous system

	Intracellular	Extracellular
Antigen targets	Nuclear, cytoplasmic	Cell surface, synaptic
Patient age	Older	Younger
Neoplasm	Common	Variable
Best antibody sensitivity	Serum and CSF	CSF
Prognosis	Unfavorable	Favorable

Abbreviation: CSF, cerebrospinal fluid
Data from Bradshaw MJ, Linnoila JJ. An Overview of Autoimmune and Paraneoplastic Encephalitides. Semin Neurol. 2018;38(3):330-343. https://doi.org/10.1055/s-0038-1660821.

Autoantibody-associated encephalitis may result in a variety of typical neurologic syndromes, including limbic encephalitis, cerebellar degeneration, stiff person syndrome, and encephalomyelitis, among others (**Table 2**). Although there is substantial overlap in the diseases associated with these clinical syndromes, there are still certain presentations that should immediately raise suspicion for a particular antibody. For example, neuromyotonia is strongly associated with Caspr2 antibodies (Isaac syndrome).[5] Faciobrachial dystonic seizures are nearly always associated with anti-Lgl1 encephalitis.[6] Extreme delta brush on electroencephalogram is highly specific for NMDA-R encephalitis.[5] Although in many cases clinicians will send a panel of autoantibodies in patients with suspected autoimmune encephalitis, recognizing characteristic presentations and sending targeted testing for single antibodies can be cost- and time-efficient and should be done when possible. Many excellent review articles have been written that organize and characterize neural autoantibody

Table 2
Typical syndromes caused by autoantibody-associated encephalitides

Syndrome	Intracellular Antibodies	Extracellular Antibodies
Limbic encephalitis	Anti-GAD65, Anti-Ma2	Anti-NMDAR, Anti-AMPAR, Anti-LGI1, Anti-GABA(B), Anti-mGluR5
Cerebellar degeneration	Anti-Yo, Anti-Ri, Anti-GAD65, Anti-Ma1	Anti-mGluR1, Anti-Tr, Anti-VGCC
Stiff person syndrome	Anti-GAD65, Anti-amphiphysin	Anti-GlyR, Anti-GABA(A)
Encephalomyelitis	Anti-Hu, Anti-CV2/CRMP5, anti-GFAP	
Opsoclonus-myoclonus	Anti-Ri	
Refractory seizures		Anti-GABA(A), Anti-GABA(B), Anti-LGI1 (faciobrachial dystonic)
Diencephalic	Anti-Ma1, Anti-Ma2	Anti-Aqp4
Brainstem syndrome	Anti-Hu, Anti-Ri, Anti-Ma1, Anti-Ma2	Anti-IgLON5, anti-Aqp4, anti-GQ1b
CNS hyperexcitability	Anti-DPPX	
PNS hyperexcitability (neuromyotonia)		Anti-Caspr2
Sensory neuronopathy	Anti-Hu	

Data from Refs.[6,15,58,59]

syndromes; these may be used to gauge the likelihood of specific antibodies and identify their associated malignancies.[5–7]

Nonautoantibody-Associated Meningitis and Encephalitis

Autoimmune causes of meningitis and encephalitis without an associated antibody are diverse (**Table 3**). These diseases are often diagnosed pathologically and can be categorized as such, including granulomatous/histiocytic, demyelinating, vasculitic, and amyloid-related conditions. Several systemic rheumatologic diseases also can have meningeal and/or parenchymal neurologic manifestations and are more often diagnosed by positive serum studies and exclusion of alternative diseases.

Granulomatous/histiocytic diseases

Neurosarcoidosis is by far the most common granulomatous autoimmune CNS disease and can affect a multitude of structures including cranial nerves, parenchyma, meninges, vasculature, and spinal cord (**Fig. 1**). CSF abnormalities can include elevated opening pressure, pleocytosis, hypoglycorrhachia, and occasionally OCBs or high IgG index.[3] Neurosarcoidosis has a predilection for the hypothalamus and pituitary axis, a characteristic it shares with other histiocytic disorders including Erdheim-Chester disease (ECD) and Langerhans cell histiocytosis (LCH). However, where sarcoidosis can indiscriminately affect any segment of the nervous system, ECD and LCH more commonly cause meningitis without encephalitis. Brain parenchymal involvement is instead often limited to circumscribed enhancing masses, although ECD can cause more infiltrative lesions and LCH is associated with degenerative changes of the posterior fossa.[8] Morbidity of brain biopsy may be avoided by use of body PET computed tomography (CT) as a sensitive study to identify systemic targets in suspected cases of neurosarcoidosis, ECD, or LCH.[3,9]

Vogt-Koyanagi-Harada (VKH) disease is a histiocytic disorder common in Asian, Hispanic, and Indigenous populations that primarily causes panuveitis but is accompanied by meningitis in up to 80% of cases.[10] CSF pleocytosis is typically lymphocytic although may be neutrophilic early in presentation.[11] Associated encephalitis is extremely rare and is still accompanied by ophthalmologic involvement.[11,12] Unlike the histiocytic disorders described earlier, VKH does not require a tissue diagnosis and may be made as a diagnosis of exclusion in patients with appropriate ophthalmologic findings and clinical presentation.

Chronic lymphocytic inflammation with pontine perivascular enhancement responsive to steroids (CLIPPERS) causes autoimmune encephalitis with a distinctive radiographic signature and pathology demonstrating perivascular lymphohistiocytic infiltration without granuloma or demyelination. Stereotypical brain imaging should demonstrate punctate and curvilinear enhancing lesions of the pons and/or cerebellum involving white and deep gray matter but sparing cortex and CSF may demonstrate mild pleocytosis and/or OCBs.[13] Although diagnosis can be made by observing the signature radiographic pattern without biopsy, caution should be used in those with linear, nodular, ring-shaped, or larger (>3 mm) areas of enhancement, and mimics such as CNS lymphoma or glial fibrillar acidic protein astrocytopathy should be considered and excluded.[14]

Fulminant demyelinating diseases

Acute disseminated encephalomyelitis (ADEM) and acute hemorrhagic leukoencephalitis (AHLE) are 2 fulminant demyelinating diseases that cause autoimmune encephalitis or meningoencephalitis. ADEM typically presents as a monophasic illness in younger patients with acute encephalopathy and multifocal enhancing edematous lesions of the

Table 3
Clinical and radiographic characteristics of autoimmune diseases that cause meningitis or encephalitis without an associated neural autoantibody.
3,8–10,13–17,19,20,22,23,28,31,32,37,38,40,41,44–47,50,79

	Syndrome	Described MRI patterns	Helpful systemic workup
Granulomatous/histiocytic			
• Sarcoidosis	M, E, ME	HPA, meningeal, vascular, parenchymal	CT → PET
• Erdheim Chester	M	HPA, infiltrative, mass lesions, meningeal	PET/CT
• Langerhans cell histiocytosis	M	HPA, mass lesions, cerebellar	Skeletal x-ray, skin exam → PET/CT
• Vogt-Koyanagi-Harada	M > E, ME	Often unremarkable; rare brainstem lesions	Ophthalmologic exam with FA
• CLIPPERS	E, ME	Punctate/curvilinear <3mm posterior fossa enhancement	
Fulminant demyelinating			
• ADEM	E, ME	Multifocal enhancing and edematous grey/white	
• AHLE	E, ME	Hemispheric enhancing hemorrhagic edematous lesions	
Vasculitic			
• PACNS	M > E, ME	Discrete or diffuse, ischemia, hemorrhage, enhancement	
• Behçet	M > E, ME	Patchy or confluent brainstem, basal ganglia lesions	Oral/genital skin, ophthalmologic exams, pathergy test
• GPA	M > E, ME	Pachymeningeal > leptomeningeal enhancement	ENT and ophthalmologic exam, ANCA
• EGPA	M	Ischemia, hemorrhage, optic neuropathy	Serum eosinophils, ANCA
• Cogan	M > E, ME	Ischemia, vestibular labyrinth obliteration	TTE, otologic & ophthalmologic exams
• Kawasaki	M	Ischemia, atrophy, subdural effusion, MERS	TTE, ophthalmologic & skin exams
Amyloid related			
• CAARI	E, ME	White matter, leptomeninges, edema, hemorrhage, infarct	Amyloid PET
• ABRA	E, ME	Similar to CAARI	Amyloid PFT
Systemic autoimmune disease			
• Sjogrens	M > E, ME	White matter, grey matter, microhemorrhages	SSA/B, Labial or salivary gland biopsy
• RA	M > E, ME	Infarcts, pachymeningitis, dural nodules, rare vasculitis	Anti-RF, CCP

(continued on next page)

	Syndrome	Described MRI patterns	Helpful systemic workup
• Susac syndrome	M, E, ME	Callosal, periventricular, meningeal enhancement	Ophthalmologic exam with FA
• HLH	E, ME	Meningeal, nodular, ring-enhancing, cortical, subcortical	Ferritin, SIL-2R, NK activity, bone marrow
• Localized scleroderma	M, E, ME	Unilateral hyperintensity, atrophy, cysts, calcifications	ANA, Skin biopsy
• Sweet syndrome	M > E, ME	White matter, grey matter, enhancement	Skin biopsy
• Still's disease	M > E, ME	Linear enhancement, infarction, demyelination	Peripheral neutrophilia, ferritin
• IgG 4 related hypertrophic pachymeningitis	M	Thick enhancing leptomeninges and/or pachymeninges	IgG4 level
Other			
• HANDL	M, ME	Often unremarkable; nonspecific T2 hyperintensities	

Table 3 (continued)

Abbreviations: ABRA, amyloid beta related angiitis; ADEM, acute disseminated encephalomyelitis; AHLE, acute hemorrhagic leukoencephalitis; CAARI, cerebral amyloid angioopathy with related inflammation; CLIPPERS, Chronic lymphocytic inflammation with pontine perivascular enhancement responsive to steroids; CT, computed tomography; E, encephalitis; EGPA, eosinophilic granulomatosis with polyangiitis; ENT, ear nose and throat; FA, fluorescein angiography; GPA, granulomatosis with polyangiitis; HaNDL, Headache with neurologic deficits and CSF lymphocytosis; HLH, hemophagocytic lymphohistiocytosis; HPA, hypothalamic pituitary axis; IgG, immunoglobulin G; M, meningitis; ME, meningoencephalitis; MERS, mild encephalopathy with reversible splenial lesion; NK, natural killer cell; PACNS, primary angiitis of the central nervous system; PET, Positron emission tomography; RA, rheumatoid arthritis; SIL-2R, soluble IL-2 receptor; TTE, transthoracic echocardiogram

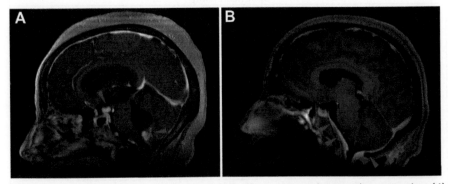

Fig. 1. T1-weighted sagittal postcontrast magnetic resonance images demonstrating (*A*) suprasellar and fourth ventricular enhancing masses and associated hydrocephalus in a patient with probable neurosarcoidosis based on lymph node biopsy and (*B*) pachymeningitis and marked smooth dural thickening at the craniocervical junction in a different patient with biopsy-proven IgG4 disease.

white and deep gray matter without cortical involvement.[15] CSF demonstrates lymphocytic or monocytic pleocytosis, typically without independent OCB or elevated IgG index. In classic presentations, brain biopsy is not typically required after reasonable exclusion of alternative diagnoses. AHLE is a severe variant of ADEM with similar demographic and radiographic features except with the addition of cerebral hemorrhages, progressive edema, and often rapid progression to herniation and death. CSF may also be more polymorphonuclear-predominant, and brain biopsy is frequently performed.[16]

Vasculitic disorders

Although autoimmune vasculitides involving the CNS typically result in ischemia, hemorrhage, or other vascular pathology, patients may also have an accompanying meningitis or less often encephalitis. PACNS is a medium- to small-vessel vasculitis strictly limited to the CNS that can also be associated with meningitis.[17,18] Imaging findings are highly variable and may show discrete or diffuse lesions often involving white matter, potentially with areas of infarct, hemorrhage, enhancement, or mass effect (**Fig. 2**).[19] Although PACNS does not cause a classic encephalitis per se, patients do have focal deficits including weakness, visual impairment, aphasia, and ataxia due to parenchymal disease. Diagnosis of PACNS can be challenging, as CSF demonstrates pleocytosis in only 60% of biopsy-proven cases, and catheter angiography is normal in almost half. Furthermore, brain biopsies performed for suspected PACNS reveal alternative diagnoses in greater than 30% of cases. The diagnosis is therefore best made via brain tissue sampling.[18]

Behçet syndrome is the only systemic autoimmune vasculitis that commonly causes not only meningitis but also encephalitis. Neuro-Behçet syndrome is typically divided into parenchymal (80%) and nonparenchymal (20%) disease, the former of which results in meningoencephalitis and the latter solely in vascular abnormalities. Parenchymal neuro-Behçet syndrome primarily affects the brainstem and less often basal ganglia, centrum semiovale, spinal cord, and cranial nerves, and biopsy is typically required for diagnosis.[19,20] CSF is inflammatory in 60% of parenchymal cases with an early neutrophil predominance that transitions to lymphocytes over days.[21]

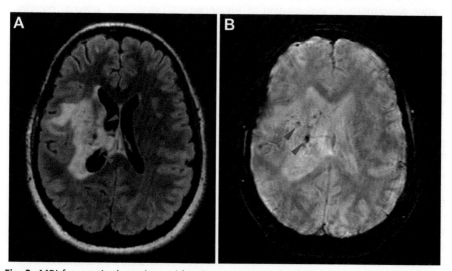

Fig. 2. MRI from a single patient with primary angiitis of the CNS that required 3 brain biopsies to diagnose, demonstrating a masslike T2 hyperintense lesion with interspersed punctate foci of susceptibility artifact on axial (*A*) T2 fluid attenuated inversion recovery (FLAIR) and (*B*) susceptibility weighted imaging (SWI) sequences.

Several systemic vasculitides may occasionally be associated with a meningitis, often in addition to vascular complications of the CNS such as hemorrhage or ischemia. Eosinophilic granulomatosis with polyangiitis is a small-vessel vasculitis nearly always associated with peripheral eosinophilia; approximately 50% of cases are ANCA-positive. CNS manifestations include ischemia, hemorrhage, meningitis, cranial neuropathies, and more uncommonly myelitis or nonspecific T2 lesions.[22] Granulomatosis with polyangiitis involves the nervous system in approximately 33% of patients, most commonly with peripheral or cranial neuropathies, but a small percentage may have a mild neutrophilic meningitis or even more rarely encephalitis.[23-25] Cogan syndrome is a variable-sized vasculitis that causes hearing loss, vertigo, and uveitis and predominantly affects young men; it may be associated with a lymphocytic meningitis.[17,19] Finally, although primarily seen in infants and children, Kawasaki disease can rarely present in adults, and approximately 10% of patients may have a mixed neutrophilic and lymphocytic pleocytosis at presentation.[26-28]

Other autoimmune systemic vasculitides typically do not cause meningitis or encephalitis although case reports have been published describing rare associations. For example, isolated meningitis has been associated with giant cell arteritis, and polyarteritis nodosa has been rarely reported to cause meningoencephalitis.[29,30]

Amyloid-related

Cerebral amyloid angiopathy (CAA) is a vasculopathy characterized by amyloid beta-peptide deposits in small-to medium-sized cortical and meningeal vessels of older adults. Although often noninflammatory, CAA can also be associated with 2 different autoimmune responses, termed (1) CAA-related inflammation (CAARI) when inflammation involves the perivascular space and (2) Amyloid beta–related angiitis (ABRA) when inflammation leads to a destructive, transmural vasculitis.[31-33] Both CAARI and ABRA cause encephalitis with or without associated meningitis; approximately half of the patients demonstrate a cerebrospinal fluid pleocytosis occasionally accompanied by OCBs or elevated IgG index.[31] Imaging findings are heterogeneous with substantial overlap between CAARI and ABRA but often demonstrate white matter abnormalities, leptomeningeal enhancement, vasogenic edema, microhemorrhages, superficial siderosis, and occasional infarction (**Fig. 3**).[32] PET imaging using the amyloid-binding Pittsburgh compound B may be helpful to demonstrate amyloid deposits with the caveat that these may be found in other conditions such as Alzheimer disease.[33] Diagnosis of CAARI and ABRA often requires brain biopsy, but given hemorrhagic potential in these patients, when imaging findings are typical, CSF demonstrates clear inflammation, and amyloid PET is positive, empirical therapy may be considered without tissue diagnosis.[34]

Systemic autoimmune diseases associated with meningitis or encephalitis

Rheumatoid arthritis (RA), Sjögren syndrome, Susac syndrome, and systemic lupus erythematosus (SLE) are 4 systemic autoimmune conditions that have been associated with meningitis and extremely rarely with encephalitis. RA can lead to lymphocyte-predominant meningitis and/or MRI enhancement involving the leptomeninges, pachymeninges, or both.[35,36] Imaging may also reveal infarcts related to an associated vasculitis. Meningoencephalitis associated with RA has very rarely been reported, and diagnosis typically requires brain biopsy.[37] CNS involvement occurs in 2% to 5% of patients with Sjögren syndrome and can include aseptic meningitis, cerebellar syndromes, movement disorders, demyelination, and very rarely encephalitis and/or vasculitis.[38-40] CSF may reveal lymphocytic meningitis, elevated IgG index, or OCBs, and MRI typically shows nonspecific T2 abnormalities.[39,40] Susac syndrome is typically clinically

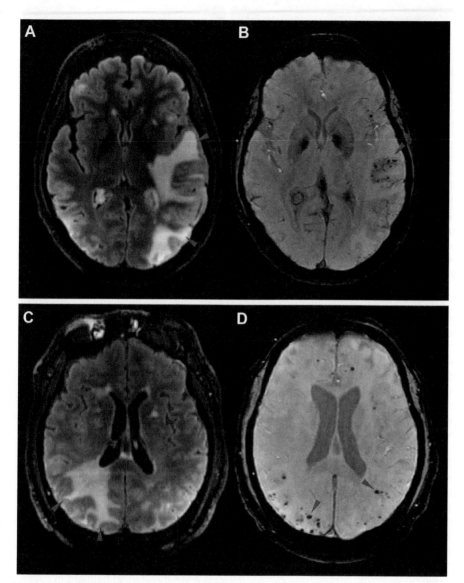

Fig. 3. (*A*) Axial MRI FLAIR and (*B*) SWI sequences in a patient with biopsy-proven cerebral amyloid angiopathy with related inflammation, demonstrating white matter-predominant confluent T2 hyperintensities with associated cortical microhemorrhages. (*C*) Axial FLAIR and (*D*) SWI sequences in a different patient with biopsy-proven amyloid beta–related angiitis demonstrating very similar white matter-predominant T2 hyperintensities and more diffuse cortical microhemorrhages.

diagnosed by its characteristic triad of hearing loss, branch retinal artery occlusions, and CNS dysfunction and may be associated with a modest CSF pleocytosis.[41] MRI nearly always shows callosal and periventricular T2 lesions, sometimes with leptomeningeal enhancement (**Fig. 4**). Finally, although SLE has been associated with a wide spectrum of neuropsychiatric presentations, meningitis occurs in no more than 3% of patients and in those cases is often better attributed to a drug or infection.[42]

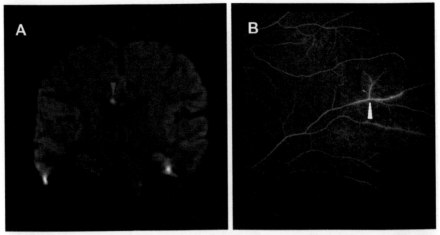

Fig. 4. (*A*) MRI coronal diffusion-weighted image demonstrating a small callosal infarct in a patient with clinically diagnosed Susac syndrome (*red arrow*). (*B*) Ophthalmologic fluorescein angiography demonstrating hyperfluorescent vasculitic changes (*white arrow*) and branch retinal artery occlusion (*black arrow*).

Localized scleroderma affecting the scalp commonly also involves the CNS and is associated with a progressive, relapsing meningitis or encephalitis.[43,44] CNS involvement is classified into 2 overlapping subtypes: linear scleroderma "en coup de sabre" characterized by a linear, thickened patch of skin typically over the scalp, and progressive hemifacial atrophy (Parry-Romberg syndrome) with sparing of overlying skin but involvement of dermis and deeper tissue.[44] Both may lead to epilepsy, and MRI abnormalities are common, including gyral T2 hyperintensities with associated atrophy, calcifications, microhemorrhage, cysts, and parenchymal and/or meningeal enhancement, usually ipsilateral to skin involvement (**Fig. 5**).[44,45] CSF may be normal or shows modest lymphocytic pleocytosis or independent OCBs.[44]

Relative to other systemic rheumatologic disorders, the dermatologic Sweet syndrome is somewhat more commonly associated with meningitis and encephalitis, frequently preceded by fever, peripheral neutrophilia, and erythematous painful nodules, blisters, or plaques. Sweet syndrome may be seen following an infection, during pregnancy, or in the context of hematologic malignancy or a different systemic autoimmune condition.[44] CSF may be normal or show a lymphocytic or neutrophilic predominance with or without OCBs. MRI may demonstrate nonspecific T2 hyperintensities of the cortex, white matter, and basal ganglia, with parenchymal or meningeal enhancement.

Hemophagocytic lymphohistiocytosis (HLH) is a life-threatening multiorgan inflammatory syndrome involving dysregulation of macrophages, natural killer cells, and cytotoxic lymphocytes as triggered by an infectious, malignant, or iatrogenic event.[46] HLH may involve CNS in approximately 10% of patients, and MRI findings are heterogeneous but may include meningeal enhancement, diffuse white matter changes, or focal cortical or subcortical lesions with variable enhancement patterns; only a minority of patients demonstrate CSF pleocytosis.[47] Patients presenting with CNS HLH should always have systemic involvement, and thus diagnosis usually does not require brain biopsy and can be made using scoring tools supplemented by systemic biopsy such as bone marrow, liver, spleen, or lymph nodes.[46]

Common symptoms of adult-onset Still's disease include fever, arthritis, and evanescent rash; neurologic involvement is present in approximately 7% of patients and can include meningitis and less often encephalitis or infarction. CSF may show

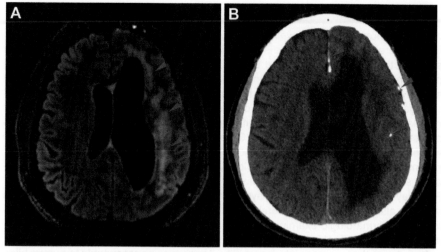

Fig. 5. (*A*) Axial fluid-attenuated inversion recovery MRI of a patient with clinically diagnosed focal scleroderma, demonstrating white-matter predominant T2 hyperintensities with associated hemispheric atrophy and ex-vacuo ventricular dilation. (*B*) Axial computed tomography demonstrates associated calcification.

neutrophilic or lymphocytic pleocytosis and potentially elevated intracranial pressure. Peripheral neutrophilia, hyperferritinemia, transaminitis, and lymphadenopathy may all be helpful systemic disease indicators.[48,49]

Finally, IgG4-related disease may be associated with meningitis, and imaging demonstrates dural thickening with smooth pachymeningeal and/or leptomeningeal enhancement with potential to cause underlying mass effect (see **Fig. 1**).[50] CSF shows lymphocytic meningitis in more than half of patients with CNS involvement, nearly always with elevated IgG index or OCBs. When performed, CSF IgG4 levels may also be markedly increased.[51] Diagnosis of IgG4-related disease often requires biopsy.

Other autoimmune meningitis

Headache with neurologic deficits and CSF lymphocytosis (HaNDL) describes a characteristic clinical syndrome of acute onset headache, lymphocytic meningitis, and temporary neurologic deficits often preceded by a viral-like illness.[52] As biopsy is not performed in these patients due to the very self-limited nature of symptoms, the pathophysiology of HaNDL has been debated but is generally favored to be autoimmune.

Diagnostic Approach

When evaluating patients with meningitis or encephalitis, clinicians must simultaneously consider potential autoimmune, infectious, and neoplastic causes. Important serum testing in most patients will include human immunodeficiency virus serologies, rapid plasma reagin, and rheumatologic screening testing including erythrocyte sedimentation rate, C-reactive protein, and antinuclear antibodies. In cases with higher suspicion for autoimmune diseases, rheumatologic testing should be expanded, especially to include those tests identified in **Table 3**. Workup should also include a brain MRI scan with and without contrast, and lumbar puncture for cell count, differential, protein, glucose, Gram stain and culture, OCBs, and IgG index.[53] Clinicians must use caution interpreting CSF OCBs or IgG index, as both are nonspecific markers for intrathecal antibody production and may be abnormal in both autoimmune and infectious causes of meningitis and encephalitis.[54] Targeted CSF testing for treatable, common organisms such as herpesviruses and cryptococcus should be done in most patients, as well as CSF cytology and flow cytometry when neoplasm is considered. Finally, given the substantial etiologic overlap between autoimmune and infectious pathologies, broad testing for CNS infections such as metagenomic next-generation sequencing or universal polymerase chain reaction should be strongly considered where available to help broadly evaluate likelihood of infection.[55]

Regardless of whether meningitis or encephalitis is of autoimmune, infectious, or neoplastic origin, systemic workup with imaging and possible biopsy may be helpful and should be aggressively pursued. CT of the chest, abdomen, and pelvis is useful in identifying systemic malignancy and/or sites of extracranial disease involvement, potentially providing opportunity for biopsy. In undifferentiated meningitis or encephalitis, such biopsies should almost always be performed when feasible and low-risk. PET may add sensitivity for finding systemic involvement of malignancy or sarcoidosis and can also identify specific cerebral pathologies such as amyloid.[3,33] Ophthalmologic and dermatologic examinations can reveal suggestive or even diagnostic findings, and vitreal and skin biopsies should be pursued when abnormalities are found. In fact, due to the low associated morbidity, it may even be reasonable to pursue blind skin biopsy when considering certain causes of meningitis or encephalitis.[56] Additional testing for systemic diagnostic clues should be pursued as targeted to the most likely diseases (see **Table 3**), such as transvaginal or scrotal ultrasound in patients with suspected NMDA-R encephalitis.[6]

Narrowing the Autoimmune Differential Diagnosis

It is helpful for clinicians to recognize features that increase the likelihood of an antibody-mediated disorder and thereby defer brain biopsy.[57] Patients presenting with subacute classic syndromes such as cerebellar degeneration or limbic encephalitis should raise suspicion (see **Table 2**).[58] Similarly, MRI scans with abnormalities that demonstrate a particular functional tropism, such as for the temporal lobes, diencephalon, or specific white matter tracts, suggest an antibody-mediated process. In addition, normal MRI scans in patients who nevertheless have a clinical syndrome consistent with a particular functional tropism are also suspicious for an antibody-mediated process.[5,59] CSF for patients with neuroantibodies typically shows either absent or modest CSF lymphocytic pleocytosis (median 4–8 cells/mm^3), normal glucose, and often independent OCBs or elevation in IgG index with some variability.[60–62] Anti-NMDA-R and antiglutamic acid decarboxylase (GAD) encephalitis in particular are associated with oligoclonal bands, which are seen less often in VGKC-complex antibody syndromes.[62,63] In contrast, marked CSF pleocytosis, neutrophilic pleocytosis, and/or hypoglycorrhachia are more typical of several nonautoantibody associated autoimmune causes of meningitis such as sarcoidosis.[3] Finally, patients with a preexisting history or new diagnosis of systemic malignancy, particularly those such as small cell lung cancer, are at particular risk for a paraneoplastic autoantibody.[6]

High likelihood of an antibody-mediated process

When clinical features strongly suggest an autoantibody-mediated process, clinicians should make every effort to maximize the yield of autoantibody testing and await results before pursuing higher risk testing such as brain biopsy.[57] Autoantibody panels should be sent from both serum and CSF, with consideration for simultaneous targeted testing for individual antibodies to hasten diagnosis. Plasmapheresis, intravenous immunoglobulin (IVIG), and steroids may all reduce the yield of antibody assays and thus should be avoided before testing whenever clinically feasible.[58] However, because plasmapheresis and IVIG are unlikely to reduce diagnostic yield of biopsy, either may be used as empirical therapy in patients for whom there is high suspicion of an antibody-mediated process even before antibody results return. In contrast, initiation of steroids before brain biopsy is strongly associated with a non-diagnostic sample, and so empirical corticosteroids should be avoided until a definitive diagnosis is established whenever possible.[64]

Low likelihood of an antibody-mediated process

In patients with undifferentiated autoimmune meningitis or encephalitis whose disease features do not align well with an antibody-mediated process, either brain or systemic biopsy is commonly required for diagnosis, with primary exceptions including classic presentations of ADEM, Vogt-Koyanagi-Harada disease, Susac syndrome, CLIPPERS, HaNDL, and occasionally amyloid-PET positive ABRA or CAARI. Even in patients seropositive for rheumatologic diseases—for example, a patient with RA and new encephalitis—a biopsy is often critical to exclude other pathologies due to the rarity of meningitis or encephalitis associated with these illnesses. Systemic biopsy sites may be very helpful, such as skin, lymph node, bone marrow, labial, or salivary gland, and should be comprehensively assessed and pursued.[65] However, in the absence of such options, brain biopsy is often the best next step in patients without a diagnosis who are not spontaneously improving.

The choice of whether and when to pursue brain biopsy can be challenging and requires weighing risks and benefits. In patients who are rapidly deteriorating or have severe symptoms (increased intracranial pressure, cerebral edema, hydrocephalus) risks of withholding treatment are greater and brain biopsy should be pursued more aggressively. In patients with easily accessible brain abnormalities characteristic for a disease that requires tissue such as PACNS, pursuing relatively early biopsy may be cost- and time-efficient. Immune suppressed patients have a higher likelihood of diagnostic brain biopsy and of finding a dual diagnosis, and threshold for biopsy should be lower.[65] In contrast, those patients with disease only affecting eloquent brain areas, or who are otherwise at high complication risk, brain biopsy should be avoided when possible. Infratentorial lesions in particular are less likely to yield a diagnosis, perhaps due to hesitancy in obtaining sufficient tissue or due to especially challenging operative approaches.[65] Finally, patients who are already improving on empirical therapy, particularly steroids, will have lower tissue yield and biopsy should be delayed to such a time if and when symptoms recur.

Ultimately, recent evidence demonstrates that more than 70% of brain biopsy samples may provide a specific histologic diagnosis—a percentage much higher than for many solid-organ biopsies.[65] Furthermore, permanent neurologic morbidity and mortality rates are low and compare favorably to complication rates for systemic biopsies.[57,65] It is therefore reasonable for clinicians to consider brain biopsy early in the diagnostic algorithm in patients with a negative less-invasive workup, lack of systemic biopsy options, and an accessible brain lesion, particularly in those tertiary care centers with high levels of expertise and experience.

Maximizing Yield of Brain Biopsy

Once the decision is made to pursue brain biopsy, clinicians should make every effort to maximize tissue yield and minimize morbidity. Steroids should be avoided or minimized for 2 weeks before biopsy to reduce risk of a nondiagnostic sample.[64] Target site should be chosen based on the presence of an imaging abnormality balanced with anatomic eloquence; the presence of enhancement can suggest higher likelihood of yield but the association is not strong.[57,65,66] Autopsy can occasionally yield a specific tissue diagnosis where brain biopsy does not, indicating that sufficient biopsy size is also helpful.[66] It is recommended to sample 1 cubic centimeter containing whichever structures are of highest clinical interest (dura, leptomeninges, white or gray matter). The decision of where and what structures to biopsy should be a collaborative decision between neurologists, neurosurgeons, and neuroradiologists. Finally, because brain biopsy yield is lower in patients with unspecified encephalitis particularly when additional follow-up pathologic analyses are not performed, providers should discuss which disease entities are of highest suspicion with neuropathology, in order to ensure appropriate specimen handling that enables these follow-up studies.

After the biopsy, platelet count should be maintained greater than 100 G/L for a minimum of 7 days due to the association between thrombocytopenia and brain biopsy complications.[65] In those patients in whom brain biopsy does not yield a specific diagnosis, often pathology results can still be useful in narrowing the differential diagnosis and providing avenues for additional workup.[66]

Special Clinical Situations

Immune checkpoint inhibitor therapy

Immune checkpoint inhibitors (ICIs) target the regulatory steps of T-cell activation and thereby enhance the endogenous immune response against neoplastic disease. Although such therapies have revolutionized cancer therapy, 4% to 14% of patients receiving ICIs develop autoimmune disease of the nervous system.[67] Neuromuscular syndromes are the most common, but CNS manifestations occur almost as often, including hypophysitis, encephalitis, meningoencephalitis, and more rarely isolated meningitis. Brain MRI abnormalities in these patients are variable and include localized T2 hyperintensities, focal atrophy, or parenchymal or meningeal enhancement, whereas CSF will nearly always demonstrate a mild lymphocytic pleocytosis occasionally with independent OCBs. Clinicians should emphasize the evaluation for autoantibody syndromes when assessing patients with suspected ICI-associated encephalitis, as more than half have detectable, known neural-specific autoantibodies, most of which target intracellular or synaptic antigens and present with symptoms typical for the antibody.[67] However, nonantibody-mediated CNS autoimmune disease has also been associated with ICI initiation, including neurosarcoidosis, vasculitis, and Vogt-Koyanagi-Harada syndrome.[67,68] Because neurologic autoimmunity after ICI use typically arises within 3 months of treatment initiation, providers must maintain an especially high suspicion for autoimmune etiologies in patients presenting with meningitis or encephalitis within this period.[67] In fact, in these cases often testing can be abbreviated and invasive diagnostics such as brain biopsy forgone in favor of empirical steroids, IVIG, or plasmapheresis.

Autoimmune disease related to severe acute respiratory syndrome coronavirus 2

Severe acute respiratory syndrome coronavirus 2 (SARS-CoV2) has been associated with numerous neurologic complications including encephalitis, meningoencephalitis, and rarely isolated meningitis.[69–72] Some presentations resemble autoantibody syndromes, such as limbic encephalitis, seizures, brainstem dysfunction, involuntary movements, and concurrent acute peripheral nervous system disease, although specific autoantibodies are variably identified.[69,73] Other patients present with fulminant AHLE including typical multifocal white matter lesions with microhemorrhage, enhancement, and edema on MRI and often lymphocytic pleocytosis on CSF.[71] Finally, acute necrotizing encephalopathy has been associated with SARS-CoV2, specifically manifesting as bilateral T2 signal and necrosis in the deep gray matter on MRI and by definition requiring an acellular CSF.[74] It is unclear whether these processes represent direct viral injury, a hyperinflammation syndrome concurrent with acute illness, or a postinfectious autoimmune process, as SARS-CoV2 genetic material is only occasionally detected in

CSF samples.[69,75] However, many patients demonstrate improvement with corticosteroids, IVIG, or plasmapheresis, at least in part supporting an autoimmune cause.[69,74]

Unidentified neural antibodies

Because the spectrum of autoantibody-associated neurologic disease is rapidly evolving and novel antigens are regularly being discovered, it is unsurprising that occasionally a pattern of neural-specific binding may be observed that has not previously been described.[1,76] In these cases the presence of an as-yet unidentified antibody is suspected. Although evidence-based guidance for the management of these cases is lacking, when diagnostic results indicate an unidentified neural autoantibody, it is reasonable for clinicians to complete an abbreviated workup for other diagnoses, aggressively seek systemic neoplastic disease, but forgo brain biopsy and proceed with empirical therapy with corticosteroids, IVIG, or plasmapheresis. Such patients should be referred for research-based testing whenever possible, as technology for novel autoantibody discovery is continuously evolving and such patients are critical to promote ongoing progress in the field.[77]

Management

In cases of autoimmune meningitis or encephalitis, once a specific neural autoantibody is found, a tissue diagnosis made, or a characteristic syndrome identified, diagnostic testing is tapered and clinicians consider therapeutics. However, there are particular situations in which diagnostic errors are especially likely, and this transition should be made carefully to avoid diagnosis momentum.

False-positive test results

Certain autoantibodies, such as GAD-65 and VGKC complex antibodies, may be commonly found in asymptomatic individuals. Clinicians should carefully consider the possibility of a false-positive result when an autoantibody is present in the serum but not the CSF, if the autoantibody does not fit the patient's clinical syndrome, or if the autoantibody is only present at low titers (<1:80).[6] Serologic testing performed after IVIG administration may also lead to false positives.[1] When uncertainty arises, clinicians can discuss results and clinical presentation with the testing laboratory for clarification. Furthermore, although tissue pathology is the gold-standard diagnostic test for many autoimmune disorders of the CNS, results still should be interpreted with caution. For example, noncaseating granulomas suggest sarcoidosis but can also be due to other infectious and noninfectious diseases.[3]

A word of caution is also worth mentioning in the interpretation of elevated antithyroid antibodies, specifically antithyroid peroxidase and antithyroglobulin. These are antibodies that have been classically associated with the diagnosis of steroid-responsive encephalopathy associated with autoimmune thyroiditis (SREAT), originally termed Hashimoto encephalopathy. However, antithyroid antibodies are present in up to 13% of healthy individuals and are likely an indicator of an autoimmune predilection rather than a specific disease.[7] Indeed, recent evidence suggests that greater than 70% of patients with suspected SREAT have a nonimmune-mediated neurologic disorder and more than half do not have evidence of any primary neurologic disorder.[78] The presence of positive antithyroid antibodies should therefore be interpreted with significant caution and should not be used as an independent criterion to determine the presence of CNS inflammation.

Treatment and monitoring

High-dose intravenous corticosteroids are first-line therapy for most of the autoimmune causes of meningitis and encephalitis discussed in this article. In steroid-refractory fulminant demyelinating conditions and most autoantibody-mediated syndromes, steroids are combined with either IVIG or plasmapheresis as first-line therapy.[5,16] Common second-line treatments for CNS autoantibody syndromes include rituximab or cyclophosphamide.[5] Beyond corticosteroids, the management for autoimmune meningitis or encephalitis without an associated autoantibody is specific to the disease and may include cyclophosphamide, methotrexate, azathioprine, mycophenolate mofetil, tumor necrosis factor-α inhibitors, and less often rituximab.[3,17,31,38] Patients receiving long-term corticosteroids and other immune suppression should be screened for latent infections and receive up-to-date vaccines before initiation and be prescribed prophylaxis to prevent opportunistic infections, osteoporosis, or gastric ulcers as needed.[58]

Patients with autoimmune meningitis and encephalitis are also at high risk for numerous comorbid complications including seizures, hydrocephalus, and cerebral edema and should be monitored accordingly. Increased intracranial pressure may be seen in AHLE, neurosarcoidosis, HLH, various cerebral vasculitides including ABRA, and SARS-CoV2-associated CNS inflammatory syndromes.[3,16,17,32,47] In addition, although seizures may complicate most CNS disorders, patients with antibody-associated encephalitides are at particular risk for refractory seizures.[1,6]

SUMMARY

Meningitis and encephalitis are inflammatory syndromes of the meninges and brain parenchyma, respectively, and may be identified either by finding definitive evidence of inflammation on tissue pathology or by CSF analysis showing pleocytosis or intrathecal antibody synthesis. Clinicians evaluating undifferentiated meningitis or encephalitis should simultaneously consider autoimmune, infectious, and neoplastic causes, using patient risk factors, clinical syndrome, and diagnostic results including CSF and MRI findings to narrow the differential diagnosis. If an autoimmune cause is favored, an important early diagnostic question is whether a specific neural autoantibody is likely to be identified. If so, clinicians should pursue a thorough evaluation for the autoantibody concurrent with a tailored neoplastic workup and await results of autoantibody testing whenever possible before pursuing brain biopsy. Empiric IVIG or plasmapheresis may be given particularly in deteriorating patients, but if brain biopsy remains a possibility, corticosteroids are often best withheld pending definitive diagnosis. In patients for whom autoantibody-associated disease is not favored, brain or systemic biopsy is often warranted and should be pursued with efforts to maximize its yield. Finally, once the specific cause of autoimmune meningitis or encephalitis is identified and false positives are unlikely, systemic corticosteroids plus additional disease-specific treatment may be initiated.

CLINICS CARE POINTS

- The presence of inflammation in the meninges or brain parenchyma often indicates a treatable disorder, and clinicians should consider infectious, neoplastic, and autoimmune diseases in patients with undifferentiated meningitis or encephalitis. Suspicion for autoimmune disease is heightened in younger patients with subacute disease onset and/or a personal or family history of autoimmunity, but infectious and neoplastic disorders should nevertheless be simultaneously considered and evaluated.

- Early evaluation of suspected autoimmune encephalitis should include assessment for specific neural autoantibodies, as the identification of a positive antibody often precludes the need for brain biopsy and allows therapeutics to commence.

- Numerous autoimmune processes without specific associated neural autoantibodies can cause isolated meningitis, encephalitis, or both concurrently. These diseases may be categorized into histiocytic, fulminant demyelinating, vasculitic, amyloid-related, and systemic rheumatologic disorders. Although several have characteristic features and may be diagnosed clinically, many require tissue sampling to confirm.

- Although clinicians should aggressively seek alternative systemic biopsy sites when available, brain biopsy is a high-yield and relatively low-morbidity procedure in the appropriate clinical setting.

DISCLOSURE

The author has nothing to disclose.

REFERENCES

1. Tobin WO, Pittock SJ. Autoimmune neurology of the central nervous system. Contin Minneap Minn 2017;23(3):627–53.
2. Gold SM, Willing A, Leypoldt F, et al. Sex differences in autoimmune disorders of the central nervous system. Semin Immunopathol 2019;41(2):177–88.
3. Pawate S. Sarcoidosis and the nervous system. Contin Minneap Minn 2020;26(3): 695–715.
4. Powers WJ. Primary angiitis of the central nervous system: diagnostic criteria. Neurol Clin 2015;33(2):515–26.
5. Lancaster E. The diagnosis and treatment of autoimmune encephalitis. J Clin Neurol Seoul Korea 2016;12(1):1–13.
6. Bradshaw MJ, Linnoila JJ. An overview of autoimmune and paraneoplastic encephalitides. Semin Neurol 2018;38(3):330–43.
7. Graus F, Titulaer MJ, Balu R, et al. A clinical approach to diagnosis of autoimmune encephalitis. Lancet Neurol 2016;15(4):391–404.
8. Wang Y, Camelo-Piragua S, Abdullah A, et al. Neuroimaging features of CNS histiocytosis syndromes. Clin Imaging 2020;60(1):131–40.
9. Bhatia A, Hatzoglou V, Ulaner G, et al. Neurologic and oncologic features of Erdheim-Chester disease: a 30-patient series. Neuro-Oncol. 2020;22(7):979–92.
10. Diallo K, Revuz S, Clavel-Refregiers G, et al. Vogt-Koyanagi-Harada disease: a retrospective and multicentric study of 41 patients. BMC Ophthalmol 2020; 20(1):395.
11. Kato Y, Kurimura M, Yahata Y, et al. Vogt-Koyanagi-Harada's disease presenting polymorphonuclear pleocytosis in the cerebrospinal fluid at the early active stage. Intern Med Tokyo Jpn 2006;45(12):779–81.
12. Hashimoto T, Takizawa H, Yukimura K, et al. Vogt-Koyanagi-Harada disease associated with brainstem encephalitis. J Clin Neurosci 2009;16(4):593–5.
13. Pittock SJ, Debruyne J, Krecke KN, et al. Chronic lymphocytic inflammation with pontine perivascular enhancement responsive to steroids (CLIPPERS). Brain J Neurol 2010;133(9):2626–34.
14. Taieb G, Mulero P, Psimaras D, et al. CLIPPERS and its mimics: evaluation of new criteria for the diagnosis of CLIPPERS. J Neurol Neurosurg Psychiatry 2019;90(9): 1027–38.
15. Bevan CJ, Cree BA. Fulminant demyelinating diseases of the central nervous system. Semin Neurol 2015;35(6):656–66.
16. Grzonka P, Scholz MC, De Marchis GM, et al. Acute hemorrhagic leukoencephalitis: a case and systematic review of the literature. Front Neurol 2020;11:899.
17. Adams HP. Chapter 31 - Cerebral vasculitis. In: Biller J, Ferro JM, editors. Handbook of clinical Neurology. Vol 119. Neurologic aspects of systemic disease Part I. .

Elsevier; 2014. p. 475–94. Available at: https://www.sciencedirect.com/science/article/pii/B978070204086300031X. Accessed April 22, 2021.

18. Krawczyk M, Barra LJ, Sposato LA, et al. Primary CNS vasculitis: a systematic review on clinical characteristics associated with abnormal biopsy and angiography. Autoimmun Rev 2021;20(1):102714.

19. Abdel Razek AAK, Alvarez H, Bagg S, et al. Imaging spectrum of CNS vasculitis. Radiographics 2014;34(4):873–94.

20. Kidd DP. Neurological complications of Behçet's syndrome. J Neurol 2017; 264(10):2178–83.

21. Akman-Demir G, Serdaroglu P, Tasçi B. Clinical patterns of neurological involvement in Behçet's disease: evaluation of 200 patients. Brain 1999;122(11):2171–82.

22. André R, Cottin V, Saraux J-L, et al. Central nervous system involvement in eosinophilic granulomatosis with polyangiitis (Churg-Strauss): report of 26 patients and review of the literature. Autoimmun Rev 2017;16(9):963–9.

23. Nishino H, Rubino FA, DeRemee RA, et al. Neurological involvement in Wegener's granulomatosis: an analysis of 324 consecutive patients at the Mayo Clinic. Ann Neurol 1993;33(1):4–9.

24. Thiel G, Shakeel M, Ah-See K. Wegener's granulomatosis presenting as meningitis. J Laryngol Otol 2012;126(2):207–9.

25. Yajima R, Toyoshima Y, Wada Y, et al. A fulminant case of granulomatosis with polyangiitis with meningeal and parenchymal involvement. Case Rep Neurol 2015; 7(1):101–4.

26. Dengler LD, Capparelli EV, Bastian JF, et al. Cerebrospinal fluid profile in patients with acute Kawasaki disease. Pediatr Infect Dis J 1998;17(6):478–81.

27. Hu F, Shi X, Fan Y, et al. Cerebrospinal fluid changes and clinical features of aseptic meningitis in patients with Kawasaki disease. J Int Med Res 2021; 49(2). 300060520980213.

28. Wolff AE, Hansen KE, Zakowski L. Acute Kawasaki disease: not just for kids. J Gen Intern Med 2007;22(5):681–4.

29. Roelcke U, Eschle D, Kappos L, et al. Meningoradiculitis associated with giant cell arteritis. Neurology 2002;59(11):1811–2.

30. Paula De Carvalho Panzeri Carlotti A, Paes Leme Ferriani V, Tanuri Caldas C, et al. Polyarteritis nodosa with central nervous system involvement mimicking meningoencephalitis. Pediatr Crit Care Med 2004;5(3):286–8.

31. Corovic A, Kelly S, Markus HS. Cerebral amyloid angiopathy associated with inflammation: a systematic review of clinical and imaging features and outcome. Int J Stroke 2018;13(3):257–67.

32. Salvarani C, Morris JM, Giannini C, et al. Imaging findings of cerebral amyloid angiopathy, Aβ-Related Angiitis (ABRA), and cerebral amyloid angiopathy–related inflammation. Medicine (Baltimore) 2016;95(20):e3613.

33. Chwalisz BK. Cerebral amyloid angiopathy and related inflammatory disorders. J Neurol Sci 2021;424:117425.

34. Torres J, Loomis C, Cucchiara B, et al. Diagnostic yield and safety of brain biopsy for suspected primary central nervous system angiitis. Stroke 2016;47(8):2127–9.

35. Bathon JM, Moreland LW, DiBartolomeo AG. Inflammatory central nervous system involvement in rheumatoid arthritis. Semin Arthritis Rheum 1989;18(4):258–66.

36. DeQuattro K, Imboden JB. Neurologic manifestations of rheumatoid arthritis. Rheum Dis Clin North Am 2017;43(4):561–71.

37. Alexander SK, Di Cicco M, Pohl U, et al. Rheumatoid disease: an unusual cause of relapsing meningoencephalitis. BMJ Case Rep 2018;2018.

38. Pavlakis PP. Rheumatologic disorders and the nervous system. Contin Minneap Minn 2020;26(3):591–610.

39. Margaretten M. Neurologic manifestations of primary sjögren syndrome. Rheum Dis Clin North Am 2017;43(4):519–29.

40. Sophie D, Jerome de S, Anne-Laure F, et al. Neurologic manifestations in primary Sjögren syndrome: a study of 82 patients. Medicine (Baltimore) 2004;83(5):280–91.

41. Jarius S, Kleffner I, Dörr JM, et al. Clinical, paraclinical and serological findings in Susac syndrome: an international multicenter study. J Neuroinflammation 2014;11:46.

42. de Amorim JC, Frittoli RB, Pereira D, et al. Epidemiology, characterization, and diagnosis of neuropsychiatric events in systemic lupus erythematosus. Expert Rev Clin Immunol 2019;15(4):407–16.

43. Stone J, Franks AJ, Guthrie JA, et al. Scleroderma "en coup de sabre": pathological evidence of intracerebral inflammation. J Neurol Neurosurg Psychiatry 2001;70(3):382–5.

44. Wallach AI, Magro CM, Franks AG, et al. Protean neurologic manifestations of two rare dermatologic disorders: sweet disease and localized craniofacial scleroderma. Curr Neurol Neurosci Rep 2019;19(3):11.

45. Amaral TN, Peres FA, Lapa AT, et al. Neurologic involvement in scleroderma: a systematic review. Semin Arthritis Rheum 2013;43(3):335–47.

46. Griffin G, Shenoi S, Hughes GC. Hemophagocytic lymphohistiocytosis: an update on pathogenesis, diagnosis, and therapy. Best Pract Res Clin Rheumatol 2020;34(4):101515.

47. Cai G, Wang Y, Liu X, et al. Central nervous system involvement in adults with haemophagocytic lymphohistiocytosis: a single-center study. Ann Hematol 2017;96(8):1279–85.

48. Sfriso P, Priori R, Valesini G, et al. Adult-onset Still's disease: an Italian multicentre retrospective observational study of manifestations and treatments in 245 patients. Clin Rheumatol 2016;35(7):1683–9.

49. Zhao M, Wu D, Shen M. Adult onset still's disease with neurological involvement: a single center report. Rheumatol Oxf Engl 2020;60(9):4152–7.

50. Lu LX, Della-Torre E, Stone JH, et al. IgG4-related hypertrophic pachymeningitis: clinical features, diagnostic criteria, and treatment. JAMA Neurol 2014;71(6):785–93.

51. Levraut M, Cohen M, Bresch S, et al. Immunoglobulin G4-related hypertrophic pachymeningitis: a case-oriented review. Neurol Neuroimmunol Neuroinflamm 2019;6(4):e568.

52. Berg MJ, Williams LS. The transient syndrome of headache with neurologic deficits and CSF lymphocytosis. Neurology 1995;45(9):1648–54.

53. Richie MB, Josephson SA. A practical approach to meningitis and encephalitis. Semin Neurol 2015;35(6):611–20.

54. Berek K, Hegen H, Auer M, et al. Cerebrospinal fluid oligoclonal bands in Neuroborreliosis are specific for Borrelia burgdorferi. PLoS One 2020;15(9):e0239453.

55. Gu W, Miller S, Chiu CY. Clinical metagenomic next-generation sequencing for pathogen detection. Annu Rev Pathol 2019;14:319–38.

56. Sitthinamsuwan P, Chinthammitr Y, Pattanaprichakul P, et al. Random skin biopsy in the diagnosis of intravascular lymphoma. J Cutan Pathol 2017;44(9):729–33.

57. Bai HX, Zou Y, Lee AM, et al. Diagnostic value and safety of brain biopsy in patients with cryptogenic neurological disease: a systematic review and meta-analysis of 831 cases. Neurosurgery 2015;77(2):283–95 [discussion 295].

58. López-Chiriboga AS, Flanagan EP. Diagnostic and therapeutic approach to autoimmune neurologic disorders. Semin Neurol 2018;38(3):392–402.

59. Hermetter C, Fazekas F, Hochmeister S. Systematic review: syndromes, early diagnosis, and treatment in autoimmune encephalitis. Front Neurol 2018;9:706.
60. Hébert J, Gros P, Lapointe S, et al. Searching for autoimmune encephalitis: Beware of normal CSF. J Neuroimmunol 2020;345:577285.
61. Zrzavy T, Höftberger R, Wimmer I, et al. Longitudinal CSF findings in autoimmune encephalitis—a monocentric cohort study. Front Immunol 2021;12:646940.
62. Malter MP, Elger CE, Surges R. Diagnostic value of CSF findings in antibody-associated limbic and anti-NMDAR-encephalitis. Seizure 2013;22(2):136–40.
63. Jarius S, Hoffmann L, Clover L, et al. CSF findings in patients with voltage gated potassium channel antibody associated limbic encephalitis. J Neurol Sci 2008; 268(1):74–7.
64. Chabaane M, Amelot A, Riche M, et al. Efficacy of a second brain biopsy for intracranial lesions after initial negativity. J Clin Neurol Seoul Korea 2020;16(4):659–67.
65. Mathon B, Le Joncour A, Bielle F, et al. Neurological diseases of unknown etiology: brain-biopsy diagnostic yields and safety. Eur J Intern Med 2020;80:78–85.
66. Gelfand JM, Genrich G, Green AJ, et al. Encephalitis of unclear origin diagnosed by brain biopsy: a diagnostic challenge. JAMA Neurol 2015;72(1):66–72.
67. Sechi E, Markovic SN, McKeon A, et al. Neurologic autoimmunity and immune checkpoint inhibitors: Autoantibody profiles and outcomes. Neurology 2020; 95(17):e2442–52.
68. Cuzzubbo S, Javeri F, Tissier M, et al. Neurological adverse events associated with immune checkpoint inhibitors: Review of the literature. Eur J Cancer 2017;73:1–8.
69. Paterson RW, Brown RL, Benjamin L, et al. The emerging spectrum of COVID-19 neurology: clinical, radiological and laboratory findings. Brain 2020;143(10):3104–20.
70. Khodamoradi Z, Hosseini SA, Gholampoor Saadi MH, et al. COVID-19 meningitis without pulmonary involvement with positive cerebrospinal fluid PCR. Eur J Neurol 2020;27(12):2668–9.
71. Varadan B, Shankar A, Rajakumar A, et al. Acute hemorrhagic leukoencephalitis in a COVID-19 patient—a case report with literature review. Neuroradiology 2021; 63(5):653–61.
72. Romero-Sánchez CM, Díaz-Maroto I, Fernández-Díaz E, et al. Neurologic manifestations in hospitalized patients with COVID-19: the ALBACOVID registry. Neurology 2020;95(8):e1060–70.
73. Franke C, Ferse C, Kreye J, et al. High frequency of cerebrospinal fluid autoantibodies in COVID-19 patients with neurological symptoms. Brain Behav Immun 2021;93:415–9.
74. Virhammar J, Kumlien E, Fällmar D, et al. Acute necrotizing encephalopathy with SARS-CoV-2 RNA confirmed in cerebrospinal fluid. Neurology 2020;95(10):445–9.
75. Edén A, Kanberg N, Gostner J, et al. CSF biomarkers in patients with COVID-19 and neurologic symptoms: a case series. Neurology 2021;96(2):e294–300.
76. Dubey D, Pittock SJ, Kelly CR, et al. Autoimmune encephalitis epidemiology and a comparison to infectious encephalitis. Ann Neurol 2018;83(1):166–77.
77. O'Donovan B, Mandel-Brehm C, Vazquez SE, et al. High-resolution epitope mapping of anti-Hu and anti-Yo autoimmunity by programmable phage display. Brain Commun 2020;2(2):fcaa059.
78. Valencia-Sanchez C, Pittock SJ, Mead-Harvey C, et al. Brain dysfunction and thyroid antibodies: autoimmune diagnosis and misdiagnosis. Brain Commun 2021; 3(2):fcaa233.
79. Barón J, Mulero P, Pedraza MI, et al. HaNDL syndrome: correlation between focal deficits topography and EEG or SPECT abnormalities in a series of 5 new cases. Neurol Engl Ed 2016;31(5):305–10.

Diagnosis and Management of Central Nervous System Demyelinating Disorders

Lahoud Touma, MD[a], Alexandra Muccilli, MD, MEd, FRCPC[b],*

KEYWORDS

- Demyelinating disease • Multiple sclerosis • Acute disseminated encephalomyelitis
- Neuromyelitis optica spectrum disorder

KEY POINTS

- Central nervous system demyelinating disorders typically present with acute to subacute onset neurologic symptoms reflecting the location of inflammatory lesions within the brain, optic nerves, and spinal cord.
- In acute multiple sclerosis relapses, the use of high-dose intravenous or oral corticosteroids hastens recovery.
- Acute disseminated encephalomyelitis is a monophasic, multifocal central nervous system immune-mediated condition usually affecting children and often preceded by a viral infection.
- Aquaporin-4 and myelin oligodendrocyte glycoprotein antibody-mediated disorders require consideration in the presence of certain clinical, radiologic, and biological findings.

INTRODUCTION

The spectrum of central nervous system (CNS) demyelinating diseases is broad. Although many of these conditions have a chronic course, they often present with acute to subacute neurologic symptoms necessitating more urgent assessment and management. Multiple sclerosis (MS) is the most common inflammatory disorder affecting the CNS and serves as a prototype to inform the diagnosis and treatment of more rare conditions. This article reviews the clinical features of the CNS demyelinating diseases commonly encountered in the inpatient setting, with a particular emphasis on acute management principles.

Dr L. Touma has no conflicts of interest. Dr A. Muccilli has received speaking honoraria from Biogen, EMD Serono, and Novartis.
[a] Department of Neurosciences, Unviersity of Montreal, Centre Hospitalier de l'Université de Montréal; [b] Department of Medicine, Division of Neurology, St. Michael's Hospital, University of Toronto, Toronto, Canada
* Corresponding author.
E-mail address: Alexandra.muccilli@unityhealth.to

Neurol Clin 40 (2022) 113–131
https://doi.org/10.1016/j.ncl.2021.08.008
0733-8619/22/© 2021 Elsevier Inc. All rights reserved.

DIAGNOSIS OF MULTIPLE SCLEROSIS

MS is the most common CNS inflammatory disorder in the inpatient setting.[1] It affects women 3 times more often than men, with a mean age of diagnosis of 30 years. Although MS presents with various clinical courses, the relapsing–remitting (RRMS) phenotype is the most common, making up approximately 85% of cases at onset. Although patients occasionally require inpatient treatment of acute relapses, non–MS-related concerns (eg, digestive, genitourinary, and circulatory) now constitute a higher proportion of hospitalizations.[2]

An MS diagnosis relies on clinical history and objective examination or paraclinical findings of one or more characteristic neurologic syndromes. In one large French series, symptoms of long tract dysfunction were the most common at onset.[3] Involvement of the posterior and lateral columns resulting in sensory and motor complaints, respectively, is typical of an MS partial myelitis. Optic neuritis (ON) is also frequent and characterized by subacute monocular vision loss, color desaturation, and pain with extraocular movements. Isolated brainstem symptoms are seen in less than 10% of patients at onset, with variable presentations including internuclear ophthalmoplegia, sixth nerve palsy, gaze evoked nystagmus, and trigeminal neuralgia.[3]

In 2017, the McDonald criteria for RRMS were revised and simplified to allow for a timelier diagnosis.[4] After symptoms of a typical demyelinating attack have been identified, MRI may provide evidence of dissemination in both space and time as outlined in **Table 1**. MRI lesions must be evident in 2 of 4 locations—periventricular (**Fig. 1**), cortical or juxtacortical (**Fig. 2**), infratentorial (**Fig. 3**), and spinal cord (**Fig. 4**)—each with a distinct appearance. If criteria for dissemination in time are not met, detection of cerebrospinal fluid (CSF)-specific oligoclonal bands (OCBs) may be used as a substitute marker.

THE ACUTE MULTIPLE SCLEROSIS RELAPSE

An MS relapse, commonly called a flare or exacerbation, is characterized by the onset of new neurologic symptoms lasting more than 24 hours, in the absence of fever or infection.[4] Symptoms typically intensify over hours to days, followed by variable recovery over weeks to months. The resulting neurologic deficits reflect the location of the symptomatic lesion within the CNS. Although relapses may seem to occur randomly, studies have shown they have a propensity for previously affected neuroanatomic sites.[5,6]

An MS relapse should be distinguished from a pseudorelapse, wherein there is reemergence of symptoms of a prior attack due to an increase in core body temperature as a result of fever, infection, or, occasionally, during the mid-to-late luteal phase of a woman's menstrual cycle.[7] Several pathophysiological hypotheses have been proposed for the pseudorelapse phenomenon, with the most commonly accepted being the temperature-sensitive conduction blockade of partially demyelinated axons.[8] These recrudescent symptoms do not require treatment and should resolve when the provoking factor is removed.

Treatment of Multiple Sclerosis Relapse

The goal of treating an MS relapse is to decrease the intensity and duration of functionally limiting neurologic symptoms. Treatment, although hastening recovery, does not alter long-term disability outcomes.[9] The risks and benefits of intervention must therefore be carefully considered, and most MS experts agree pharmacotherapy is

Table 1
The 2017 McDonald criteria for the diagnosis of relapsing remitting multiple sclerosis

Clinical Attacks	Number of Lesions With Objective Clinical Evidence	Additional Data Needed for Multiple Sclerosis Diagnosis
≥2 Clinical attacks	≥2	None; MRI is encouraged
	1 (with clear-cut historical evidence of a previous attack involving a lesion in a distinct anatomic location)	
	1	DIS demonstrated by an additional clinical attack implicating a different CNS site or by MRI
1	≥2	DIT as demonstrated by one of the following: 1. An additional clinical attack 2. MRI with new lesion 3. CSF-specific oligoclonal bands
	1	DIS as demonstrated by either an additional clinical attack OR MRI lesion implicating a different CNS site AND DIT as demonstrated by one of the following: 1. An additional clinical attack 2. MRI with new lesion 3. CSF-specific oligoclonal bands

Abbreviations: CSF, cerebrospinal fluid; DIS, dissemination in space; DIT, dissemination in time.
   From Thompson AJ, Banwell BL, Barkhof F, et al. Diagnosis of multiple sclerosis: 2017 revisions of the McDonald criteria. Lancet Neurol. 2018;17(2):162–173. doi:10.1016/S1474-4422(17)30470-2; Reprinted with permission of Elsevier, Inc.

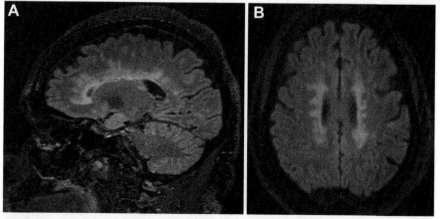

Fig. 1. Sagittal (*A*) and axial (*B*) FLAIR images showing demyelinating plaques oriented perpendicular to the body of the lateral ventricles ("Dawson fingers") typical for multiple sclerosis.

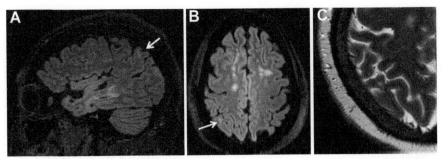

Fig. 2. Right parietal MS lesion (*arrow*) contacts the cortex and is therefore a "juxtacortical" lesion as seen on the sagittal (*A*) and axial (*B*) FLAIR images and the magnified T2-weighted image (*C*).

warranted only when neurologic symptoms are severe (eg, vision loss or pronounced motor deficits).

Corticosteroids

Steroids are the cornerstone of MS relapse management with multiple studies and meta-analyses supporting their use.[10–12] Perhaps the most well known is the Optic Neuritis Treatment Trial, which demonstrated faster recovery from acute ON in individuals treated with high-dose intravenous methylprednisolone versus treatment with oral prednisone (1 mg/kg) or placebo.[13] Although parenteral steroids accelerated improvement, no overall long-term impact on visual metrics was detected.

At present, a 3- to 5-day course of 1-gram intravenous methylprednisolone is the standard treatment of an acute MS exacerbation. Although steroids were long thought to be more effective when administered parenterally, recent work has shown

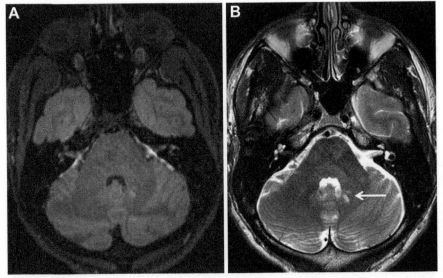

Fig. 3. Axial FLAIR (*A*) and T2-weighted (*B*) images demonstrate hyperintense left cerebellar MS lesions.

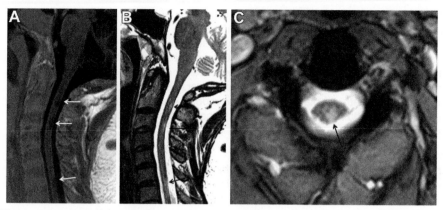

Fig. 4. Sagittal PSIR (*A*), sagittal T2 (*B*), and axial (*C*) T2-weighted images demonstrate short segment lesions with partial cord involvement and predilection for posterior columns seen on axial image in this MS patient.

noninferiority of equivalently high-dosed oral administration (**Table 2**).[14,15] Given such evidence and the obvious practical and financial advantages, most MS relapses are now managed in the outpatient setting with oral steroids. The choice to pursue a steroid taper is mostly based on physician preference, as no definitive evidence supports this practice.

Steroid use is not without adverse effects. However, given the relatively short course of treatment, most patients avoid the deleterious effects associated with chronic steroid therapy. Such complications include hypothalamic-pituitary-adrenal axis suppression, infection, cataracts, glaucoma, myopathy, metabolic syndrome, reduced bone health, and avascular necrosis, the latter of which can occur with a short-term use as well. The most frequently endorsed side effects with a 3- to 5-day steroid treatment regimen include insomnia, mood dysfunction, hyperglycemia, and gastrointestinal upset.[16]

Second-Line Treatments

Plasma exchange
Plasma exchange (PLEX) is widely used in many antibody-mediated disorders affecting the CNS. Both retrospective and prospective studies support its use in severe MS relapses, which are unresponsive to steroids. In a randomized sham-controlled trial of patients with demyelinating conditions refractory to steroids, treatment with PLEX led to significant improvement in 42% of cases, compared with 5%

Table 2 Corticosteroid dosing and equivalency		
Corticosteroid	Dose Equivalent	Appropriate Oral Dose for MS Relapse
Prednisone	1 mg	1250 mg
Methylprednisolone	0.8 mg	1000 mg
Dexamethasone	0.15 mg	200 mg

of those in the sham arm.[17] Predictors of response to PLEX include male gender, pre-served reflexes, and early initiation of treatment.[18]

PLEX is often performed via central venous access; however peripheral administra-tion is possible in cooperative patients with favourable vasculature. It remains a rela-tively low-risk procedure, with hypotension, fever, minor allergic reaction, and citrate toxicity among the more frequently reported adverse effects. Complications related to central venous catheter placement (eg, thrombosis, hemorrhage, and pneumothorax) are rare but should not be overlooked, as these can result in significant morbidity and mortality.

Intravenous immunoglobulin

Intravenous immunoglobulin (IVIG) is another alternative adjunctive treatment used in MS relapses, although no randomized trial evidence exists to support its use, either in conjunction with or over steroids.[19]

Cyclophosphamide

Cyclophosphamide is used in certain cases of fulminant MS due to its potent myeloabla-tive properties. It has, however, largely fallen out of favor due to its significant side-effect profile (eg, gonadotoxicity, myelosuppression, hemorrhagic cystitis, and cardiotoxicity) and the availability of newer more tolerable options. The gonadotoxicity is of particular relevance for women of reproductive age, who make up a large proportion of patients with MS.

Natalizumab

Because of its fairly rapid time to effect, Natalizumab is also sometimes used in the acute relapse period subsequent to steroids, although there are little data to support this practice. A 2004 study of Natalizumab administered within 4 days of relapse onset did not show superior clinical effect over placebo.[20] However, a significant decrease in gadolinium-enhancing lesion volume was noted at 1 and 3 weeks after treatment, sup-porting Natalizumab's role in rapidly halting inflammatory disease.

MULTIPLE SCLEROSIS VARIANTS
Tumefactive Multiple Sclerosis

Patients with MS-like lesions measuring greater than 2 cm and with a neoplastic appearance are diagnosed with tumefactive MS.[21] On brain MRI, tumefactive lesions are usually quite large, with surrounding vasogenic edema, variable degree of mass effect, and an open-ring enhancement pattern (**Fig. 5**). Advanced imaging techniques such as magnetic resonance spectroscopy and PET may be used to distinguish demyelination from malignancy; however, biopsy is often required for a definitive diag-nosis. Spinal cord imaging may be helpful, as asymptomatic demyelinating lesions support an MS diagnosis. Similarly, the presence of CSF OCBs may also point toward MS, although this is not definitive, as patients with a tumefactive presentation have been shown to be less likely than those with established MS (52% vs 90%) to have CSF-restricted OCBs.[22]

The clinical presentation of tumefactive MS is variable and often polysymptomatic, with motor, cognitive, sensory, and cerebellar signs most common at onset.[21] Inten-sive care unit admission is sometimes necessary, as lesions with significant mass ef-fect may result in midline shift and herniation. Management with high-dose steroids resembles that of a typical acute MS relapse. PLEX is often used in refractory cases of tumefactive MS, although only retrospective data support this practice.[23] Cyclo-phosphamide and rituximab are considered in severe treatment-refractory cases.

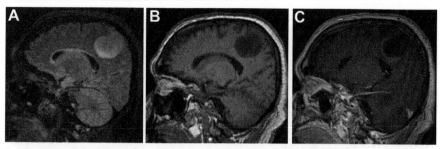

Fig. 5. Sagittal FLAIR (*A*), noncontrast T1 (*B*), and postcontrast T1-weighted (*C*) images of a left parietal lobe lesion with local mass effect demonstrating FLAIR hyperintensity, T1 hypointensity, and partial rim of enhancement ("open ring" sign) in keeping with tumefactive demyelination.

In the largest published series of biopsy-proven tumefactive MS cases, approximately half of patients went on to have a recurrent attack, thus confirming a diagnosis of RRMS.[21] Twenty-four percent had a monophasic course, with the others having a more progressive phenotype. Interestingly, those with a tumefactive presentation followed-up over 10 years had significantly better clinical outcomes compared with a cohort of patients with MS matched for disease duration.[21]

Baló Concentric Sclerosis

Patients with Baló concentric sclerosis present with acute or subacute neurologic symptoms and MRI evidence of one or more concentric multilayered ringlike lesions with alternating high and low signal intensity on T2-weighted sequences (**Fig. 6**).[24] Baló lesions are sometimes associated with peripheral gadolinium enhancement as well as evidence of restricted diffusion at the edge. Pathology demonstrates a similar whorled pattern of alternating rings of demyelination and spared myelin, often resulting in an onion bulb appearance.[24]

Baló-like lesions have been described in other diseases including neuromyelitis optica spectrum disorder (NMOSD) and progressive multifocal leukoencephalopathy, highlighting the fact that the association with MS is not absolute.[25,26] In one case series, 55% of patients with Baló lesions at presentation had concurrent evidence of typical MS lesions.[24] CSF-specific OCBs are much less common in Baló cases than in those with established MS, although their presence does perhaps predict a risk of conversion.[27,28]

Given its rarity, there is scarce high-quality evidence to guide management of Baló concentric sclerosis. First-line treatment is often with high-dose steroids, and, in refractory cases, therapeutic algorithms are similar to those used in cases of refractory MS and fulminant demyelination (eg, PLEX, cyclophosphamide, and other immunosuppressive agents). Patients with Baló concentric sclerosis were previously thought to have a universally poor prognosis, but this no longer the case as many go on to recover completely.[24]

Marburg Variant of Multiple Sclerosis

Marburg variant is a rare fulminant form of MS first described in the early 1900s. Patients typically present with an acute and unrelenting progressive course of multifocal neurologic deficits, leading to death within months. The disorder bears some clinical and radiologic overlap with tumefactive demyelination and acute disseminated encephalomyelitis (ADEM), but with a lesser tendency to cause diffuse

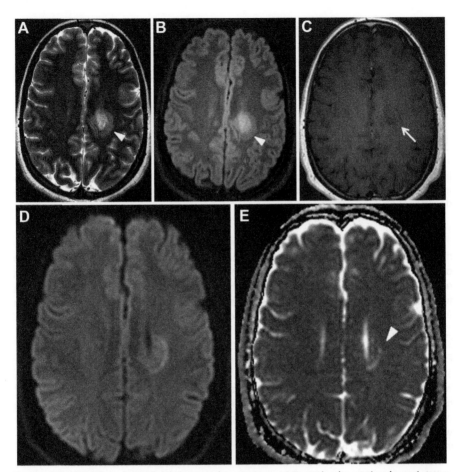

Fig. 6. Axial T2 (*A*) and FLAIR (*B*) images demonstrate concentric alternating hyperintense and iso- to hypointense areas within a lesion in left corona radiata (*arrowhead*) consistent with Balò concentric sclerosis. Postcontrast T1-weighted (*C*) images demonstrate faint enhancement (*arrow*). Axial DWI (*D*) and ADC (*E*) images demonstrate ring of mildly restricted diffusion (*arrowhead*). ADC, apparent diffusion coefficient; DWI, diffusion-weighted imaging.

encephalopathy at onset than the latter.[29] Pathologically speaking, Marburg MS gives rise to a far more acute and destructive process. Imaging demonstrates large multi-focal demyelinating lesions with associated enhancement and perilesional edema. CSF testing reveals increased protein with a normal or mildly increased cell count and absent OCBs.[30] Treatment consists of high-dose corticosteroids followed by PLEX and consideration of additional immunosuppression often with cyclophospha-mide or mitoxantrone.[29] Neuroprotective strategies are critical to reduce the risk of herniation, but prognosis is often poor.

Schilder Disease

Myelinoclastic diffuse sclerosis, also termed Schilder disease, is a rare monophasic neuroinflammatory condition more commonly affecting children. Distinguishing Schilder disease from other MS variants, ADEM, NMOSD, and certain leukodystrophies may be difficult, as imaging patterns exhibit significant overlap. With Schilder disease, MRI demonstrates 1 or 2 large, roughly symmetric demyelinating lesions involving the centrum semiovale.[31] These lesions are generally associated with minimal gadolinium enhancement, but evidence of restricted diffusion in the acute phase. OCBs are absent in most of the cases.[30]

OTHER FULMINANT DEMYELINATING DISEASES
Acute Demyelinating Encephalomyelitis

ADEM is sometimes referred to as postinfectious encephalomyelitis and is a monophasic autoimmune demyelinating disease affecting the CNS. Children are more commonly affected than adults, with a mean onset of symptoms 26 days postinfection.[32]

In 2007, the International Pediatric MS Study Group defined ADEM as the acute to subacute onset of polyfocal neurologic symptoms with accompanying encephalopathy and abnormal imaging.[33] Neurologic deficits usually attain maximal intensity within 2 to 5 days.[34] Altered consciousness not attributable to a febrile illness is a critical feature of the diagnosis and includes a broad spectrum from lethargy to coma.[34] Contrary to the pediatric population, cases of postinfectious neurologic symptoms in adults are not always associated with encephalopathy but are sometimes termed ADEM nonetheless.[35] As is the case in MS, the clinical symptomatology in ADEM reflects the areas of CNS involvement, with motor symptoms predominating at onset in adults.[35] Other common abnormalities include sensory deficits, brainstem symptoms, and ataxia. Aphasia, meningismus, seizures, and optic neuritis are rare in those aged 18 years and older.

MRI abnormalities in ADEM typically consist of multifocal, large ($\geq$1–2 cm), asymmetric, poorly demarcated lesions of the supra- and infratentorial white matter. Gray matter structures are also frequently involved, notably the basal ganglia and thalami.[33,34] Lesions with associated gadolinium enhancement are reported in up to one-third of patients, as is involvement of the spinal cord.[34] The absence of exclusively well-defined, ovoid-shaped, perpendicularly oriented lesions abutting the corpus callosum helps to differentiate ADEM from MS.[36]

CSF analysis is frequently performed in cases of ADEM, as infectious differential diagnoses are often a consideration. Findings are variable, with 50% to 80% of patients demonstrating nonspecific abnormalities including mild lymphocytic pleocytosis and elevated protein.[35] OCBs are rare in children with ADEM but have been reported in adult cases, although generally transient.[36] In one series, no OCBs or identical serum and CSF OCBs ("mirror pattern") were detected in 84% of patients with ADEM, but only 10% of those with MS.[37] The presence of matched OCBs suggests systemic autoimmune activation and is an additional paraclinical element helpful in distinguishing the 2 conditions.

Infections have been implicated as common triggers for ADEM, with a prior viral upper respiratory tract infection noted in 50% to 75% of adult cases in one series.[38] Although rare, ADEM has also been described following immunization. In a German series of 40 adults, a single patient developed ADEM after receiving the tetanus and diphtheria vaccination.[35] Most experts agree that vaccinations do not increase the risk of ADEM, given the only clear epidemiologic association exists with the Semple form of the rabies vaccine that is now discontinued.[39] ADEM has also been reported following bone marrow and solid organ transplantation.[40]

Recent studies have highlighted a subpopulation of patients with ADEM with antibodies to myelin oligodendrocyte glycoprotein (MOG); this is particularly relevant in children, in whom MOG autoantibodies have been identified in a large proportion of patients presenting with ADEM.[41,42] Those with MOG-associated ADEM have certain discernible MRI features including large and hazy bilateral lesions, absence of small and well-defined areas of signal abnormality, involvement of more anatomic areas, and an accompanying longitudinally extensive transverse myelitis (TM).[42] Initial studies suggested persistently positive MOG antibody status was associated with a propensity for relapsing disease in both children and adults.[41] However, more recent data argue this association is less definitive, with only 9% of a large Canadian cohort of MOG IgG-associated ADEM cases having a relapsing course.[43] As a result, the presence of anti-MOG antibodies should not prompt initiation of long-term immuno-modulatory therapy.

There are no randomized data to direct ADEM treatment, and current management is mostly driven by observational studies and expert opinion. Concomitant antimicro-bial coverage is often empirically initiated until an infectious cause has been excluded. Initial treatment of ADEM typically consists of 1000 mg of intravenous methylprednis-olone daily for 5 days, followed by an oral steroid taper over 4 to 6 weeks. For cases unresponsive to steroids, other treatment options include IVIG (2 g/kg) or PLEX. The latter is favored by most in fulminant cases where concurrent standard neuroprotec-tive measures are used to reduce malignant cerebral edema.

Outcomes in patients with ADEM are usually favorable, with a mortality rate ranging between 1% and 5%.[36,44] Approximately 80% of patients have little or no residual disability, with varying degrees of multidomain cognitive impairment in the remaining 20%.[44] As previously noted, ADEM is typically a monophasic illness, but relapses may occur with an identical or distinct phenotype, the latter referred to as multiphasic ADEM.[33] A subset of these cases will be diagnosed with relapsing disorders, including MS, NMOSD, and MOG antibody-associated disease (MOGAD).

Acute Hemorrhagic Leukoencephalitis or Hurst Disease

Acute hemorrhagic leukoencephalitis is a very rare and fulminant hemorrhagic form of ADEM that primarily affects adults. Patients typically present with acute and rapidly progressive multifocal neurologic symptoms and encephalopathy, evolving over days to coma and herniation. MRI lesions are similar to those noted in ADEM, but with associated hemorrhage. CSF analysis is nonspecific with elevated protein and variable pleocytosis, but polymorphonuclear cells may predominate making the distinction from an infectious process more difficult.[45] Early treatment with steroids and PLEX is recommended. Unfortunately, the mortality rate was close to 50% in one systematic review, underscoring the need for better treatment options to improve outcomes.[45]

NEUROMYELITIS OPTICA SPECTRUM DISORDER

NMOSD, also known as Devic disease, is a neuroinflammatory condition character-ized by severe and simultaneous ON and longitudinally extensive TM.[46] The under-standing of NMOSD evolved considerably in 2004 after a high proportion of patients were discovered to have aquaporin-4 (AQP4) autoantibodies. The identification of this specific biomarker allowed for a better classification of the disease, namely with the recognition of its extra-opticospinal manifestations. The diagnostic criteria for NMOSD were revised in 2015 (**Fig. 7**) and included stratification based on APQ4-IgG serostatus.[47]

The 3 cardinal manifestations of NMOSD are ON, TM, and, less frequently, area postrema syndrome (APS).[47] The clinical and imaging features of optic nerve and

NMO Spectrum Disorder

NMOSD AQP4-IgG +VE:	NMOSD AQP4-IgG -VE OR UNKNOWN STATUS :

1. ≥ 1 core clinical characteristic
2. Seropositivity for AQP4 (cell-based assay recommended)
3. Exclusion of other diagnoses
	1. ≥2 core clinical characteristics due ≥1 attack and ALL of:
	  a. ≥1 of the core clinical characteristics must be optic neuritis, LETM, or area postrema syndrome
	  b. Dissemination in space (≥2 core clinical characteristics)
	  c. Fulfillment of MRI requirements for specific syndromes
	2. Negative AQP4 testing using best available detection method, or testing unavailable
	3. Exclusion of other diagnoses

Core Clinical Characteristics:
1. Optic neuritis
2. Acute myelitis
3. Area postrema syndrome
4. Acute brainstem syndrome
5. Symptomatic narcolepsy or acute diencephalic clinical syndrome with NMOSD-typical diencephalic MRI lesions.
6. Symptomatic cerebral syndrome with NMOSD-typical MRI lesions.

Additional MRI Requirements for AQP4-IgG seronegative cases:
1. Optic neuritis: a) MRI showing normal or non-specific white matter lesions OR b) T2 hyperintense or T1-gadolinium-enhancing lesion involving > ½ optic nerve length or optic chiasm
2. Acute myelitis: associated intramedullary MRI lesion extending over ≥ 3 contiguous segments (LETM) OR focal atrophy in cases with prior history of myelitis
3. Area postrema syndrome: associated dorsal medulla/area postrema lesion
4. Acute brainstem syndrome: associated periependymal brainstem lesions.

Fig. 7. Diagnostic criteria for NMO spectrum disorder. (*Adapted from* Wingerchuk DM, Banwell B, Bennett JL, et al. International consensus diagnostic criteria for neuromyelitis optica spectrum disorders. Neurology. 2015;85(2):177-189. https://doi.org/10.1212/WNL.0000000000001729; with permission.)

spinal cord involvement in NMOSD are relatively distinct from those observed in MS (**Table 3**). Optic neuritis is generally recurrent, sequential, or bilateral, with preferential involvement of the posterior optic pathway (**Fig. 8**). Vision loss is typically severe at onset with poor recovery. The myelitis is also more disabling, with evidence of a complete spinal cord syndrome on clinical examination. In the acute phase, MRI frequently demonstrates a longitudinally extensive hyperintensity extending over 3 or more contiguous vertebral body segments, with a predilection for the central gray matter. "Bright spotty lesions" are relatively specific to AQP4-mediated disease and are characterized by prominent hyperintensity on axial T2-weighted images, typically with higher signal intensity than that of the surrounding CSF (**Fig. 9**).[48] Cervical cord lesions that extend cranially to the medulla and fourth ventricle (**Fig. 10**), sometimes with associated APS, also suggest NMOSD.

Other less common manifestations of NMOSD include diencephalic syndromes (eg, narcolepsy, endocrinopathies, hypothermia, and so forth.) and symptoms associated with brainstem or cerebral involvement.[47] Brain MRI abnormalities are detected in more than 60% of cases at onset, may increase with disease progression, and are generally nonspecific (see **Fig. 8**).[49]

The diagnosis of NMOSD is facilitated by commercial availability of cell-based assays, which offer increased sensitivity and specificity over older-generation enzyme-linked immunosorbent assays. Nonetheless, approximately 25% of patients with NMOSD remain AQP4 seronegative, with up to 10% having autoantibodies to MOG-IgG.[50]

CSF studies typically reveal a variable degree of pleocytosis, often more marked than in MS. Although lymphocytes typically predominate, neutrophils and eosinophils may also be present (see **Table 3**).[47] CSF-specific OCBs are noted in 15% to 30% of NMOSD cases.[47] More comprehensive investigations may reveal serum biomarkers of systemic autoimmunity, with or without evidence of concurrent clinical disease. In elderly individuals in particular, NMOSD may occur in a paraneoplastic context.

Table 3
Comparison of central nervous system demyelinating disorders

	MS	NMO	MOG
Demographics			
Sex (F:M)	2–3:1	9:1	1.5:1
Ethnicity	Any, mostly Caucasian	Any, African-American/Afro-Caribbean, Asian at higher risk	Any
Most affected age	20–40 y	30–50 y	0–40 y
Clinical Characteristics			
Disease course at onset	Relapsing 85%, progressive 15%	Relapsing	Monophasic 40% (more common in children); remainder relapsing
Optic neuritis	Variable severity (rarely severe), posterior, good recovery	Severe, posterior, sequential, bilateral, poor recovery (<20/200)	Unilateral or bilateral, recurrent, mainly anterior (optic disc edema common), severe at nadir but good recovery, excellent response to steroids
Myelitis	Variable severity, dorsal and lateral column dysfunction	Generally transverse myelitis with severe deficits	Transverse myelitis with frequent sphincteric dysfunction
Other common clinical manifestations	Brainstem and cerebellar symptoms	APS, diencephalic and other brainstem syndromes	ADEM (more common in children), brainstem and cerebellar syndromes

Investigations				
MRI	Brain	Ovoid periventricular lesions oriented perpendicularly to lateral ventricles, juxtacortical/cortical, infratentorial, open ring enhancement	Normal or nonspecific; with APS lesion involving dorsal inferior medulla oblongata at caudal end of fourth ventricle; callosal lesions following ependyma and diffuse callosal lesions; large hemispheric lesions; ependymal or cloud enhancement	ADEM-like lesions involving white and deep gray matter, brainstem including diffuse middle cerebellar peduncle lesions
	Orbit	Unilateral; <50% of optic nerves involved	Bilateral; >50% of optic nerve; posterior optic pathway involving chiasm and tracts	Bilateral; >50% of optic nerve; anterior optic pathway
	Spine	Multiple short segment lesions; dorsal and lateral predilection; variable peripheral enhancement	Single longitudinally extensive lesion ($\geq$3 vertebral segments); > 50% axial surface involved with predilection for central cord; < 15% short segment lesions; variable enhancement	75% of lesions are longitudinally extensive; 25% short segment lesions; involvement of conus; axial H sign with predilection for gray matter; variable enhancement
CSF		WBC up to 50/mm^3 (lymphocytic); OCBs in up to 90%	WBC variable, usually lymphocytic but may be neutrophilic or eosinophilic); OCBs in 15%–30%	WBC variable (lymphocytic); OCBs < 15%
Blood biomarker		None	AQP4-Ig	MOG-Ig
Management & Prognosis				
Acute		IV methylprednisolone	IV methylprednisolone and early adjunctive PLEX	IV methylprednisolone; IVIG or PLEX if severe
Recovery		Often complete	Often incomplete	Often complete

Abbreviations: ADEM, acute disseminated encephalomyelitis; APS, area postrema syndrome; AQP4, aquaporin-4; IV, intravenous; MOG, myelin oligodendrocyte glycoprotein; OCB, oligoclonal bands; ; WBC, white blood cell.

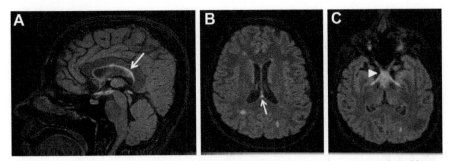

Fig. 8. Sagittal (*A*) and axial (*B*) FLAIR images in NMOSD demonstrate periependymal hyperintensity (*arrow*) and involvement of bilateral optic nerves, chiasm, and bilateral optic tracts (*arrowhead*) (*C*). Few white matter lesions in deep and subcortical white matter are also seen.

Screening for an underlying malignancy is therefore a critical consideration, with carcinomas noted as most common in one series.[51]

The management of AQP4-seropositive disease continues to evolve with new and more effective disease-modifying therapies. Unfortunately, when relapses occur, significant disability often ensues. First-line relapse treatment includes prompt initiation of a 5-day course intravenous methylprednisolone, followed by a prolonged high-dose oral prednisone taper while bridging to a steroid-sparing agent. In cases of relapse with moderate-to-severe neurologic deficits, PLEX is often used as an early adjunctive treatment and has shown improved outcomes.[52]

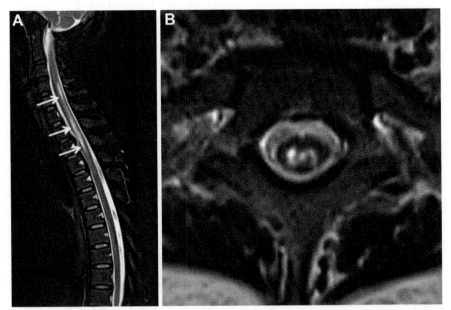

Fig. 9. Sagittal (*A*) and axial (*B*) T2-weighted spine images in NMOSD showing central T2 hyperintense lesion longer than 3 vertebral body heights with "bright spotty" lesions (*arrows*).

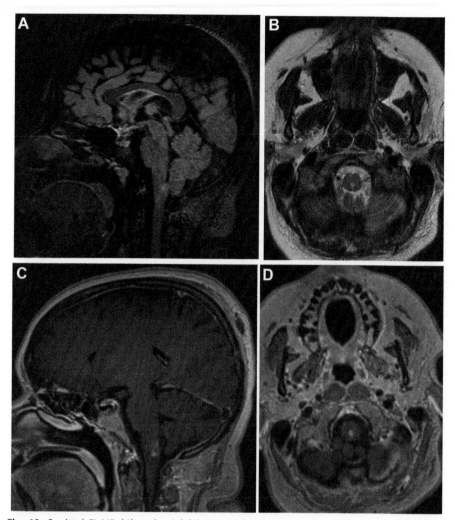

Fig. 10. Sagittal FLAIR (*A*) and axial (*B*) T2-weighted images demonstrate a hyperintense lesion in the dorsal inferior surface of the medulla in this NMOSD patient who presented with area postrema syndrome. Sagittal (*C*) and axial (*D*) postcontrast-T1 weighted images demonstrate enhancement of this lesion.

ANTIMYELIN OLIGODENDROCYTE GLYCOPROTEIN ANTIBODY DISEASE

Autoantibodies to MOG have been identified in up to 10% of adults with AQP4-negative NMOSD and in up to 40% of children with acute demyelinating syndromes (eg, ADEM).[50,53] The term MOGAD is widely used to describe the association of a positive MOG autoantibody with a relevant clinical syndrome.

MOGAD is more common in children and young adults.[54] There is a fairly equal sex distribution, with one large study noting a slight female predominance of 57% (see **Table 3**).[54] A flulike prodrome may precede symptom onset, leading to suspicion of infectious versus immune-mediated cause.

Clinical manifestations in MOGAD are varied, although ON is most common at presentation.[54] ON may be unilateral or bilateral (almost half of cases), monophasic, or recurrent with a median of 3 attacks noted in one study.[55] Optic nerve involvement tends to be more anterior, with optic disc edema detected in 86% of patients.[55] Orbital MRI findings common in MOGAD include perineural enhancement with extension to the surrounding orbital tissues, noted in approximately 50% of cases.[55] As is the case in AQP4-mediated disease, visual acuity may be severely impaired at the nadir in MOGAD, but there is often good response to steroids with an average final visual acuity of 20/30.[55]

In one series, spinal cord involvement was reported in 18% of cases at the time of onset.[54] A severe clinical myelitis with evidence of a longitudinally extensive lesion on MRI is typical of both AQP4 and MOG antibody–mediated spinal cord disease. However, the presence of other short segment lesions and a tendency to affect the conus medullaris suggest MOGAD as is confinement of T2-signal abnormality to gray matter ("H-sign") and lack of enhancement.[56]

As noted earlier, ADEM-like presentations are quite common in those with MOG autoantibodies, especially in children. Brainstem or cerebellar involvement may also occur, although APS is rare. MRI findings of diffuse middle cerebellar peduncle lesions may distinguish MOGAD from MS and NMOSD, as noted in one study.[57]

Testing for MOGAD should be performed in patients presenting with typical clinical and radiological phenotypes, as false positives are not infrequent, notably in those with a borderline titer. Serum testing for MOG-antibody by cell-based assay should be performed over CSF studies, as the latter remain of uncertain significance even when positive. Those with high and persistent serum MOG-IgG titers are at higher risk of relapse, although the autoantibody may decrease with treatment and between relapses.[58] CSF findings in MOGAD are similar to those in NMOSD (ie, variable white blood cell count and infrequent OCBs).

Relapses are typically treated with high-dose intravenous corticosteroids, PLEX, or IVIG. As is the case with AQP4-IgG seropositive NMOSD, a prolonged oral prednisone taper is often prescribed to mitigate the risk of an early relapse. A high proportion of patients with MOGAD have a monophasic course and may not require long-term immunosuppression. A variety of factors should be considered in making the decision to start maintenance treatment in MOGAD, including recovery from the attack, number of prior relapses, and patient preference.

SUMMARY

The various CNS demyelinating diseases outlined in this review demonstrate significant overlap. However, several distinct clinical and radiologic features exist helping to differentiate the disorders. Diagnostic discrimination has long-term treatment and prognostic implications but should not delay acute phase management, as prompt initiation of steroids is central to each. If there is no response to initial treatment, other immunosuppressive strategies are often considered.

REFERENCES

1. Lampl C, Klingler D, Deisenhammer E, et al. Hospitalization of patients with neurological disorders and estimation of the need of beds and of the related costs in Austria's non-profit hospitals. Eur J Neurol 2001;8(6):701–6.
2. Marrie RA, Elliott L, Marriott J, et al. Dramatically changing rates and reasons for hospitalization in multiple sclerosis. Neurology 2014;83(10):929–37.
3. Confavreux C, Vukusic S. Natural history of multiple sclerosis: a unifying concept. Brain 2006;129(Pt 3):606–16.

4. Thompson AJ, Banwell BL, Barkhof F, et al. Diagnosis of multiple sclerosis: 2017 revisions of the McDonald criteria. Lancet Neurol 2018;17(2):162–73.

5. Mowry EM, Deen S, Malikova I, et al. The onset location of multiple sclerosis predicts the location of subsequent relapses. J Neurol Neurosurg Psychiatry 2009; 80(4):400–3.

6. Tsantes E, Leone MA, Curti E, et al. Location of first attack predicts the site of subsequent relapses in multiple sclerosis. J Clin Neurosci 2020;74:175–9.

7. Wingerchuk DM, Rodriguez M. Premenstrual multiple sclerosis pseudoexacerbations: role of body temperature and prevention with aspirin. Arch Neurol 2006; 63(7):1005–8.

8. Guthrie TC, Nelson DA. Influence of temperature changes on multiple sclerosis: critical review of mechanisms and research potential. J Neurol Sci 1995; 129(1):1–8.

9. Brusaferri F, Candelise L. Steroids for multiple sclerosis and optic neuritis: a meta-analysis of randomized controlled clinical trials. J Neurol 2000;247(6): 435–42.

10. Sellebjerg F, Christiansen M, Jensen J, et al. Immunological effects of oral high-dose methylprednisolone in acute optic neuritis and multiple sclerosis. Eur J Neurol 2000;7(3):281–9.

11. Burton JM, O'Connor PW, Hohol M, et al. Oral versus intravenous steroids for treatment of relapses in multiple sclerosis. Cochrane Database Syst Rev 2012; 12:Cd006921.

12. Barnes D, Hughes RA, Morris RW, et al. Randomised trial of oral and intravenous methylprednisolone in acute relapses of multiple sclerosis. Lancet 1997; 349(9056):902–6.

13. Beck RW, Cleary PA, Anderson MM Jr, et al. A randomized, controlled trial of corticosteroids in the treatment of acute optic neuritis. The Optic Neuritis Study Group. N Engl J Med 1992;326(9):581–8.

14. Le Page E, Veillard D, Laplaud DA, et al. Oral versus intravenous high-dose methylprednisolone for treatment of relapses in patients with multiple sclerosis (COPOUSEP): a randomised, controlled, double-blind, non-inferiority trial. Lancet 2015;386(9997):974–81.

15. Morrow SA, Fraser JA, Day C, et al. Effect of treating acute optic neuritis with bioequivalent oral vs intravenous corticosteroids: a randomized clinical trial. JAMA Neurol 2018;75(6):690–6.

16. Gensler LS. Glucocorticoids: complications to anticipate and prevent. Neurohospitalist 2013;3(2):92–7.

17. Weinshenker BG, O'Brien PC, Petterson TM, et al. A randomized trial of plasma exchange in acute central nervous system inflammatory demyelinating disease. Ann Neurol 1999;46(6):878–86.

18. Keegan M, Pineda AA, McClelland RL, et al. Plasma exchange for severe attacks of CNS demyelination: predictors of response. Neurology 2002;58(1):143–6.

19. Sorensen PS, Haas J, Sellebjerg F, et al. IV immunoglobulins as add-on treatment to methylprednisolone for acute relapses in MS. Neurology 2004;63(11):2028–33.

20. O'Connor PW, Goodman A, Willmer-Hulme AJ, et al. Randomized multicenter trial of natalizumab in acute MS relapses: clinical and MRI effects. Neurology 2004; 62(11):2038–43.

21. Lucchinetti CF, Gavrilova RH, Metz I, et al. Clinical and radiographic spectrum of pathologically confirmed tumefactive multiple sclerosis. Brain 2008;131(Pt 7): 1759–75.

22. Altintas A, Petek B, Isik N, et al. Clinical and radiological characteristics of tume-factive demyelinating lesions: follow-up study. Mult Scler 2012;18(10):1448–53.

23. Magaña SM, Keegan BM, Weinshenker BG, et al. Beneficial plasma exchange response in central nervous system inflammatory demyelination. Arch Neurol 2011;68(7):870–8.

24. Hardy TA, Miller DH. Baló's concentric sclerosis. Lancet Neurol 2014;13(7):740–6.

25. Masuda H, Mori M, Katayama K, et al. Anti-aquaporin-4 antibody-seronegative NMO spectrum disorder with Baló's concentric lesions. Intern Med 2013; 52(13):1517–21.

26. Markiewicz D, Adamczewska-Goncerzewicz Z, Dymecki J, et al. A case of primary form of progressive multifocal leukoencephalopathy with concentric demyelination of Baló type. Neuropatol Pol 1977;15(4):491–500.

27. Seewann A, Enzinger C, Filippi M, et al. MRI characteristics of atypical idiopathic inflammatory demyelinating lesions of the brain : a review of reported findings. J Neurol 2008;255(1):1–10.

28. Kira J. Astrocytopathy in Balo's disease. Mult Scler 2011;17(7):771–9.

29. Hardy TA, Reddel SW, Barnett MH, et al. Atypical inflammatory demyelinating syndromes of the CNS. Lancet Neurol 2016;15(9):967–81.

30. Capello E, Mancardi GL. Marburg type and Baló's concentric sclerosis: rare and acute variants of multiple sclerosis. Neurol Sci 2004;25(Suppl 4):S361–3.

31. Poser CM, Goutières F, Carpentier MA, et al. Schilder's myelinoclastic diffuse sclerosis. Pediatrics 1986;77(1):107–12.

32. de Seze J, Debouverie M, Zephir H, et al. Acute fulminant demyelinating disease: a descriptive study of 60 patients. Arch Neurol 2007;64(10):1426–32.

33. Krupp LB, Banwell B, Tenembaum S. Consensus definitions proposed for pediatric multiple sclerosis and related disorders. Neurology 2007;68(16 Suppl 2): S7–12.

34. Tenembaum S, Chamoles N, Fejerman N. Acute disseminated encephalomyelitis: a long-term follow-up study of 84 pediatric patients. Neurology 2002;59(8): 1224–31.

35. Schwarz S, Mohr A, Knauth M, et al. Acute disseminated encephalomyelitis: a follow-up study of 40 adult patients. Neurology 2001;56(10):1313–8.

36. Pohl D, Alper G, Van Haren K, et al. Acute disseminated encephalomyelitis: Updates on an inflammatory CNS syndrome. Neurology 2016;87(9 Suppl 2):S38–45.

37. Franciotta D, Columba-Cabezas S, Andreoni L, et al. Oligoclonal IgG band patterns in inflammatory demyelinating human and mouse diseases. J Neuroimmunol 2008;200(1–2):125–8.

38. Koelman DL, Chahin S, Mar SS, et al. Acute disseminated encephalomyelitis in 228 patients: A retrospective, multicenter US study. Neurology 2016;86(22): 2085–93.

39. Hemachudha T, Griffin DE, Giffels JJ, et al. Myelin basic protein as an encephalitogen in encephalomyelitis and polyneuritis following rabies vaccination. N Engl J Med 1987;316(7):369–74.

40. Lindzen E, Gilani A, Markovic-Plese S, et al. Acute disseminated encephalomyelitis after liver transplantation. Arch Neurol 2005;62(4):650–2.

41. López-Chiriboga AS, Majed M, Fryer J, et al. Association of MOG-IgG serostatus with relapse after acute disseminated encephalomyelitis and proposed diagnostic criteria for MOG-IgG-associated disorders. JAMA Neurol 2018;75(11): 1355–63.

42. Baumann M, Hennes EM, Schanda K, et al. Children with multiphasic disseminated encephalomyelitis and antibodies to the myelin oligodendrocyte

glycoprotein (MOG): extending the spectrum of MOG antibody positive diseases. Mult Scler 2016;22(14):1821–9.

43. Waters P, Fadda G, Woodhall M, et al. Serial anti-myelin oligodendrocyte glyco-protein antibody analyses and outcomes in children with demyelinating syn-dromes. JAMA Neurol 2020;77(1):82–93.

44. Menge T, Hemmer B, Nessler S, et al. Acute disseminated encephalomyelitis: an update. Arch Neurol 2005;62(11):1673–80.

45. Grzonka P, Scholz MC, De Marchis GM, et al. Acute hemorrhagic leukoencepha-litis: a case and systematic review of the literature. Front Neurol 2020;11:899.

46. Miyazawa I, Fujihara K, Itoyama Y. Eugène Devic (1858-1930). J Neurol 2002; 249(3):351–2.

47. Wingerchuk DM, Lennon VA, Lucchinetti CF, et al. The spectrum of neuromyelitis optica. Lancet Neurol 2007;6(9):805–15.

48. Salama S, Levy M. Bright spotty lesions as an imaging marker for neuromyelitis optica spectrum disorder. Mult Scler 2021;26. 1352458521994259.

49. Pittock SJ, Lennon VA, Krecke K, et al. Brain abnormalities in neuromyelitis op-tica. Arch Neurol 2006;63(3):390–6.

50. Sato DK, Callegaro D, Lana-Peixoto MA, et al. Distinction between MOG antibody-positive and AQP4 antibody-positive NMO spectrum disorders. Neurology 2014;82(6):474–81.

51. Pittock SJ, Lennon VA. Aquaporin-4 autoantibodies in a paraneoplastic context. Arch Neurol 2008;65(5):629–32.

52. Abboud H, Petrak A, Mealy M, et al. Treatment of acute relapses in neuromyelitis optica: steroids alone versus steroids plus plasma exchange. Mult Scler 2016; 22(2):185–92.

53. Reindl M, Waters P. Myelin oligodendrocyte glycoprotein antibodies in neurolog-ical disease. Nat Rev Neurol 2019;15(2):89–102.

54. Jurynczyk M, Messina S, Woodhall MR, et al. Clinical presentation and prognosis in MOG-antibody disease: a UK study. Brain 2017;140(12):3128–38.

55. Chen JJ, Flanagan EP, Jitprapaikulsan J, et al. Myelin oligodendrocyte glycopro-tein antibody-positive optic neuritis: clinical characteristics, radiologic clues, and outcome. Am J Ophthalmol 2018;195:8–15.

56. Dubey D, Pittock SJ, Krecke KN, et al. Clinical, radiologic, and prognostic fea-tures of myelitis associated with myelin oligodendrocyte glycoprotein autoanti-body. JAMA Neurol 2019;76(3):301–9.

57. Banks SA, Morris PP, Chen JJ, et al. Brainstem and cerebellar involvement in MOG-IgG-associated disorder versus aquaporin-4-IgG and MSJournal of Neurology. Neurosurgery & Psychiatry 2021;92:384–90.

58. Hennes EM, Baumann M, Schanda K, et al. Prognostic relevance of MOG anti-bodies in children with an acquired demyelinating syndrome. Neurology 2017; 89(9):900–8.

Approach to Myelopathy and Myelitis

Anne G. Douglas, MD[a], Denise J. Xu, MD[a], Maulik P. Shah, MD, MHS[b],*

KEYWORDS

- Spinal cord ischemia • Autoimmune inflammatory myelitis • Infectious myelitis
- Subacute combined degeneration • Paraneoplastic myelitis

KEY POINTS

- Myelopathy may be structural, vascular, metabolic, toxic, inflammatory, infectious, or neoplastic in etiology.
- MRI and cerebrospinal fluid analysis help distinguish myelopathy from myelitis.

INTRODUCTION

First used to describe spinal cord disorder nearly 150 years ago, the term myelopathy remains a clinical diagnosis with elusive causes.[1] In the late 1800s, pathologists used the term to describe vascular and inflammatory pathologic changes.[2] Studies in the early 1900s explored whether myelitis occurred as a primarily inflammatory, postinfectious process, as with cases related to smallpox and rabies vaccinations, or a directly infectious process, as with measles, mycoplasma, and rubella infections.[3–6] Closer to 1950, the term transverse myelitis was coined to emphasize the sensory level on examination, and the term continues to be used to underscore the bandlike sensory symptoms, rather than the pathologic or radiographic appearance of underlying lesions.[7] Although knowledge has been gained of additional potential causes in the subsequent decades, in recent case series, patients transferred to academic neurologic centers with transverse myelitis were discharged with an idiopathic diagnosis in more than one-quarter of cases.[8]

Myelopathy ranges from an insidious illness to an acute, neurologic emergency with a range of therapeutic options depending on cause from antimicrobials to immunomodulatory treatments. Although increasingly more serologic and cerebrospinal fluid (CSF) assays are available to identify pathogens and antibodies, prolonged turnaround times can lead to significant delays in care with resultant increases in morbidity and mortality. Patterns on imaging may help narrow the differential diagnosis and

[a] Department of Neurology, Perelman School of Medicine, University of Pennsylvania, 3 West Gates Building, 3400 Spruce Street, Philadelphia, PA 19104, USA; [b] Department of Neurology, University of California San Francisco, 505 Parnassus Avenue, Box 0114, San Francisco, CA 94143, USA
* Corresponding author.
E-mail address: maulik.shah@ucsf.edu

Neurol Clin 40 (2022) 133–156
https://doi.org/10.1016/j.ncl.2021.08.009
0733-8619/22/© 2021 Elsevier Inc. All rights reserved.

allow more focused diagnostic evaluation, as well as earlier initiation of empiric therapy. Accordingly, this article highlights pertinent radiologic findings to help neurohospitalists in their approach to myelopathy on the inpatient service (**Table 1**).

COMPRESSIVE MYELOPATHY

In patients presenting with acute myelopathic signs and symptoms, compressive myelopathy should remain at the top of the differential diagnosis, because prompt referral for decompressive procedures may spare patients significant morbidity. From a localization standpoint, evidence may emerge from the history and physical examination that could suggest spinal cord compression, including radicular and vertebral pain, early upper motor neuron signs, or a Brown-Sequard syndrome.[9] From an etiology standpoint, history may reveal clues to suggest trauma or infection, but malignant and neurovascular causes may present more insidiously. More specifically, the differential diagnosis includes trauma, epidural hematoma, epidural abscess, epidural metastases, or intradural neoplasms such as meningioma or neurofibroma. MRI, with contrast administration when there is particular concern for epidural processes, should detect most disorder; but computed tomography (CT) modalities, including myelogram with contrast, can be used to evaluate the spinal canal and extramedullary spaces when MRI is not available or feasible.

Cervical spondylotic arthropathy is the most common cause of myelopathy in adults older than 55 years. Some studies report an incidence of nearly 90% of degenerative skeletal changes in at least 1 level of the cervical spine in adults older than 60 years, with C5 to C6 being the most common level.[10,11] The mechanisms underlying cervical spondylotic myelopathy and associated imaging findings may involve mechanical compression, dynamic forces,[12] and ischemia.[13]

Interestingly, although timely diagnosis may lead to improved outcomes in cervical spondylotic myelopathy, recent studies have found that imaging features may not initially be appreciated as showing external compression, and diagnosis is often delayed because further testing is often pursued. A 2017 analysis of patients with cervical myelopathy showed a correlation between degree of disability and MRI changes ranging from no cord signal abnormality to T2-weighted signal hyperintensity to T1-weighted signal hypointensity, with the last of these being associated with worse recovery potential.[14] Another review of a series of 56 patients in whom spondylotic myelopathy was suspected and spine surgery was performed found that, in many of these patients, presurgical spinal imaging showed longitudinal, spindle-shaped T2 hyperintensity with cord enlargement and a characteristic pancakelike transverse band of gadolinium enhancement (**Fig. 1**). Seventy percent of the patients in this cohort were misdiagnosed initially with neoplastic or inflammatory myelopathy, and surgical decompression was delayed on the order of months to years.[15] Optimal management of cervical spondylotic myelopathy is complex, and studies suggests that both operative and nonoperative treatment plans can be successful, and a multidisciplinary approach factoring in medical comorbidities and surgical risk should be pursued for each individual patient.[16–18]

VASCULAR CAUSES OF MYELOPATHY

Spinal cord ischemia should be considered in patients presenting with acute, progressive weakness; sensory changes; and bowel and bladder dysfunction without evidence of trauma or structural cord compression. Given extensive collateralization of the vascular supply to the spinal cord, ischemia here is much less common than in the brain but can occur in patients with underlying thoracoabdominal aortic disorder.[19]

Table 1
Causes of myelopathy and associated clinical and radiological characteristics

	Disorder/Disease	Key History/Examination Findings	Compartment	Imaging Key Findings	Diagnostic Considerations
Compressive	Cervical spondylotic arthropathy	Neck pain, paresthesias, weakness and spasticity, gait instability, ± bowel/bladder dysfunction, often developing insidiously; examination also with hyperreflexia ± Lhermitte and atrophy of intrinsic hand muscles	Extradural	Longitudinal, spindle-shaped T2 hyperintensity with cord enlargement and a pancakelike transverse band of enhancement[15], T1 hypointensity correlates with myelomalacia and poor recovery[14]	Presence of vertebral spondylosis, congenital canal stenosis, and/or degenerative changes leading to cord compression, commonly at C5–C6[10,11]
Vascular	Infarct	Acute, progressive weakness; sensory changes; and bowel/bladder dysfunction in the setting of aortic proceduralization or cardiopulmonary bypass; examination with leg weakness and a sensory level to pain/temperature with spared vibration/proprioception (if involving the anterior spinal artery)	Intramedullary	Restricted diffusion seen on DWI sequences; anterior predominant, pencillike longitudinally extensive T2 hyperintensity with associated edema and (subacute) enhancement, as well as T2-hyperintense owl's eyes of the anterior horn cells[21]; findings can be subtle, and MRI may appear normal	DWI sequences may be more sensitive for acute spinal cord ischemia

(continued on next page)

Table 1
(continued)

Disorder/Disease	Key History/Examination Findings	Compartment	Imaging Key Findings	Diagnostic Considerations
Dural arteriovenous fistula	Subacute progressive back pain, leg weakness, sensory changes, and bladder dysfunction, typically in a male patient >50 y old	Intramedullary	Central T2-hyperintense signal changes, usually longitudinally extensive and involving the conus; there may be associated flow voids along the surface of the cord[28]	Spinal catheter angiogram can confirm the diagnosis
Cavernous malformation	Discrete episodes of back pain, extremity weakness, and sensory changes with interval recovery (caused by acute hemorrhage from the cavernoma) or progressive accumulation of deficits	Intramedullary	Popcornlike lesions with heterogeneous T1 and T2 signal changes, minimal/no contrast enhancement, and blooming artifact seen on gradient echo sequences; commonly involves the thoracic cord[25]	Can be associated with genetic syndromes and presence of vascular malformations elsewhere in the neural axis
Nutritional/toxic — Vitamin B$_{12}$ deficiency	Progressive gait dysfunction/imbalance, paresthesias, and behavioral/cognitive changes in a patient with recent bariatric surgery or history of malabsorption; examination with hyperreflexia, leg > arm weakness and spasticity, distal vibratory/proprioceptive loss, and sensory ataxia	Intramedullary	T2-hyperintense signal changes of the posterior and/or lateral columns with an inverted V appearance of the posterior funiculus,[32] often involving contiguous segments of the cervical and thoracic cord[31]	Low serum cobalamin and/or increased plasma homocysteine and methylmalonic acid levels; EMG/NCS with evidence of length-dependent axonal neuropathy; may have associated megaloblastic anemia with hypersegmented neutrophils
Nitrous oxide toxicity	Identical to vitamin B$_{12}$ deficiency; patients may have a history of recreational use (whippets) or recent procedures necessitating anesthesia	Intramedullary	Identical to vitamin B$_{12}$ deficiency	Increased plasma homocysteine and methylmalonic acid levels

Copper deficiency	Intramedullary	Similar to vitamin B$_{12}$ deficiency clinically; history of bariatric surgery or excess use of zinc-containing products	T2-hyperintense signal changes of the posterior columns ± involvement of the lateral columns, commonly in the cervical cord, without enhancement[36]	Low serum copper and ceruloplasmin levels (with increased serum zinc levels in the setting of zinc toxicity); EMG/NCS with evidence of length-dependent axonal neuropathy
Vitamin E deficiency	Intramedullary	Spinocerebellar syndrome and visual difficulties; examination with depressed or absent reflexes, vibratory/proprioceptive loss, sensory and cerebellar ataxia, and +Babinski sign	Cerebellar atrophy ± T2-hyperintense signal changes of the posterior columns[37,38]	Low plasma α-tocopherol level; eye examination with pigmentary retinopathy; genetic testing may reveal abetalipoproteinemia or mutations of α-tocopherol transfer protein; may have associated anemia
Autoimmune/inflammatory Multiple sclerosis	Intramedullary	Incomplete/asymmetric hemiparesis with sensory deficits and bowel/bladder involvement (in the setting of relapsing-remitting events or progressive accumulation of disability)	Multiple short-segment, asymmetric, eccentric T2-hyperintense lesions with associated enhancement in the setting of active demyelination; longer segments may be caused by the confluence of multiple small cord lesions[39]	Dissemination of lesions in space and time as per the 2017 revised McDonald criteria; CSF often reveals unique oligoclonal bands and an increased IgG index caused by intrathecal protein synthesis
NMOSD	Intramedullary	Symmetric and severe paraparesis or quadriparesis with bowel/bladder dysfunction and a sensory level (in the setting of relapsing events, often including bilateral optic neuritis, with variable recovery and rapid accumulation of deficits)	Longitudinally extensive T2-hyperintense lesions spanning >3 vertebral segments, typically involving the central cord with diffuse enhancement and cord edema[40,41]	Positive serum or CSF AQP4-IgG antibody (best detected via cell-based assay), although patients can have seronegative NMOSD; CSF may show a pleocytosis with increased protein but absent oligoclonal bands

(continued on next page)

Table 1
(continued)

Disorder/Disease	Key History/Examination Findings	Compartment	Imaging — Key Findings	Diagnostic Considerations
MOG-associated myelitis	Similar clinical presentation of myelitis as NMOSD, although typically with a monophasic course (may be associated with bilateral optic neuritis and acute disseminated encephalomyelitis)	Intramedullary	Longitudinally extensive T2-hyperintense lesions spanning >3 vertebral segments with patchy or lack of enhancement; may present with multiple cord lesions and involvement of the conus medullaris; may exclusively involve the gray matter in an H pattern[40,41]	Positive serum or CSF MOG-IgG antibody (best detected via cell-based assay)
Neurosarcoidosis	Can be the first presentation of systemic sarcoidosis, manifesting with headache, cranial neuropathies, radicular pain, and focal deficits from intracranial lesions, in addition to weakness, sensory loss, and bowel/bladder dysfunction sustained from transverse myelitis	Intramedullary and leptomeningeal	Central canal and dorsal-subpial enhancement (trident sign)[42], may present variably with longitudinally extensive > short-segment or anteriorly isolated T2-hyperintense lesions[43]	May see evidence of multifocal spinal and/or intracranial leptomeningeal enhancement, mediastinal/hilar adenopathy, and bony lesions; biopsy with noncaseating granulomas; CSF may show pleocytosis, increased protein level, and hypoglycorrhachia
Paraneoplastic	Depending on involved tracts, patients may have rapidly progressive weakness and spasticity, sensory loss and sensory ataxia, and/or bowel/bladder dysfunction in the setting of known or occult malignancy (often small cell lung cancer) or exposure to immunotherapy	Intramedullary	Longitudinally extensive, symmetric T2-hyperintense tract-specific lesions with contrast enhancement[75,76]	Detection of systemic malignancy or known prior treatment with immunotherapy with positive paraneoplastic antibodies (eg. anti-CRMP5, anti-Hu, antiamphiphysin antibodies); CSF may show evidence of inflammation with negative cytology

Infectious				
Herpesviruses (eg, HSV-1/2, VZV, CMV)	Depending on the spinal compartment involved, may present with acute to subacute progression of asymmetric weakness, sensory changes, and/or radicular pain, often in immunocompromised patients	Variably intramedullary and/or leptomeningeal	Variable, but includes expansile T2hyperintense signal of cord parenchyma (which can be longitudinally extensive), cord and multifocal nerve root enhancement (including of the cauda equina)	CSF with lymphocytic pleocytosis, presence of viral DNA via PCR, and/or positive CSF viral serologies
Retroviruses (eg, HIV, HTLV-1)	Can cause a chronic symmetric spastic paraparesis with weakness, vibratory and proprioceptive loss, hyperreflexia, and bowel/bladder dysfunction	Intramedullary	Initial intrinsic T2 hyperintensities involving the posterolateral columns, with progression over time to cord atrophy, most frequently involving the thoracic cord[51]	HTLV-1: serum or CSF with HTLV-1 viral DNA or positive serologies HIV vacuolar myelopathy: more likely than HTLV-1 to have associated cognitive dysfunction
Flaviviruses (eg, WNV), pcliovirus, and enteroviruses (eg, D68 and 71)	Typically presents as acute flaccid myelitis with asymmetric flaccid weakness and depressed reflexes without sensory changes; often accompanied by respiratory dysfunction	Typically intramedullary	T2 hyperintensities of the anterior horns, which can correlate with severity of clinical disease ± nerve root enhancement	CSF with pleocytosis (may initially be neutrophilic predominant with a subsequent shift to lymphocytes) and presence of serum or CSF serologies, which can be negative in the first weeks after onset of neurologic symptoms

(continued on next page)

Table 1
(continued)

Disorder/Disease		Key History/Examination Findings	Compartment	Imaging Key Findings	Diagnostic Considerations
Neoplastic	Ependymoma	Back or radicular pain and sensory dysesthesias that can slowly progress over time to weakness, gait instability, and bowel/bladder dysfunction	Intramedullary	Centrally located, well-defined, expansile lesions that are T1 hypointense, T2 hyperintense, and strongly enhance; can have associated cystic change and cap sign (caused by hemorrhage)[58-60]	Compared with astrocytomas, ependymomas are more common in adults
	Astrocytoma	Localized pain and slowly progressive sensory dysesthesias and weakness, which may be consistent with a Brown-Séquard syndrome	Intramedullary	Eccentrically located (but can come to involve the entire cord), ill-defined lesions that are T1 hypointense, T2 hyperintense, and have variable and patchy enhancement[60,61]	Compared with ependymomas, astrocytomas are more common in children
	Meningioma	Back or radicular pain with slow accumulation of other neurologic deficits, including sensory changes, weakness, and gait instability	Intradural extramedullary	T1 hypointense or isointense with strong and homogeneous enhancement; associated dural tail[62,63]	Schwannomas may have dumbbell morphology and a cystic or hemorrhagic component, whereas neurofibromas classically are peripherally T2 hyperintense and centrally T2 hypointense[60], associated with neurofibromatosis
	Metastasis	Most commonly in the setting of metastatic lung, breast, prostate, thyroid, and renal malignancies[9], patients can present with back pain and vertebral compression fractures	Typically extradural but can involve any spinal compartment	Multifocal extradural vertebral masses that are T1 hypointense with variable T2 signal, may have a rim of bright signal (halo sign),[64] and can cause mass effect with local cord signal abnormality; intramedullary cord metastases can have rim of enhancement	Evidence of primary malignancy and/or other metastatic lesions; spinal metastases may be FDG avid on PET/CT

Methotrexate toxicity	Recent exposure to methotrexate, in particular, via intrathecal administration	Intramedullary	Bilateral T2 hyperintensities of the posterior and lateral columns[71]	Known exposure to methotrexate
Radiation induced	Exposure to radiation in proximity to the cord lesion; can manifest acutely (within the first year after therapy) or more commonly, in a delayed, chronic, progressive pattern	Intramedullary	Longitudinally extensive T2-hyperintense lesions that over time progress to cord atrophy/myelomalacia; associated T1-hyperintense vertebral marrow changes[67–69]	Ancillary testing (eg, PET/CT and methionine accumulation) can help distinguish radiation-induced myelopathy from neoplastic disease progression

Abbreviations: AQP4, aquaporin-4; CMV, cytomegalovirus; CRMP5, collapsing response mediator protein-5; CT, computed tomography; DWI, diffusion-weighted imaging; EMG/NCS, electromyogram and nerve conduction studies; FDG fluorodeoxyglucose; HIV, human immunodeficiency virus; HSV, herpes simplex virus; HTLV, human T-cell lymphotropic virus; IgG, immunoglobulin G; MOG, myelin oligodendrocyte glycoprotein; NMOSD, neuromyelitis optica spectrum disorder; PCR, polymerase chain reaction; VZV, varicella-zoster virus; WNV, West Nile virus.

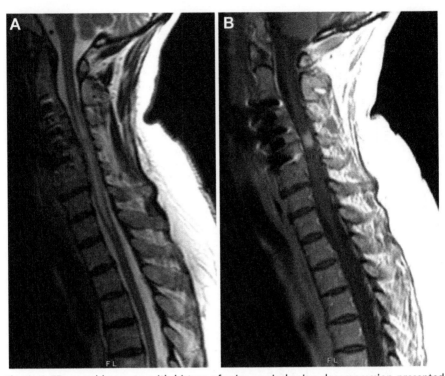

Fig. 1. A 75-year-old woman with history of prior cervical spine decompression presented with progressive neck pain, asymmetric hand tingling, and neuropathic pain, followed by urinary incontinence and gait difficulty. Sagittal T2-weighted MRI (*A*) showed longitudinally extensive hyperintense signal and T1 postgadolinium contrast imaging (*B*) showed a short area of pancakelike contrast enhancement in an area of arthritic changes and compression. She was diagnosed with cervical spondylotic compressive myelopathy and underwent recurrent decompression.

Embolism or hypoperfusion may lead to spinal cord ischemia during aortic surgeries or cardiopulmonary bypass. If spinal cord ischemia is suspected outside of these clinical contexts, work-up should include evaluation for cardioembolic sources, aortic or vertebral dissection, systemic vasculitis (including infectious causes such as varicella-zoster virus [VZV] and syphilis), hypercoagulable states, and fibrocartilaginous embolism related to adjacent vertebral body disease or antecedent trauma.

The anterior spinal artery and the lower thoracic cord are involved most frequently.[20] Patients typically present with lower extremity weakness caused by ischemia in the corticospinal tracts. Initially, there may be flaccid tone and absent deep tendon reflexes of the limbs, and weakness may be asymmetric. Later, upper motor neuron signs usually develop. Patients report abnormal pain and temperature sensation, often with a thoracic sensory level, caused by injury of the spinothalamic tracts. Proprioception and vibratory sense are typically spared, because the dorsal column pathways are supplied by the posterior spinal arteries.

In the first few hours to days following spinal cord ischemia, MRI may be normal. Diffusion-weighted imaging may show evidence of ischemic changes before development of clear abnormalities on other sequences, but sensitivity is limited because of the small size of the spinal cord. After several days, imaging may show anterior-predominant, pencillike, longitudinally extensive cord signal change with edema on

T2 sequences; subacute contrast enhancement on T1 postgadolinium sequences; and so-called owl's eyes pattern of T2 hyperintensity within the anterior horn cells on axial imaging.[21] Adjacent disc bulge and disease may suggest fibrocartilaginous embolism as the cause in appropriate clinical situations.[22] In some patients, there is evidence of secondary enhancement of adjacent ventral nerve roots.[23] Myelomalacia develops over time.

Acute management involves early blood pressure augmentation and consideration of spinal fluid drainage to reduce CSF counterpressure and promote spinal cord perfusion, with gradual weaning of these therapies depending on clinical response and improvement. As with patients with myelopathy of other causes, prevention of associated medical problems, including venous clots, infections, and pressure ulcers, is important to prevent further morbidity.[19]

In contrast with the subtle initial imaging abnormalities associated with acute ischemia, the presence of flow voids and mixed T1 and T2 cord signal abnormalities on MRI suggests hemorrhage and should prompt catheter spinal angiography to confirm arteriovenous malformation (AVM).[24] Heterogenous, well-demarcated, popcornlike lesions on MRI suggest cavernous malformations, which are occult on catheter angiography and may be associated with genetic syndromes.[25]

However, the most common vascular malformation involving the spine often presents subacutely. Spinal dural arteriovenous (AV) fistulas are thought to be acquired disorders, perhaps caused by remote local trauma or hypercoagulable state. An abnormal direct connection between the dural branch of a radicular artery and a radicular vein leads to venous hypertension, congestion, and subsequent spinal cord dysfunction.[26] The typical presentation involves a male patient more than 50 years of age with progressive back pain, leg weakness, and sensory changes, and urinary dysfunction caused by involvement of the lower thoracic cord and conus.[27] In 1 case series, all patients had either central cord T2 cord signal change, usually involving the conus and spanning more than 3 vertebral segments, or flow voids seen along dorsal or ventral aspect of the spinal cord, indicating dilated veins[28] (**Fig. 2**). Despite abnormal MRI, diagnosis is often delayed, on average greater than 18 months after first symptom onset.[27] After MRI, catheter spinal angiography should be pursued to confirm diagnosis and guide therapeutic decisions, specifically consideration of endovascular chemoembolization or open surgical resection. Most patients who are successfully treated experience clinical stabilization or improvement, highlighting the importance of recognition of this cause of progressive myelopathy.[27,28]

METABOLIC, NUTRITIONAL, AND TOXIC MYELOPATHY

Noncompressive, subacute progressive myelopathies can be noninflammatory or inflammatory. Of noninflammatory causes, metabolic/nutritional disorders and toxic exposures can lead to spinal cord disorder with characteristic clinical and radiographic findings. Identifying nutritional causes of myelopathy is crucial, because treatment is readily available, and prompt management can prevent further neurologic impairment.

Subacute combined degeneration (SCD) refers to the pattern of myelopathy seen in vitamin B_{12} deficiency, wherein the lateral and posterior columns of the spinal cord are preferentially damaged (**Fig. 3**). Vitamin B_{12} is an essential cofactor in methylation reactions necessary for DNA and myelin synthesis; deficiency causes swelling and breakdown of myelin sheaths and, eventually, gliosis and axonal degeneration.[29] SCD presents as a slowly progressive spastic paraparesis with hyperreflexia caused by corticospinal tract dysfunction, as well as distal vibratory and proprioceptive sensory loss caused by dorsal column involvement. Affected individuals develop gait

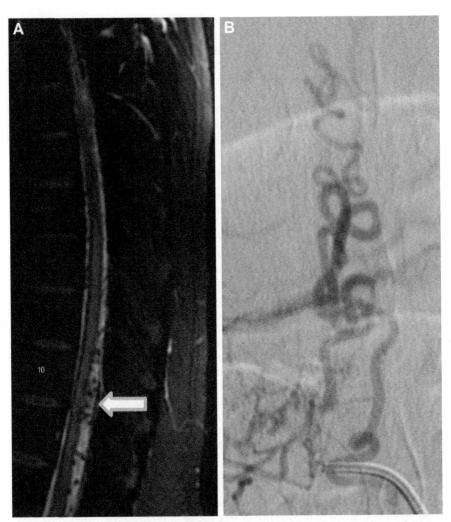

Fig. 2. A 31-year-old man presented with acute onset of paraparesis, numbness with T8 sensory level, and urinary retention. Sagittal T2-weighted MRI (*A*) showed diffuse longitudinally extensive cord signal change spanning from midthoracic spine to conus as well as prominent dark flow voids along surface of cord (*white arrow*). Subsequent spinal catheter angiogram (*B*) revealed dural arteriovenous fistula at the T10 level, which was treated with endovascular chemoembolization.

abnormality from sensory ataxia. Vitamin B_{12} deficiency can also cause concomitant peripheral axonal polyneuropathy, and thus patients may report distal symmetric paresthesias. Other associated neurologic deficits include autonomic dysfunction, optic atrophy, and behavioral and cognitive changes, which help distinguish this cause from structural causes of myelopathy.[30] Patients can also develop a megaloblastic anemia with increased mean corpuscular volumes and hypersegmented neutrophils.

Diagnosis is made with a low serum cobalamin level or increased plasma homocysteine and methylmalonic acid levels. Neuroimaging in B_{12} deficiency can be characteristic, demonstrating T2 hyperintensities in the posterior and/or lateral columns, often in

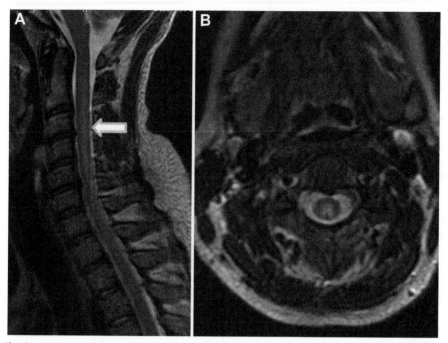

Fig. 3. A 47-year-old woman who had undergone gastric bypass surgery 5 years prior presented with progressive numbness of her arms and legs and difficulty balancing. Sagittal (*A*) and axial (*B*) T2-weighted MRI of the cervical spinal cord showed hyperintense signal of the dorsal columns in an inverted V appearance, extending contiguously from C2 to C7 (*white arrow*), consistent with subacute combined degeneration caused by vitamin B$_{12}$ deficiency.

contiguous segments of the cervical and thoracic spinal cord.[31] Because of involvement of the posterior funiculus, these MRI abnormalities have been described as having an inverted V or inverted rabbit ears appearance.[32]

Causes of vitamin B$_{12}$ deficiency include chronically low intake, inherited malabsorption syndromes such as pernicious anemia, autoimmune gastritis,[33] and inflammatory bowel disease, and acquired malabsorption secondary to gastric or small bowel surgery. Nitrous oxide (N$_2$O) toxicity–induced SCD resembles B$_{12}$ deficiency both clinically and radiographically. N$_2$O is a dissociative anesthetic commonly used in dental and surgical procedures and can also be inhaled recreationally (colloquially referred to as whippets). N$_2$O oxidizes methylcobalamin into an inactivated form of B$_{12}$, causing a functional vitamin B$_{12}$ deficiency and leading to loss of myelin cohesion and spinal cord vacuolization.[30] As with B$_{12}$ deficiency–associated SCD, imaging in N$_2$O toxicity shows posterior and lateral column T2-hyperintense lesions that are often longitudinally extensive.[34] Treatment of B$_{12}$ deficiency and N$_2$O exposure involves high-dose B$_{12}$ supplementation, although, in the case of the latter, repletion is ineffective without concomitant abstinence from further N$_2$O exposure.

Copper deficiency and zinc excess are also implicated in nutritional myelopathies. Copper is a trace metal essential for mitochondrial metabolism and nervous system functioning.[35] Myelopathy caused by copper deficiency is virtually indistinguishable from the subacute combined degeneration seen with vitamin B$_{12}$ deficiency. Copper absorption occurs primarily in the stomach and duodenum; deficiency can result from low intake, malabsorption following bariatric surgery, and zinc toxicity. Zinc upregulates the expression of a chelator, metallothionein, which has higher binding affinity for copper than for zinc. Copper bound to metallothionein remains in enterocytes and is ultimately eliminated, leading to decreased copper absorption with risk of hypocupremia. Excess consumption of over-the-counter supplements or denture pastes that contain zinc can thus lead to toxicity.[29,30]

Diagnostic work-up for copper deficiency reveals low serum copper and ceruloplasmin levels. Although MRI can be normal, radiographic abnormalities associated with copper deficiency include increased T2 signal of the posterior columns, most commonly in the cervical cord. Lateral segments may also be involved, and contrast enhancement is usually not seen.[36] These changes resemble those seen in B_{12} deficiency–associated SCD. Treatment of copper deficiency involves oral copper gluconate supplementation.

Vitamin E deficiency can cause a range of neurologic deficits, including spinocerebellar syndromes, peripheral neuropathy, and retinopathy. Vitamin E is absorbed in the gastrointestinal tract, binds the alpha-tocopherol transfer protein (ATTP), and is ultimately incorporated into lipoproteins. As a result, low serum levels may result from malabsorption, genetic defects of ATTP, and abetalipoproteinemia.[30] MRI findings include T2-hyperintense signal changes of the posterior columns and cerebellar atrophy.[37,38]

INFLAMMATORY MYELITIS

Inflammatory myelitis occurs at a rate of 1 to 8 cases per million per year.[39] Intramedullary or leptomeningeal contrast enhancement on MRI and increased levels of CSF inflammatory markers, including presence of pleocytosis, unique oligoclonal bands, or increased immunoglobulin (Ig) G index, are nonspecific but suggest inflammatory causes of myelitis. Transverse myelitis has a broad differential diagnosis, including autoimmune, infiltrative, and infectious causes. Basic CSF studies are unlikely to discriminate between causes, and newer laboratory studies can test for many antibodies and pathogens but the results take many weeks. Although clinical practice has not changed drastically in terms of acute treatment of noninfectious causes of myelitis in the last decade, with corticosteroids as the gold standard empiric therapy, followed by plasmapheresis and possibly longer-acting immunomodulating therapies such as rituximab for refractory cases, identifying patterns on imaging may narrow the differential diagnosis, focus further diagnostic evaluation, and allow earlier initiation of empiric therapy.

Evaluation of the longitudinal extent of myelitis on sagittal plane imaging and horizontal extent, including tract-specific involvement on axial imaging, can help distinguish between common causes of autoimmune myelitis. In multiple sclerosis, spinal cord lesions tend to span less than 2 vertebral segments, often involve the periphery of the spinal cord, and are often asymmetric, involving the dorsal and lateral columns. Acute flares enhance on postgadolinium contrast imaging, but multifocal nonenhancing lesions are often seen, suggesting prior disease. In terms of clinically isolated syndromes, acute partial transverse myelitis is associated with a higher risk of recurrent disease compared with acute complete transverse myelitis.[39]

Longitudinally extensive T2-hyperintense lesions spanning greater than 3 vertebral segments are more commonly seen in neuromyelitis optica (NMO) spectrum disorder (often associated with aquaporin-4-antibody) and myelin oligodendrocyte glycoprotein (MOG) IgG antibody–associated myelitis. In NMO, the central cord is usually involved, along with both gray and white matter structures, and acute disease is usually associated with diffuse postgadolinium contrast enhancement and cord edema. Multiple spinal cord lesions are more commonly seen with MOG-IgG myelitis, and conus involvement is more common than in multiple sclerosis or NMO. Acute lesions may not enhance on imaging despite presence of CSF pleocytosis, and, in 1 retrospective analysis, 30% of patients had exclusive gray matter involvement on axial imaging, showing an H pattern on T2 sequences.[40,41]

A recent case series suggests that the presence of central canal enhancement associated with dorsal-subpial enhancement, which has been dubbed the trident sign for its appearance on axial imaging, suggests spinal sarcoidosis[42] (**Fig. 4**). Another retrospective analysis also underscores the frequency of dorsal subpial enhancement in patients with sarcoidosis-associated myelitis, as well as an increased prevalence of sarcoidosis disease involvement and enhancement at locations of spondylosis, making it at times challenging to distinguish from compressive causes. This analysis identified 4 patterns of morphology on spine MRI for patients with sarcoidosis-associated myelopathy: longitudinally extensive myelitis, short tumefactive myelitis, spinal meningitis, and anterior myelitis associated with degenerative disc disease, further highlighting sarcoidosis as one of the great masqueraders of medicine, and the importance of having a high index of suspicion and initiation of more systemic diagnostic evaluation to look for extraneural disease involvement.[43]

Myelitis associated with systemic lupus erythematosus is often longitudinally extensive on imaging and there may be overlap with other autoimmune syndromes, including NMO. Recent studies have described 2 distinct subtypes: gray and white matter myelitis. Gray matter myelitis presents more acutely, often with flaccid severe weakness; is associated with a CSF profile that may initially suggest infectious causes, including marked neutrophilic predominant pleocytosis and hypoglycorrhachia; and carries a poor prognosis even with early initiation of immunomodulatory therapy

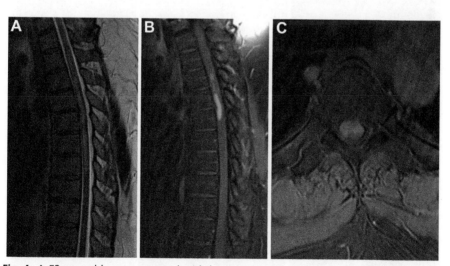

Fig. 4. A 53-year-old man presented with lower extremity numbness, weakness, falls, and urinary incontinence. Sagittal T2-weighted MRI (*A*) showed hyperintense cord signal abnormality spanning from T1 to T8 with an epicenter at T4 to T5 interdisc space with slight cord expansion at this level. Sagittal (*B*) and axial (*C*) T1 postgadolinium contrast imaging showed intramedullary enhancement predominantly involving the anterior two-thirds of the cord at T4 to T5. Hilar lymph node biopsy showed fragmented lymphoid tissue with a few nonnecrotizing granulomas, consistent with diagnosis of sarcoidosis.

such as cyclophosphamide. White matter myelitis tends to present more subacutely with lesser degree of CSF inflammation and has better prognosis, although recovery is often incomplete.[44]

INFECTIOUS MYELITIS

Accurate diagnosis of infection as the cause of myelopathy can crucially guide testing and empiric treatment. Neuroimaging can help narrow the differential, because certain pathogens have tropism for the cord parenchyma, nerve roots, tracts, gray and/or white matter, and adjacent structures. Although several infections, including neurocysticercosis, schistosomiasis, aspergillosis, tuberculosis, and pyogenic epidural abscess, typically present with abnormal radiographic findings, unremarkable imaging does not rule out infection, especially when considering viral causes, such as herpes simplex virus (HSV), Epstein-Barr virus (EBV), VZV, human T-lymphotropic virus 1 (HTLV-1), and West Nile virus (WNV).[45]

When abnormalities are present on MRI, any of several patterns may manifest. Intramedullary, central T2 signal hyperintensity with variable transverse and longitudinal cord involvement can be seen in EBV, Lyme, and hepatitis C virus–associated myelitis. Pathogens that cause acute flaccid myelitis, including Enterovirus-71 and D68, WNV, and poliomyelitis, may show pronounced signal abnormality in the anterior horns. A primary extramedullary pattern with enhancement of the meninges, extra-axial spaces, and spinal nerve roots can be seen in a variety of infectious and noninfectious disorders. Smooth and linear enhancement of the surface of the spinal cord and cauda equina is more suggestive of viral causes such as HSV, Zika, WNV, and cytomegalovirus (CMV) (**Fig. 5**). A cystic appearance may suggest neurocysticercosis or

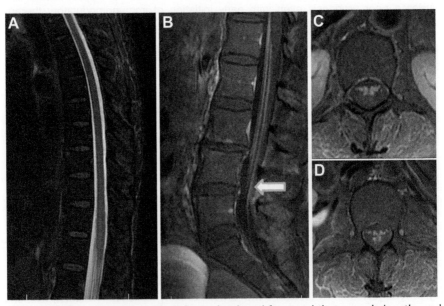

Fig. 5. A 46-year-old woman with diabetes developed fever and then encephalopathy and asymmetric flaccid weakness in her legs with urinary retention. Sagittal T2-weighted MRI (*A*) was normal but sagittal T1-weighted postgadolinium imaging (*B*) revealed smooth, linear enhancement of lumbosacral nerve roots (*white arrow*). Axial postcontrast imaging (*C*) and (*D*) showed ventral-predominant nerve root enlargement and enhancement. CSF analysis revealed lymphocytic pleocytosis, and West Nile virus serologies were positive.

coccidioidomycosis, whereas nodular or nonuniform enhancement can indicate infiltrative processes such as metastatic disease.[46] Indolent tract-specific myelitis (manifesting both radiographically and clinically) can occur with human immunodeficiency virus (HIV) vacuolar myelopathy, which affects the dorsal and lateral columns, often with associated cord atrophy but without contrast enhancement; tabes dorsalis caused by neurosyphilis; and rare presentations of progressive multifocal leukoencephalopathy, which can involve the fasciculus gracilis.[47,48]

Pathogens within the herpesvirus family of DNA viruses can affect the spinal cord in myriad ways and often with multifocal involvement. VZV remains latent in neurons of cranial nerves, dorsal roots, and autonomic ganglia and can reactivate in the setting of reduced cell-mediated immunity, whether caused by increasing age and immunosenescence, exposure to immunosuppressant therapy, or acquired immunodeficiency syndrome. With reactivation, the virus can cause isolated myelitis, radiculomyelitis, and spinal cord infarction, with or without antecedent dermatologic manifestations.[49] MRI may reveal multiple findings depending on the spinal compartment involved, including enhancement of the spinal nerve roots and cauda equina and longitudinally extensive expansile intramedullary T2-hyperintense lesions, which may be diffuse or ipsilateral to the affected dermatome.[45,50,51] CMV infection can also cause polyradiculitis, myeloradiculitis, and isolated myelitis in immunocompromised individuals, particularly those with a cluster of differentiation (CD) 4 count of less than 100 cells/μL or who have undergone hematopoietic stem cell or solid organ transplant. Imaging may reveal enhancement of the leptomeninges and nerve roots, including the cauda equina.[52,53] HSV-2 is another important pathogen implicated in spinal cord disorder for both immunocompetent and immunosuppressed individuals. Clinical presentations may vary, with the ascending necrotizing subtype being most aggressive.[54] MRI in HSV-2–associated myeloradiculitis can show hyperintensity in the cord parenchyma on T2-weighted images with enhancement of the meninges and nerve roots, including the cauda equina.[54] Lumbosacral radicular fibers and the cord itself may appear edematous.[55,56] Diagnosis of herpesvirus infections is made via CSF detection of serologies, especially for VZV, or presence of viral DNA via polymerase chain reaction testing. Empiric antiviral therapy should be considered in high-risk patients with suggestive clinical and imaging syndromes.

NEOPLASTIC MYELOPATHY

Recognition of neoplastic myelopathies is paramount, because accurate diagnosis helps guide decisions around intervention and management. The history often suggests progressive spinal cord dysfunction, although more acute presentations can occur, especially if the neoplasm is prone to hemorrhage. Determining via MRI which spinal cord compartment (namely, the intramedullary, intradural extramedullary, and extradural spaces) is involved can help narrow the differential.[9]

Of the primary intramedullary tumors, ependymomas and astrocytomas occur most commonly in adults. Spinal ependymomas are thought to arise from ependymal cells lining the central canal and thus are centrally located.[57] These slow-growing tumors first cause sensory symptoms related to compression of the anterior commissure; over time and with enlargement, they may result in motor deficits.[58] Radiographically, they classically are described as T1-hypointense and T2-hyperintense lesions that enhance strongly and homogeneously with gadolinium; however, they can include areas of cystic change or hemorrhage that lead to heterogeneous signal.[58,59] Because of the propensity to bleed, these neoplasms have also been shown to have a cap sign: a rim of extreme T1 and T2 hypointensity at the margins caused by hemosiderin content.[58,60] As with other intramedullary tumors, local cord expansion is a key finding. Ependymomas usually present with a plane between the tumor and normal cord tissue, so total resection is feasible.

In contrast, astrocytomas arise from astrocytic glial cells in the cord parenchyma and thus tend to be eccentrically located. Over time, these tumors can come to involve the entire cord and then appear more central on axial images.[61] Because of their lateral tendency, they may present with local pain or an insidiously progressive Brown-Séquard syndrome.[9] These tumors are also T1 hypointense and T2 hyperintense on MRI. However, compared with ependymomas, low-grade astrocytomas variably enhance, and, when there is enhancement, it is usually nodular or ill-defined[60,61] (Fig. 6). Despite their less aggressive nature, low-grade astrocytomas have a propensity to infiltrate, making effective resection challenging.

Intradural, extramedullary malignancies, including meningiomas and nerve sheath tumors, exist in the subarachnoid space. Meningiomas, thought to arise from meningothelial cells of the arachnoid mater, are the most common primary spinal cord

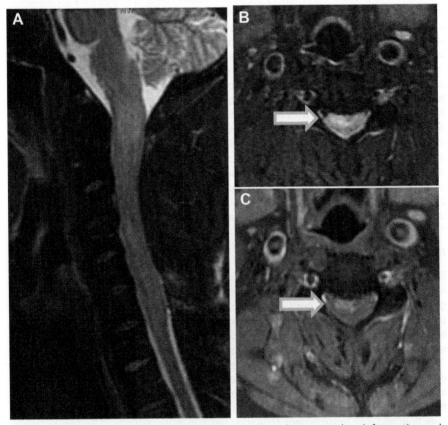

Fig. 6. A 27-year-old man with progressive asymmetric right greater than left spastic quadriparesis. Sagittal T2-weighted MRI (A) showed cord expansion from cervicomedullary junction to lower cervical spine with subtle areas of hyperintensity. Axial T2-weighted imaging (B) showed eccentric right-sided anterior cord signal change and axial T1-weighted postgadolinium imaging (C) showed focal enhancement at C2 level (white arrows). Biopsy revealed infiltrative grade II spine astrocytoma.

neoplasm in adults. Patients usually become symptomatic because of compression of the spinal cord. MRI shows lesions that are isointense or hypointense on T1-weighted sequences with robust, homogeneous enhancement after contrast administration.[62] About 60% to 70% of meningiomas have a dural tail on postcontrast scans, referring to an enhancing margin of reactive fibrovascular tissue.[46,63] Surgery—with the goal of complete resection—can be curative.

Of all spinal cord neoplasms, extradural masses are most common and typically represent bony metastatic disease from systemic malignancy. Extradural metastases are most likely to originate from lung, breast, prostate, thyroid, and renal cancers.[9] Metastatic lesions are typically T1 hypointense and may feature a rim of high T2 signal intensity, called a halo sign; this can be difficult to appreciate when the metastasis is itself diffusely T2 hyperintense.[64] High-dose corticosteroids are often initiated to acutely decrease edema, whereas surgical treatment, including cord decompression and tumor debulking, should be considered when clinically appropriate. Recent advances have led to the development of stereotactic body radiotherapy, which delivers precise, high-dose radiation for pain control and local reduction of tumor burden.[65]

Disease-directed neoplastic therapy can also cause spinal cord disorder. Radiation-induced myelopathy is a dose-dependent consequence of injury to myelinated white matter tracts and blood vessels.[66] Subtypes include acute transient radiation myelopathy, which occurs within the first year after irradiation, and the more common chronic progressive radiation myelopathy, which manifests, on average, 9 to 18 months after completion of radiation therapy, although there can be a latency period of several years.[66,67] Although MRI can be normal, characteristic radiographic abnormalities include a longitudinally extensive T2-hyperintense intramedullary lesion and associated T1-hyperintense vertebral marrow changes in the field of prior radiation.[67,68] Both tract-specific and patchy involvement, including of the central cord, have been described.[60,67] There may be initial evidence of cord edema or expansion and focal enhancement that subsequently resolves over serial scans, and later cord atrophy and myelomalacia may develop.[69]

Intrathecal and systemic oncologic treatment can also cause myelopathy. Methotrexate, a commonly used chemotherapeutic agent that disrupts the folic acid pathway and inhibits DNA synthesis, can cause severe neurotoxicity. Onset of symptoms ranges from acute to subacute to chronic; myelopathy, a rare complication, tends to present over hours to days, especially following intrathecal methotrexate administration.[70] MRI resembles subacute combined degeneration, with bilateral T2 hyperintensities of the posterior and lateral columns, suggesting a shared pathophysiology with vitamin B_{12} deficiency.[71] An intact folic acid pathway is necessary for metabolism of cobalamin, which is used in the synthesis of methionine, a cofactor crucial to maintenance of myelin sheaths, and histopathologic findings of methotrexate myelopathy have shown demyelination of the posterior columns.[71]

In the setting of known metastatic disease and/or exposure to immune checkpoint inhibitors, paraneoplastic autoimmune myelopathy should additionally be a consideration, although symptoms of these syndromes often begin before detection of occult malignancy. As such, diagnosis of a paraneoplastic phenomenon warrants a thorough and expeditious cancer screen. Paraneoplastic disorders result when innate immunologic mechanisms are directed at antigens in tumor cells that are also present in cells of the nervous system.[72] Anti-CRMP5, anti-Hu, and anti-amphiphysin antibodies are most commonly associated with paraneoplastic myelopathy[73,74] (**Fig. 7**). Hallmark radiographic findings of paraneoplastic myelopathy include a longitudinally extensive, symmetric, T2-hyperintense tractopathy that enhances with contrast.[75] There can be disorder involving the lateral columns, dorsal columns, and gray matter,[76] but it is

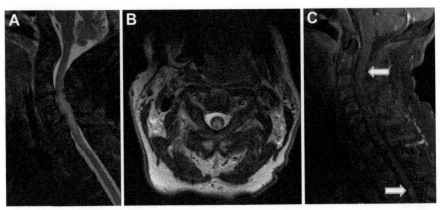

Fig. 7. A 57-year-old man with small cell lung cancer presented with profound ataxia and proprioceptive sensory loss following initiation of checkpoint inhibitor immunotherapy. Sagittal (*A*) and axial (*B*) T2-weighted MRI showed cord edema and hyperintense lesions involving the posterior columns, and sagittal T1-weighted postgadolinium contrast MRI (*C*) showed multifocal areas of hazy enhancement within the posterior cord (*white arrows*). Imaging was consistent with longitudinally extensive symmetric tractopathy, and CSF testing revealed CRMP5 IgG antibodies.

important to recognize that MRI can also be normal.[77] As such, in the setting of tract-specific disorder, CSF analysis showing increased levels of inflammatory markers may suggest a paraneoplastic cause rather than a nutritional deficiency, which may have similar imaging findings.

SUMMARY

Myelopathy encompasses a range of conditions from compression requiring acute surgical intervention to inflammatory processes at the crossroads of neurology, oncology, and infectious diseases. Although clinical suspicion remains critical to identify myelopathy, MRI can narrow the differential diagnosis and guide empiric therapy. Future work is needed to further identify imaging patterns and other novel diagnostic tools to expedite work-up and treatment to minimize morbidity and mortality moving forward.

CLINICS CARE POINTS

- Myelopathy has a broad differential diagnosis, and neurohospitalists must use historical clues and the neurologic examination, MRI, and CSF analysis to distinguish between noninflammatory (including compressive, vascular, neoplastic, metabolic, and toxic) and inflammatory (including infectious and autoimmune) causes.

- Spondylotic cervical myelopathy is a common cause of progressive myelopathy in patients more than 60 years of age and imaging may show focal enhancement, which may initially be interpreted as suggesting inflammatory myelitis.

- Vascular causes of myelopathy include spinal cord ischemia, which typically involves the anterior spinal artery and is most commonly associated with abdominal aortic disorder or procedures.

- Vitamin B$_{12}$ deficiency, copper deficiency, and nitrous oxide toxicity can lead to dorsal column and corticospinal tract dysfunction and subacute progressive myelopathy.

- Patterns of imaging, including the extent of T2 MRI abnormality on sagittal imaging and axial imaging characteristics, can help distinguish between common causes of autoimmune myelitis, including multiple sclerosis, neuromyelitis optica, and MOG IgG antibody–associated myelitis.
- Spinal neoplasms are uncommon, but the compartment of involvement within the spinal canal can help with differential diagnosis. Neurohospitalists should also be aware of the myelopathic complications of radiation and chemotherapy.

DISCLOSURE

The authors have nothing to disclose.

REFERENCES

1. Power H, Sedgwick LW. The New Sydenham Society's lexicon of medicine and the allied sciences, vol. 4. London: The New Sydenham Society; 1892.
2. Bastian HC. Special diseases of the spinal cord. In: Quain R, editor. A dictionary of medicine: including general pathology, general therapeutics, hygiene, and the diseases peculiar to women and children/by various writers. London: Longmans, Green; 1882. p. 1479–83.
3. Rivers TM. Viruses. JAMA 1929;92:1147–52.
4. Ford FR. The nervous complications of measles: with a summary of literature and publications of 12 additional case reports. Bull Johns Hopkins Hosp 1928;43: 140–84.
5. Milton MD, Morris MH, Robbins A. Acute infectious myelitis following rubella. J Pediatr 1943;23(3):365–7.
6. Senseman LA. Myelitis complicating measles. Arch Neuropsych 1945;53(4): 309–10.
7. Suchett-Kaye AI. Acute transverse myelitis complicating pneumonia. Lancet 1948;255:417.
8. Beh SC, Greenberg BM, Frohman T, et al. Transverse Myelitis. Neuro Clin 2013; 31(1):79–138.
9. Bican O, Minagar A, Pruitt AA. The spinal cord: a review of functional neuro-anatomy. Neurol Clin 2013;31(1):1–18.
10. Toledano M, Bartleson JD. Cervical spondylotic myelopathy. Neurol Clin 2013; 31(1):287–305.
11. Boden SD, McCowin PR, Davis DO, et al. Abnormal magnetic-resonance scans of the cervical spine in asymptomatic subjects. A prospective investigation. J Bone Joint Surg Am 1990;72(8):1178–84.
12. Ichihara K, Taguchi T, Sakuramoto I, et al. Mechanism of the spinal cord injury and the cervical spondylotic myelopathy: new approach based on the mechanical features of the spinal cord white and gray matter. J Neurosurg 2003;99(3 Suppl):278–85.
13. Kalsi-Ryan S, Karadimas SK, Fehlings MG. Cervical spondylotic myelopathy: the clinical phenomenon and the current pathobiology of an increasingly prevalent and devastating disorder. Neuroscientist 2013;19:409–21.
14. Nouri A, Martin AR, Kato S, et al. The Relationship Between MRI Signal Intensity Changes, Clinical Presentation, and Surgical Outcome in Degenerative Cervical Myelopathy: Analysis of a Global Cohort. Spine (Phila Pa 1976) 2017;42(24): 1851–8.

15. Flanagan EP, Krecke KN, Marsh RW, et al. Specific pattern of gadolinium enhancement in spondylotic myelopathy. Ann Neurol 2014;76(1):54–65.

16. Wang T, Tian XM, Liu SK, et al. Prevalence of complications after surgery in treatment for cervical compressive myelopathy: A meta-analysis for last decade. Medicine (Baltimore) 2017;96(12):e6421.

17. Rhee J, Tetreault LA, Chapman JR, et al. Nonoperative Versus Operative Management for the Treatment Degenerative Cervical Myelopathy: An Updated Systematic Review. Glob Spine J 2017;7(3 Suppl):35S–41S.

18. Tetreault LA, Karadimas S, Wilson JR, et al. The Natural History of Degenerative Cervical Myelopathy and the Rate of Hospitalization Following Spinal Cord Injury: An Updated Systematic Review. Glob Spine J 2017;7(3 Suppl):28S–34S.

19. McGarvey ML, Cheung AT, Szeto W, et al. Management of neurologic complications of thoracic aortic surgery. J Clin Neurophysiol 2007;24(4):336–43.

20. Robertson CE, Brown RD, Wijdicks EF, et al. Recovery after spinal cord infarcts: long-term outcome in 115 patients. Neurology 2021;78(2):114–21.

21. Vargas MI, Gariani J, Sztajzel R, et al. Spinal cord ischemia: practical imaging tips, pearls, and pitfalls. AJNR Am J Neuroradiol 2015;36(5):825–30.

22. Mateen FJ, Monrad PA, Hunderfund AN, et al. Clinically suspected fibrocartilagenous embolism: clinical characteristics, treatments, and outcomes. Eur J Neurol 2011;18(2):218–25.

23. Diehn FE, Hunt CH, Lehman VT, et al. Vertebral body infarct and ventral cord equina enhancement: Two confirmatory findings of acute spinal cord infarct. J Neuroimaging 2015;25(1):133–5.

24. Patsalides A, Knopman J, Santillan A, et al. Endovascular Treatment of Spinal Arteriovenous Lesions: Beyond the Dural Fistula. AJNR Am J Neurol 2011; 32(5):798–808.

25. Hegde AN, Mohan S, Lim CC. CNS cavernous hemangioma: "popcorn" in the brain and spinal cord. Clin Radiol 2012;67(4):380–8.

26. Fugate JE, Lanzino G, Rabinstein AA. Clinical presentation and prognostic factors of spinal dural arteriovenous fistula: an overview. Neurosurg Focus 2012; 32(5):E17.

27. Narvid J, Hetts SW, Larsen D, et al. Spinal dural arteriovenous fistulae: clinical features and long-term results. Neurosurgery 2008;62(1):159–67.

28. Toossi S, Josephson SA, Hetts SW, et al. Utility of MRI in spinal arteriovenous fistula. Neurology 2012;79(1):25–30.

29. Parks NE. Metabolic and Toxic Myelopathies. Continuum (Minneap Minn) 2021; 27(1):143–62.

30. Schwendimann RN. Metabolic, nutritional, and toxic myelopathies. Neurol Clin 2013;31(1):207–18.

31. Hemmer B, Glocker FX, Schumacher M, et al. Subacute combined degeneration: clinical, electrophysiological, and magnetic resonance imaging findings. J Neurol Neurosurg Psychiatry 1998;65(6):822–7.

32. Narra R, Mandapalli A, Jukuri N, et al. Inverted V sign" in Sub-Acute Combined Degeneration of Cord. J Clin Diagn Res 2015;9(5):TJ01.

33. Ota K, Yamaguchi R, Tsukahara A, et al. Subacute Combined Degeneration of the Spinal Cord Caused by Autoimmune Gastritis. Intern Med 2020;59(17):2113–6.

34. Yuan JL, Wang SK, Jiang T, et al. Nitrous oxide induced subacute combined degeneration with longitudinally extensive myelopathy with inverted V-sign on spinal MRI: a case report and literature review. BMC Neurol 2017;17(1):222.

35. Jaiser SR, Winston GP. Copper deficiency myelopathy. J Neurol 2010;257(6): 869–81.

36. Kumar N, Ahlskog JE, Klein CJ, et al. Imaging features of copper deficiency myelopathy: a study of 25 cases. Neuroradiology 2006;48(2):78–83.

37. Vorgerd M, Tegenthoff M, Kühne D, et al. Spinal MRI in progressive myeloneuropathy associated with vitamin E deficiency. Neuroradiology 1996;38(Suppl 1): S111–3.

38. Mariotti C, Gellera C, Rimoldi M, et al. Ataxia with isolated vitamin E deficiency: neurological phenotype, clinical follow-up and novel mutations in TTPA gene in Italian families. Neurol Sci 2004;25(3):130–7.

39. Scott TF, Frohman EM, De Seze J, et al. Therapeutics and Technology Assessment Subcommittee of American Academy of Neurology. Evidence-based guideline: clinical evaluation and treatment of transverse myelitis: report of the Therapeutics and Technology Assessment Subcommittee of the American Academy of Neurology. Neurology 2011;77(24):2128–34.

40. Loos J, Pfeuffer S, Pape K, et al. MOG encephalomyelitis: distinct clinical, MRI and CSF features in patients with longitudinal extensive transverse myelitis as first clinical presentation. J Neurol 2020;267(6):1632–42.

41. Dubey D, Pittock SJ, Krecke KN, et al. Clinical, Radiologic, and Prognostic Features of Myelitis Associated With Myelin Oligodendrocyte Glycoprotein Autoantibody. JAMA Neurol 2019;76(3):301–9.

42. Zalewski NL, Krecke KN, Weinshenker BG, et al. Central canal enhancement and the trident sign in spinal cord sarcoidosis. Neurology 2016;87(7):743–4.

43. Murphy OC, Salazar-Camelo A, Jimenez JA, et al. Clinical and MRI phenotypes of sarcoidosis-associated myelopathy. Neurol Neuroimmunol Neuroinflamm 2020; 7(4):e722.

44. Birnbaum J, Petri M, Thompson R, et al. Distinct subtypes of myelitis in systemic lupus erythematosus. Arthritis Rheum 2009;60(11):3378–87.

45. Richie MB, Pruitt AA. Spinal cord infections. Neurol Clin 2013;31(1):19–53.

46. Koeller KK, Shih RY. Intradural Extramedullary Spinal Neoplasms: Radiologic-Pathologic Correlation. Radiographics 2019;39(2):468–90.

47. Chong J, Di Rocco A, Tagliati M, et al. MR findings in AIDS-associated myelopathy. AJNR Am J Neuroradiol 1999;20(8):1412–6.

48. Talbott JF, Narvid J, Chazen JL, et al. An Imaging-Based Approach to Spinal Cord Infection. Semin Ultrasound CT MR 2016;37(5):411–30.

49. Gilden D, Nagel MA, Cohrs RJ. Varicella-zoster. Handb Clin Neurol 2014;123: 265–83.

50. Cortese A, Tavazzi E, Delbue S, et al. Varicella zoster virus-associated polyradiculoneuritis. Neurology 2009;73(16):1334–5.

51. Montalvo M, Cho TA. Infectious Myelopathies. Neurol Clin 2018;36(4):789–808.

52. Bazan C 3rd, Jackson C, Jinkins JR, et al. Gadolinium-enhanced MRI in a case of cytomegalovirus polyradiculopathy. Neurology 1991;41(9):1522–3.

53. Guiot HM, Pita-García IL, Bertrán-Pasarell J, et al. Cytomegalovirus polyradiculomyelopathy in AIDS: a case report and review of the literature. P R Health Sci J 2006;25(4):359–62.

54. Ellie E, Rozenberg F, Dousset V, et al. Herpes simplex virus type 2 ascending myeloradiculitis: MRI findings and rapid diagnosis by the polymerase chain method. J Neurol Neurosurg Psychiatry 1994;57(7):869–70.

55. Tavanaei R, Oraee-Yazdani M, Allameh F, et al. Cauda equina syndrome due to herpes simplex virus type 2-associated meningoradiculitis (Elsberg syndrome) after posterior lumbar spinal fusion surgery: Case report and review of literature. Clin Neurol Neurosurg 2021;205:106624.

56. Eberhardt O, Küker W, Dichgans J, et al. HSV-2 sacral radiculitis (Elsberg syndrome). Neurology 2004;63(4):758–9.

57. Epstein FJ, Farmer JP, Freed D. Adult intramedullary spinal cord ependymomas: the result of surgery in 38 patients. J Neurosurg 1993;79(2):204–9.

58. Kobayashi K, Ando K, Kato F, et al. MRI Characteristics of Spinal Ependymoma in WHO Grade II: A Review of 59 Cases. Spine (Phila Pa 1976) 2018;43(9):E525–30.

59. Fanous AA, Jost GF, Schmidt MH. A Nonenhancing World Health Organization Grade II Intramedullary Spinal Ependymoma in the Conus: Case Illustration and Review of Imaging Characteristics. Glob Spine J 2012;2(1):57–64.

60. Diehn FE, Krecke KN. Neuroimaging of Spinal Cord and Cauda Equina Disorders. Continuum (Minneap Minn) 2021;27(1):225–63.

61. Kim DH, Kim JH, Choi SH, et al. Differentiation between intramedullary spinal ependymoma and astrocytoma: comparative MRI analysis. Clin Radiol 2014; 69(1):29–35.

62. De Verdelhan O, Haegelen C, Carsin-Nicol B, et al. MR imaging features of spinal schwannomas and meningiomas. J Neuroradiol 2005;32(1):42–9.

63. Alorainy IA. Dural tail sign in spinal meningiomas. Eur J Radiol 2006;60(3): 387–91.

64. Schweitzer ME, Levine C, Mitchell DG, et al. Bull's-eyes and halos: useful MR discriminators of osseous metastases. Radiology 1993;188(1):249–52.

65. Nater A, Sahgal A, Fehlings M. Management - spinal metastases. Handb Clin Neurol 2018;149:239–55.

66. Okada S, Okeda R. Pathology of radiation myelopathy. Neuropathology 2001; 21(4):247–65.

67. Khan M, Ambady P, Kimbrough D, et al. Radiation-Induced Myelitis: Initial and Follow-Up MRI and Clinical Features in Patients at a Single Tertiary Care Institution during 20 Years. AJNR Am J Neuroradiol 2018;39(8):1576–81.

68. Maranzano E, Bellavita R, Floridi P, et al. Radiation-induced myelopathy in long-term surviving metastatic spinal cord compression patients after hypofractionated radiotherapy: a clinical and magnetic resonance imaging analysis. Radiother Oncol 2001;60(3):281–8.

69. Wang PY, Shen WC, Jan JS. MR imaging in radiation myelopathy. AJNR Am J Neuroradiol 1992;13(4):1049–58.

70. Tariq H, Gilbert A, Sharkey FE. Intrathecal Methotrexate-Induced Necrotizing Myelopathy: A Case Report and Review of Histologic Features. Clin Med Insights Pathol 2018;11. 1179555718809071.

71. Pinnix CC, Chi L, Jabbour EJ, et al. Dorsal column myelopathy after intrathecal chemotherapy for leukemia. Am J Hematol 2017;92(2):155–60.

72. McKeon A, Pittock SJ. Paraneoplastic encephalomyelopathies: pathology and mechanisms. Acta Neuropathol 2011;122(4):381–400.

73. Keegan BM, Pittock SJ, Lennon VA. Autoimmune myelopathy associated with collapsin response-mediator protein-5 immunoglobulin G. Ann Neurol 2008;63(4): 531–4.

74. Pittock SJ, Lucchinetti CF, Parisi JE, et al. Amphiphysin autoimmunity: paraneoplastic accompaniments. Ann Neurol 2005;58(1):96–107.

75. Madhavan AA, Carr CM, Morris PP, et al. Imaging Review of Paraneoplastic Neurologic Syndromes. AJNR Am J Neuroradiol 2020;41(12):2176–87.

76. Flanagan EP, McKeon A, Lennon VA, et al. Paraneoplastic isolated myelopathy: clinical course and neuroimaging clues. Neurology 2011;76(24):2089–95.

77. Flanagan EP, Keegan BM. Paraneoplastic myelopathy. Neurol Clin 2013;31(1): 307–18.

Recognition and Management of Neuromuscular Emergencies

Arun S. Varadhachary, MD, PhD

KEYWORDS

- Neuromuscular • Acute neuropathy • Neuromuscular junction disorders
- Inflammatory myopathy

KEY POINTS

- Neuromuscular disorders can be confidently diagnosed and localized by obtaining a time-line of symptom history combined with a hypothesis-driven physical exam.
- Laboratory testing and electrodiagnostics assist with defining the underlying disease state and help determine treatment strategies.
- Many neuromuscular emergencies are immune disorders that often respond to immuno-modulatory therapy. Which immune therapies to use and under what conditions is an area of active investigation.
- Management of neuromuscular emergencies requires close communication between a consulting neurologist and critical care specialists to alert the ICU to unique features of neuromuscular respiratory failure.

APPROACH TO NEUROMUSCULAR WEAKNESS

Consulting neurologists begin with understanding the history of present illness. For a patient with a suspected neuromuscular disorder, understanding the characteristics of the patient's weakness, including time of onset, evolution, waxing or waning of symptoms, distribution, symmetry, and association with sensory and cranial nerve symptoms, is paramount (**Table 1**). As basic as these features seem, the fundamental definitions of neuromuscular disorders are based on these clinical characteristics, and failure to correctly identify these symptoms is a continuing source of error for trainees and experienced clinicians alike.[1,2] Using first principles helps avoid delays in diagnosis and unnecessary testing.

Department of Neurology, Washington University in St. Louis, Campus Box 8111, 660 South Euclid Ave, St. Louis, MO 63110, USA
E-mail address: varadhacharya@wustl.edu

Neurol Clin 40 (2022) 157–174
https://doi.org/10.1016/j.ncl.2021.08.010
0733-8619/22/© 2021 Elsevier Inc. All rights reserved.

Table 1
Neuromuscular localization tips

	Anterior Horn Cell	Acute Nerve	Neuromuscular Junction	Muscle	CNS/Upper Motor Neuron
Pattern of Weakness	Variable pattern developing over hours to days to months depending on cause (eg, West Nile virus vs ALS)	Typically ascending. Occasionally facial/bulbar involvement over span of hours to days	Proximal limb, extraocular, bulbar, and respiratory muscles with waxing and waning pattern beginning weeks to months before culminating in crisis	Shoulder and hip girdle, and proximal limb	Variable pattern developing acutely, subacutely, or chronically
Reflexes	Reduced (can also be increased in ALS if UMN predominates)	Reduced	Unchanged in myasthenia; reduced in botulism; facilitation in LEMS	Reduced proportional to weakness	Increased
Sensory Symptoms	No	Sensory loss and pain	No	Myalgia rather than neuropathic	Variable
Electrodiagnostic Features	Reduced recruitment early; fibrillation potentials and positive sharp waves subacutely on EMG. Normal NCS	Conduction block; prolonged latency; temporal dispersion; slowed CV on NCS. Reduced recruitment early, and fibrillation potentials and positive sharp waves subacutely on needle EMG	Decrement on 2-Hz repetitive nerve stimulation for postsynaptic defect/myasthenia. Standard NCS and EMG typically unaffected early in disease	Normal NCS. Early recruitment on needle EMG with variable signs of membrane instability (ie, fibrillation potentials and positive sharp waves)	Reduced activation. Nonspecific sign seen with altered level of consciousness, pain, and effort
Blood Work	Mildly increased CK level	Mild to moderately increased CK level	Normal CK level	Moderately to markedly increased CK and aldolase levels	Normal CK level

Abbreviations: ALS, amyotrophic lateral sclerosis; CK, creatine kinase; CNS, central nervous system; CV, conduction velocity; EMG, electromyogram; LEMS, Lambert-Eaton myasthenic syndrome; NCS, nerve conduction studies; UMN, upper motor neuron.

MANAGEMENT OF SPECIFIC NEUROMUSCULAR DISORDERS
Acute and Subacute Myopathies

Myopathies are disorders in which a primary functional or structural impairment of the skeletal muscle exists. Weakness caused by myopathies is distinguished from disorders of peripheral nerve and neuromuscular junction by characteristic patterns of weakness and laboratory tests. Distinguishing between myopathy and nonmyopathic muscle pain or weakness is the first step in evaluating patients with muscle-related complaints. Several conditions share muscle-related symptoms, but frank muscle damage is not always present.

The terms myalgia, myopathy, and myositis should not be used interchangeably. Myalgia is reserved for conditions characterized by pain without weakness; myopathy refers to disorders of muscle with weakness and abnormal pathology; and myositis refers to disorders with weakness and inflammatory changes on histopathology. It is rare that patients with isolated myalgia require hospitalization. Although patients with known genetic causes of myopathy are occasionally admitted for complications related to their disorders, most myopathic cases encountered by inpatient clinicians are associated with systemic illness, toxic exposure, endocrine abnormalities, and/or autoimmune/inflammatory conditions. Of these possibilities, the former conditions require removal of offending agents and supportive care, whereas the autoimmune/inflammatory conditions require specific immunomodulatory treatment.

Rhabdomyolysis

Rhabdomyolysis is a syndromic disorder characterized by acutely developing very high increase in creatine kinase (CK) level, generally more than 10,000 U/L and commonly more than 30,000 U/L. Rather than referring to a specific condition, rhabdomyolysis is caused by any number of muscle traumas, such as a crush injury, muscle ischemia, sepsis, medication or toxic ingestions, and unaccustomed physical exertion (**Box 1**).[3–5] Some cases of rhabdomyolysis may be caused by unrecognized glycogen storage and metabolic disorders of muscle.[6]

In contrast with the inflammatory myopathies described further later, patients with rhabdomyolysis principally complain of muscle pain and varying degrees of generalized weakness. Muscles are tender to palpation and can appear swollen.

Markedly increased CK levels may lead to myoglobinuria and renal failure. Treatment is supportive and includes discontinuing the offending agent, hydration, and pain control. Alkalization of the urine is an option if myoglobinuria is present. CK can be tracked every few days to confirm that the supportive care strategy is working. It is common to observe that, with initiation of hydration, the CK level increases before trending downward.

Evaluation of the cause of rhabdomyolysis is geared at determining an underlying cause for the myopathy. If the cause of the rhabdomyolysis cannot be determined by history, the decision for diagnostic testing can be deferred to the outpatient setting after the CK level has returned to normal. It is important to recognize that muscle biopsies obtained immediately after the insult only highlight final common pathways of tissue injury, rather than pinpointing the causal pathophysiology. Electromyography (EMG) and muscle biopsy are not necessary for the diagnosis of rhabdomyolysis but may be helpful in diagnosing an underlying inflammatory or metabolic myopathy. These possibilities can be considered in situations of recurrent rhabdomyolysis or if the CK level fails to trend downward after allowing for CK's half-life, hydration, and supportive care.

Box 1
Substances implicated in rhabdomyolysis

Drugs and toxins

Toxins

Intravenous
　Cocaine: ischemia caused by vasoconstriction
　Heroin

Ingestion
　Haff disease: fish ingestion (United States, buffalo fish; northern Europe, burbot)
　Mushrooms: *Amanita phalloides*; *Tricholoma equestre* (*Tricholoma flavovirens*)
　Small birds that have previously eaten water hemlock (*Conium maculatum*)
　Ethanol
　Monensin
　Chromium picolinate
　Kidney beans
　Peanut oil
　Methylenedioxypyrovalerone
　Mephedrone
　Phencyclidine

Venoms
　Snake
　　Cobra, coral, viper, rattlesnake
　Insect
　　Hornet
　　Redback spider
　Wasp
　African bee
　　Blowpipe dart poison

Chemical exposure
　Chlorophenoxy insecticides
　Pentaborane
　Toluene

Medications
　Acetaminophen
　Amiodarone
　Amoxapine
　Anticholinergics
　Arsenic
　Azathioprine
　Baclofen
　Barbiturates
　Benzodiazepines
　Butyrophenones
　Caffeine
　Carbon monoxide
　Chloral hydrate
　Chlorpromazine
　Colchicine
　Corticosteroids
　Daptomycin
　Diphenhydramine
　Doxylamine
　e-Amino caproic acid
　Emetine
　Ephedra
　Fenfluramine

Glutethimide
Hydroxyzine
Isoniazid
Ketamine
Lamotrigine
Lysergic acid diethylamide
Methanol
Minocycline
Morphine
Nicotinic acid
Phencyclidine
Phenothiazines
Phentermine
Phenytoin
Propofol
Proton pump inhibitors
Quinolones
Salicylate
Serotonin antagonists
Statins
Succinylcholine
Sympathomimetics
Theophylline
Trimethoprim-sulfamethoxazole
Valproic acid
Vasopressin
Vincristine
Zidovudine

(*Data from* Pestronk A. MYOGLOBINURIA - RHABDOMYOLYSIS 2021, June 30 [Available from: https://neuromuscular.wustl.edu/index.html; and Coco TJ, Klasner AE. Drug-induced rhabdomyolysis. Curr Opin Pediatr. 2004;16(2):206-10)

Inflammatory Myopathy

In contrast with rhabdomyolysis, where inpatient care is supportive, inflammatory muscle disorders often require specific immunomodulatory treatment. Inflammatory myopathy or myositis is suspected when a patient complains of subacute-onset weakness affecting proximal greater than distal muscles. A viral prodrome or fatigue may precede frank loss of strength.

The treatable forms of myositis typically affect proximal muscle groups symmetrically. Patients voice difficulty with tasks requiring proximal muscles, such as rising from a chair, climbing steps, stepping onto a curb, and lifting overhead. Falls are a common complaint and may be the symptom that precipitates the hospitalization and request for neuromuscular consultation. Fine motor movements such as buttoning a shirt, sewing, knitting, or writing are generally minimally affected. Similarly, ocular muscles typically are unaffected and, if involved, should prompt reevaluation of the diagnosis.

Assessment of hip extension and abduction, shoulder girdle muscles, and paraspinal strength should be included in the neurologic examination, because casual bedside strength testing may miss weakness in those muscle groups. A simple examination maneuver is to observe the patient attempting to turn over in the bed.

In most cases, the diagnostic evaluation of a patient with suspected myopathy can occur in the outpatient setting. However, when there are concerns for respiratory status or swallowing function or ability to care for oneself at home, hospitalization is appropriate. Furthermore, evidence suggests that, in severe myositis, atrophy and fatty replacement of muscle tissue can occur early in the disease, and, thus, delayed treatment can lead to long-term disability.

The goals of inpatient management of myopathies are to confirm a suspected diagnosis, stabilize the patient, initiate high-potency therapeutics in a controlled environment, and begin planning for longitudinal care and immunosuppression. It is an unproven assumption that specific types of myositis respond better to various treatments. The difficulty relates to the rarity of myositis and the evolving field of myositis classification.

There are currently 5 broadly recognized subtypes of inflammatory myopathies: dermatomyositis, immune-mediated necrotizing myopathy, overlap myositis (including antisynthetase syndrome), polymyositis, and sporadic inclusion body myositis.[7,8] Ongoing efforts are attempting to define inflammatory myopathies by their unique myopathologic features.[9] Developing a consistent classification scheme is necessary to design clinical trials that can assess long-term treatment efficacy.[10] From the acute management perspective, the most important aspect of the evolving classification schemes is to distinguish those disorders that respond to treatment from those that do not (inclusion body myositis).

The initial evaluation of a patient with myositis should include serologic testing for CK level, aldolase level, and rheumatologic autoantibodies. These tests have a rapid turnaround time, and thus are vital for inpatient clinical decision making. Testing myositis-associated antibody panels is recommended; however, these antibody panels have a long turnaround time, thus their role is suited for informing outpatient or longitudinal care decisions. These antibodies are used for their ability to predict skin, lung, and malignant disorders associated with the myositis.[7]

Well before the current interest in the prognostic and pathogenic association of myositis-associated antibodies, it was recognized that a sizable percentage of patients with myositis have multisystemic and comorbid diseases that require monitoring and treatment.[11] Thus, inpatient management should include computed tomography (CT) imaging of the chest, abdomen, and pelvis to evaluate for interstitial lung disease (ILD), malignancy, and lymphadenopathy. Note that development of ILD and malignancy and myositis can be separated temporally,[12] thus a benign CT scan should not be taken as definitive exclusion of future comorbid disease, and follow-up PET scan can be considered.[12] It is this situation where the myositis-specific antibodies play a particularly useful role in surveillance of future disease.

Next, electrodiagnostics should be obtained. EMG is an important ancillary investigation in the evaluation of neuromuscular diseases because it guides subsequent testing and diagnostic procedures. EMG also allows widespread sampling of potentially affected muscle. Muscles revealing moderate EMG changes are ideal targets for subsequent biopsy.

EMG features of inflammatory myopathies include spontaneous activity on initial needle insertion, and short-duration motor unit potentials with early recruitment patterns during volitional muscle contraction. Electrodiagnostic features are sensitive but are not specific predictors of pathologic findings. For example, fibrillation potentials correlate with atrophic, necrotic, and regenerating fibers and inflammation but can be observed in situations of muscle membrane instability or neurogenic denervation.[13] It is important to recognize the limitations of needle EMG in patients with disturbances in consciousness because it is the changes in the volitional motor unit action potential morphology that are the basis of EMG localization as a myopathy.[14]

After electrodiagnostics confirm a myopathic localization, a muscle biopsy can be pursued. Muscle biopsy is sensitive and specific for myopathic disorders.[15] The selected muscle for biopsy should be clinically weak but not end stage. A moderately weak muscle is best. Selecting a very weak muscle can result in obtaining end-stage muscle with fatty and fibrotic replacement with few pathologic features to help define the type of myositis. Clinicians should be aware of pitfalls with muscle biopsies, particularly patchy representation of the underlying process and small sample size. This problem is an inherent disadvantage of muscle biopsy that can only be addressed by correct sampling site selection and adequate sample size.

Open and needle biopsies both have advantages and disadvantages. Procedure selection should be based on consideration of the prebiopsy probability of a muscle-based disorder, experience at the center with either procedure, potential need for repeat biopsy, and cost.[16,17] Turnaround time on muscle tissue samples submitted to pathology varies, but it can easily take more than 2 weeks for a complete analysis of the sample. Occasionally a specific diagnosis can be made based on the hematoxylin-eosin–stained sample, but, more typically, a full complement of histochemical and immunochemical stains are necessary to define the myopathology.

Some clinicians use muscle MRI to help confirm a diagnosis of myositis. MRI seems be helpful to identify patterns of muscle involvement and improve muscle selection for biopsy.[18,19] MRI techniques are rapidly evolving and may soon be able to match the gold standard of histopathology.[20]

A common dilemma is striking the balance between achieving diagnostic certainty and initiating treatment to prevent further patient morbidity. As mentioned earlier, most cases of myositis can be managed in the outpatient setting; however, when the clinical situation warrants and the patient requires urgent stabilization, it is worth recalling that muscle biopsy serves to distinguish treatable from untreatable forms of myositis and to assist in prognosis. Of the forms of myositis that do not respond to immunosuppression, the key pathologic findings do not change after initiation of steroids. In addition, for the more severe forms of inflammatory myopathy, such as dermatomyositis and immune-mediated necrotic myopathy, the pathognomonic features do not resolve after a few days of steroid therapy.

INPATIENT TREATMENT

Therapies for inflammatory myopathies are broadly immunosuppressive rather than targeting specific pathogenic pathways.[7] The management of myositis is not guideline based; however, despite the lack of controlled clinical trials, it is generally agreed that glucocorticoids coupled with a steroid-sparing agent are the mainstay of myositis treatment. The choice and combination are largely based on expert opinion.[21] Randomized controlled trials are seeking evidence for specific treatment in subsets of patients, but the various types of myositis, which are rare and heterogeneous, complicate enrolling adequate numbers of patients and designing appropriate studies.[22]

The initial steroid dose depends on various factors, but, in adults with muscle weakness sufficient to warrant inpatient treatment, a course of methylprednisolone 1000 mg for 3 to 5 days is a common regimen. Thereafter, and depending on the response of the patient's serologic parameters, further inpatient treatment options can be considered. It is important to recognize that clinical improvement does not occur immediately and patients should be counseled in advance that strength gains will occur gradually. Checking CK and aldolase levels daily during inpatient care is unnecessary, but checking these tests at the start and end of a treatment cycle can help assess response and guide further decisions.

For patients that have failed a course of intravenous steroids, intravenous immunoglobulin (IVIg) is a common next step. The mechanism of action of IVIg is unknown but the efficacy of IVIg is shown by a controlled trials of patients with resistant disease.[23,24] IVIg is administered in a variety of manners, with the dose or interval of administration varying depending on the disease severity and subsequent therapeutic response of the patient. IVIg therapy may be helpful in patients with dysphagia and when used in combination with other immunosuppressive agents, and particularly in settings of infection or malignancy. However, IVIg is expensive and has a long administration time. Hydration, cardiac tolerance of the intravascular volume load, and risk of hyperviscosity-related thrombotic events should be considered for each patient. Infusion-related headaches or chemical meningitis can occur.

Rituximab has been studied in patients with myositis.[25] Rituximab targets cluster of differentiation (CD) 20–positive cells leading to rapid depletion of B cells after administration. The precise regimen and dosing vary across the oncologic and the rheumatology literature. Original reports relied on a 325-mg/m^2 dosing, whereas more recent studies use a fixed 1000-mg dose. Rituximab and cyclophosphamide are being compared for patients with connective disease–associated ILD.[26]

Cyclophosphamide is an alkylating agent that interferes with the growth of cells and is generally reserved for the treatment of patients with severe myositis, patients with rapidly progressive ILD or overlapping systemic vasculitis, or for patients refractory to several other second-line or third-line agents. Cyclophosphamide can be administered orally or intravenously, but its use is limited owing to myelosuppression, myeloproliferative disorders, hemorrhagic cystitis, bladder cancer, infections, and infertility. A typical regimen is intravenous 0.5 to 1 g/m^2/mo or 10 to 15 mg/kg/mo for 6 to 12 months. Careful monitoring of the white blood cell count 10 days following each infusion is necessary to assess the degree of myelosuppression. It is often administered with mesna to prevent hemorrhagic cystitis.

ACUTE NEUROPATHY

The differential diagnosis for acute neuropathy is broad. Obtaining a clear symptom history can be challenging. Preexisting chronic neuropathies can make interpretation of electrodiagnostic tests difficult. Distinguishing between a monophasic illness and a chronic disorder is critical to developing the appropriate inpatient treatment plan (**Table 2**).

The immune-mediated neuropathies are a heterogeneous group of disorders with wide-ranging clinical presentations. The immunologic process may be directed at

Table 2 Treatment options for inpatient management of acute neuromuscular disorders				
	GBS	**Vasculitic Neuropathy**	**Myasthenia Gravis**	**Inflammatory Myopathy**
IVIg	2 g/kg in divided dosing	1–2 g/kg in divided dosing	2 g/kg in divided dosing	1–2 g/kg in divided dosing
Plasma Exchange	5 exchanges over span of ~1 wk	Variable benefit; dependent on vasculitis type	5 exchanges over span of ~1 wk	Limited data available
Solumedrol/ Steroids	NA	1 g/d × 3–5 d	Initiate low-dose prednisone and titration after IVIg or Plex	1 g/d × 3–5 d
Rituximab	NA	325 mg/m^2	No acute indication	325 mg/m^2
Cyclophosphamide	NA	1 g/m^2	NA	1 g/m^2

Abbreviations: GBS, Guillain-Barré syndrome; NA, not available; Plex, plasma exchange.

either the nerves or the supporting vasculature. The resulting neuropathic syndromes are defined by the target and specificity of the autoimmune response.[27]

GUILLAIN-BARRÉ SYNDROME AND VARIANTS

Guillain-Barré syndrome (GBS) is a monophasic illness and the most common cause of acute flaccid paralysis, with an annual global incidence of approximately 1 to 2 per 100,000 person-years, and is classically described as an acute-onset ascending sensorimotor neuropathy.

Several clinical patterns of GBS are appreciated, including a pure motor variant, bifacial palsy with distal paresthesia, pharyngeal-cervical-brachial weakness, lower extremity paretic variant, and the Miller-Fisher syndrome. In addition to clinical patterns of involvement, there are electrophysiologic subtypes termed acute inflammatory demyelinating polyneuropathy (AIDP), acute motor axonal neuropathy, and acute motor-sensory axonal neuropathy.[28] The AIDP subtype is most common in the United States and Europe, whereas the axonal subtypes are more frequently seen in Asia and South America.

Although the pathogenesis is incompletely understood, GBS is thought to be a post-infectious, macrophage-associated, inflammatory polyradiculoneuropathy. About two-thirds of patients who develop GBS report infectious symptoms in the weeks preceding the onset of the symptoms. In many cases, damage is humoral and complement mediated, and thought to be caused by an immune response to infections that result in collateral damage to the peripheral nerves caused by molecular mimicry. A more recent relationship between immunobiologic agents such as tumor necrosis factor inhibitors and immune checkpoint inhibitors and development of GBS has emerged.[29,30]

A diagnosis of GBS should be considered in patients who have rapidly progressive bilateral weakness of the arms and/or legs in the absence of central nervous system involvement. The classic form of the disorder presents with distal sensory abnormalities followed by weakness that starts in the legs and progresses to the arms and bulbar muscles. Reflexes are decreased at presentation and absent in almost all patients by the time the clinical nadir is reached at between 2 and 3 weeks. Autonomic dysfunction is common and can include blood pressure or heart rate instability, pupillary dysfunction, and constipation and urinary retention. Pain is frequently reported at symptom onset and can be muscular, radicular, or neuropathic.

There is currently no sufficiently sensitive or specific disease biomarker; thus, diagnosis for GBS is based on the patient's history and neurologic examination, and supported by electrophysiologic evaluation and cerebrospinal fluid (CSF) analysis.

Acute neuropathic weakness has a differential diagnosis beyond GBS, and certain key symptoms should raise suspicion for an alternative diagnosis to GBS. Features that warrant reevaluation of the diagnosis include but are not limited to: increased CSF pleocytosis, persistent and marked asymmetric weakness, fever at onset, and nadir within 24 hours of symptom onset.

In almost every instance of GBS, the malaise, fever, and respiratory or gastrointestinal symptoms of the preceding viral illness, if such occurred, have subsided by the time neuropathic symptoms appear. Therefore, manifestations of systemic illness (vomiting, abdominal pain, anemia, renal failure, eosinophilia) or constitutional symptoms (fever, anorexia, weight loss) or both, either preceding or coinciding with evolution of neuropathy, strongly suggest a primary diagnosis of a systemic illness or intoxication with concomitant polyneuropathy, and not GBS. Possibilities include vasculitis, porphyria, and acute intoxication with arsenic, lead, or disulfiram.

Laboratory testing is guided by the differential diagnosis to exclude other causes of acute flaccid paralysis. Testing for preceding infections does not typically add direct support to the diagnosis but might provide useful epidemiologic data during outbreaks of infectious diseases such as Zika,[31] *Campylobacter jejuni*, and the evolving coronavirus disease 2019 (COVID-19) pandemic.

CSF analysis is used primarily to exclude other causes of weakness during the initial evaluation of the patient. The classic finding in GBS is known as cytoalbuminemic dissociation with normal CSF cell count and increased CSF protein level. However, normal CSF protein levels are observed in 30% to 50% of patients during the first week of symptom onset. Thus, normal CSF protein level should not be used to exclude a diagnosis of GBS or delay treatment if other clinical features are present. In contrast, CSF pleocytosis greater than 50 cells/μL should suggest other disorders, including leptomeningeal malignancy, infections, or inflammatory processes of the spinal cord and nerve roots.

Electrodiagnostic evaluation of patients with GBS is not required for diagnosis; however, most commentators recommend these studies to be performed whenever possible to help support the diagnosis, particularly in situations where atypical features are present.

Electrodiagnostics performed very early in a patient's disease course may only show reduced recruitment on needle EMG to show the neuropathic localization of weakness. However, within a week or two of symptoms, nerve conduction studies will show a sensorimotor polyradiculoneuropathy characterized by conduction velocity slowing, reduced sensory and motor evoked amplitude potentials, temporal dispersion, and/or conduction block and denervation on EMG.

The results of electrodiagnostic studies assist with localization, differentiate between the 3 electrophysiologic subtypes of GBS, and may improve prognostication for recovery. About 80% of patients with GBS regain the ability to walk independently at 6 months after disease onset. The probability of regaining walking can be calculated using the modified Erasmus GBS outcome score prognosticator tool.[32] Nonetheless, 3% to 10% of patients with GBS die of cardiovascular and pulmonary complications in the acute and recovery stages of their disease. Risk factors for poor outcome include elderly age and severe disease at the outset.

VASCULITIC NEUROPATHY

In contrast with GBS and its variants, which are monophasic, subacute illnesses, the vasculitic neuropathies are a group of diseases that can acutely affect the peripheral nerves and typically require ongoing active immunomodulatory treatment. They can be associated with variety of systemic autoimmune and inflammatory diseases.

Primary vasculitic disorders are classified by the size of the blood vessels affected by the immune attack. Secondary vasculitic disorders are associated with connective tissue disorders, inflammatory bowel disease and idiopathic inflammatory disorders, malignancy, and some viral infections. This group of disorders can be among the most challenging to diagnose because of their multiple patterns of nerve involvement, described further later.

Vasculitic involvement of peripheral nerves leads to multiple focal areas of ischemic injury. Pain is a common feature of vasculitic neuropathy; patients complain of burning, tingling sensation in the distribution of the involved nerve.

The clinical presentations of vasculitic neuropathies form 3 anatomic patterns.[27] The most common is an acute onset of single or multiple mononeuropathies with sensory and motor deficits in the distribution of the involved nerves. The onset of the neuropathic symptoms may be sudden, with deficits such as wrist drop, finger drop, or foot drop appearing with a few hours. This pattern can be confused with deficits seen with the transient compressive neuropathies such as so-called Saturday night palsy or peroneal nerve compression from crossing a leg over a knee.

The second pattern is that of overlapping mononeuropathies. The onset is less acute, and patients present with bilateral but asymmetric involvement of the arms or legs.

The third pattern is a subacute distal symmetric sensorimotor polyneuropathy. This pattern is the least specific syndrome, and the symmetric pattern of sensory and motor deficits can easily be misinterpreted as more common chronic length-dependent axonal neuropathy if the timeline and physical examination are not carefully reviewed.

TREATMENT

Immunomodulatory therapy for acute neuropathies should be started if patients are unable to walk independently. It is uncertain whether patients who have milder forms of GBS derive any benefit from treatment. Clinical trials have shown a treatment effect for IVIg when started within 2 weeks of the onset of weakness[33] and a treatment effect for plasma exchange started within 4 weeks of symptoms.[34]

The definitive trials by The Guillain-Barré syndrome Study Group, published in 1985 and 1988, showed that treatment with either plasmapheresis or IVIg, respectively, did not cure the syndrome, prevent progression, or improve end-point disability but did reduce the time to gain 1 point on the GBS disability scale, speed time to independent walking, and decrease the time to weaning off the ventilator in severe cases. The studies also showed that treatment at more than 4 weeks from symptom onset had no benefit.

Over the years, there have been multiple studies attempting to determine whether combinations of IVIg or plasmapheresis could further improve results. Most recently, the role of a second dose of IVIg in the treatment of GBS was studied and failed to show any benefit beyond that gained from a single course.[35] Small-scale studies investigating whether complement inhibition can improve GBS outcomes have shown safety with the combination of IVIg and eculizumab,[36] but efficacy studies are still required. Multiple studies over the years have shown that corticosteroids do not improve outcomes in GBS and may even be associated with a negative effect. Ultimately, more work is needed to improve understanding of long-term prognosis and develop effective treatments.

In contrast with GBS, treatment of the vasculitic neuropathies requires chronic management that begins in the inpatient setting and carries on into the outpatient setting. IVIg[37] and several immunosuppressive agents have been used, including all those mentioned earlier in relation to myositis. In particular, for vasculitic neuropathy associated with positive antineutrophil cytoplasmic antibodies, the combination of corticosteroids with cyclophosphamide or rituximab is commonly used[38–40]

NEUROMUSCULAR JUNCTION DISORDERS

Myasthenia gravis (MG) is an autoimmune disorder affecting neuromuscular transmission, leading to generalized or localized weakness and characterized by fluctuating, fatigable weakness of extraocular, bulbar, truncal, and limb muscles. MG warranting emergent hospitalization is among the most common neuromuscular emergencies encountered by inpatient clinicians.

About 80% to 90% of patients with myasthenia have antibodies targeting the acetylcholine receptors (AChRs) in the postsynaptic motor end plate. The second most common antibody found is muscle-specific kinase (MuSK) antibody. In general, about one-fourth of all patients negative for AChR are positive for MuSK. Antibodies against low-density lipoprotein receptor–related protein 4 (LRP4) and agrin are occasionally detected in the remaining patients with clinical evidence of myasthenia. The presentations of these postsynaptic autoimmune myasthenic syndromes vary slightly, but the primary features of severe manifestations of the disease are the same.

In contrast, Lambert-Eaton myasthenic syndrome (LEMS) is exceedingly rare and severe respiratory symptoms are uncommon. It is a presynaptic disease characterized by chronic fluctuating weakness of proximal limb muscles and a small degree of bulbar involvement. The autoantibodies are directed against presynaptic P/Q-type voltage-gated calcium channels at cholinergic nerve terminals, resulting in reduced presynaptic calcium concentration and reduced quanta release of acetylcholine. The antibodies may also inhibit cholinergic synapses of the autonomic nervous system. Frequently associated with an underlying malignancy, especially small cell lung cancer, LEMS can produce symptoms 1 to 2 years before detection of the malignancy.

Typical examination features of myasthenia include combinations of ptosis; diplopia caused by paresis of extraocular muscles; facial, jaw, or tongue weakness; neck flexion/extension weakness; and dysarthric speech. Clinicians should also consider myasthenia when bulbar or neck flexion/extension weakness or respiratory dysfunction presents in isolation. Sensation is unaffected, and reflexes are affected only in proportion to muscular weakness.

The differential diagnosis of myasthenia (and LEMS) includes other neuromuscular junction disorders such as botulism, and pure motor disorders such as myopathy, amyotrophic lateral sclerosis, and the Miller-Fisher syndrome. Sometimes conditions such as chronic fatigue syndrome, migraine headaches with ocular features, and mood disorders are considered.

Diagnosis of MG can be confirmed with electrophysiologic testing. Neuromuscular junction transmission failure can be identified using slow, 2-Hz to 3-Hz repetitive nerve stimulation. This test has a sensitivity of 80% in patients with generalized MG but less than 50% in isolated ocular symptoms (patients who, by definition, would not be in myasthenic crisis). Single-fiber EMG is more sensitive than repetitive stimulation but is technically challenging and usually not well suited to the intensive care unit or other inpatient settings. The hallmark of electrophysiologic testing for LEMS is marked facilitation of the Compound muscle action potential (CMAP) amplitude after brief exercise. At high rates of repetitive stimulation, there is also an incremental response.

The most common precipitants of myasthenic crisis are infections of the upper and lower respiratory tract. Other precipitants include aspiration pneumonitis, surgery, pregnancy, perimenstrual state, some medications, and tapering of immune-modulating medications. Approximately one-third to one-half of patients may have no obvious cause for their myasthenic crisis.

Mortalities from myasthenic crisis have decreased to approximately 5% over the past decades.[41] This improvement is caused by the combination of increased recognition of the disorder, availability of rapid-acting therapies, and advances in critical care. Nonetheless, complications from infection and cardiac dysfunction continue to affect survival rates.

TREATMENT

Inpatient and acute treatment principles for myasthenic crises are similar to those described earlier for GBS. Patients with rapidly worsening symptoms, moderate to severe dysphagia, or dyspnea should be evaluated and admitted urgently. A key distinction between management in myasthenia and GBS is that corticosteroids play an important role in management in myasthenia, even in the acute setting.

Most patients show improvement in symptoms within a week of receiving standard 2-g/kg dosing of IVIg. Patients receiving plasmapheresis typically show improvement by the third to fourth treatment. Steroids should be initiated after the patient has received IVIg or undergone a few apheresis sessions. This sequence is recommended in order to prevent the paradoxic worsening of weakness that can be precipitated by steroids in myasthenic patients whose acute symptoms have not yet been stabilized. Prednisone can be initiated at 15 mg/d and conservatively titrated up by 5 mg every 3 days to a goal of 60 to 80 mg/d. Assuming the initial management of the crisis went smoothly, most patients report improved symptoms within a week or two of prednisone initiation.

More recent strategies for inpatient management of myasthenic crises include use of the anti-CD20 B cell–depleting monoclonal antibody rituximab and the complement inhibitor eculizumab. There is strong evidence for rituximab's use in cases of MuSK myasthenia[42]; however, the success rate of treating patients with AChR myasthenia is more limited, especially[43] compared with the dramatic responses observed in patients with MuSK myasthenia. In the case of eculizumab, studies investigating its effect on treatment-refractory myasthenia suggest no significant difference between eculizumab and placebo in terms of the primary end point in an activities of daily living score. However, MG exacerbations were seen less frequently in the eculizumab-treated group compared with the placebo,[44] and it has been approved by the United States Food and Drug Administration.

Treatment options for LEMS include treatment of the underlying malignancy when present; use of cholinesterase inhibitors such as pyridostigmine; use of voltage-gated potassium channel blockers such as amifampridine[45]; and, for severe and refractory patients, treatment with immunotherapy. As indicated earlier, because symptoms from LEMS are milder and rarely present with respiratory failure, compared with classic myasthenia, inpatient use of IVIg or plasmapheresis is generally not required.

SUPPORTIVE CARE
Respiratory Function

Patients presenting with neuromuscular weakness require assessment of respiratory status. Respiratory function in neuromuscular patients is characterized by impaired bellows function rather than intrinsic lung abnormalities. When present, abnormalities in oxygenation should prompt a search for a second disease process, such as pneumonia or ILD. In addition, muscles controlling swallowing and speech are frequently affected. Symptoms of neuromuscular respiratory failure include dyspnea and orthopnea, tachypnea, hypophonia, shortened sentence length, weak cough, use of accessory respiratory muscles, and paradoxic breathing. Oropharyngeal dysfunction and neck extension weakness often precede frank collapse of respiratory function. A history of weight loss and poor appetite is a frequent complaint from patients with subacute to chronic respiratory compromise.

Pulse oximetry and nasal cannula oxygen are frequently applied to hospitalized patients, but, for neuromuscular patients, these tools should be used cautiously because they can contribute to respiratory failure. Pulse oximeter measurement is important to detect hypoxemia but it does not identify the CO_2 retention typical of neuromuscular respiratory failure. Indiscriminate use of nasal cannula oxygen can lead to iatrogenic respiratory failure related to chemoreceptor signaling imbalance between O_2 and CO_2 ratios.

Arterial blood gasses are usually not informative either, because Pa_{O_2} decline and Pa_{CO_2} increase are late features of respiratory failure caused by neuromuscular weakness. A normal arterial P_{CO_2} in a tachypneic patient should be interpreted circumspectly. This finding may be a herald of impending fatigue; mechanical failure prevents the patient from reducing arterial P_{CO_2} as would be expected in an individual with normal respiratory mechanics.

Patients with neuromuscular weakness frequently complain of anxiety and air hunger, but these neuropsychiatric symptoms must be interpreted with extreme caution. It is the unfortunate experience of neuromuscular consultants to have witnessed the inappropriate use of anxiolytics and subsequent triggering of frank respiratory failure when the patient no longer was able to compensate for the respiratory muscle weakness.

Vital capacity, maximal inspiratory pressure, and maximal expiratory pressure are better bedside measures of respiratory muscle function. However, significant variability can occur between trials, which are both patient and operator dependent, with degree of cooperation and seal around the testing device affecting the reliability of measurements. Serial monitoring of vital capacity is a well-studied ancillary tool for the prediction of neuromuscular respiratory failure.[46] Measurement can be performed 2 to 4 times daily, depending on the level of concern, recent patient trends, and access to respiratory therapist support. The often-cited 20/30/40 rule (vital capacity in milliliters per kilogram; maximal inspiratory pressure in centimeters of H_2O; and maximal expiratory pressure in centimeters of H_2O) can be easily remembered and serves as a guide to when intubation should be strongly considered.[47]

The single breath count (SBC) is a proxy for vital capacity and is easily incorporated into bedside rounds. To obtain an SBC, the patient is asked to maximally inhale and then count up from 1 on a single breath. Demonstrating the technique to the patient beforehand helps improve the reproducibility and reliability of the measurement. The SBC correlates with vital capacity and maximal inspiratory pressure. Each number counted on the SBC corresponds with roughly 100 mL of vital capacity. Patients who are unable to count to 20 in a single breath should be closely observed and considered for elective intubation.

Prolonged periods of mechanical ventilation can be observed in GBS and myasthenia. Pathophysiologic factors range from deconditioning to phrenic nerve demyelination to critical illness myopathy. One-half of intubated patients with GBS ultimately require tracheostomy,[48] but the optimal timing and ultimate utility of tracheostomy is debated.[49] Delaying tracheostomy past 1 or 2 weeks after intubation may or may not be associated with higher ventilator-associated pneumonia risk and longer duration of mechanical ventilation.[49,50] Earlier intervention results in some patients getting an unnecessary tracheostomy.

Neuropathic Pain

Pain is an often-overlooked feature of GBS and vasculitic neuropathies because attention is mostly paid to motor symptoms. However, pain frequently heralds the development of weakness and persists long after motor recovery. The reported frequency of pain in GBS is highly variable, and most studies have evaluated pain only during the acute phase of illness. Longitudinal follow-up studies have shown persistence of neuropathic symptoms even a decade after illness from GBS.[51]

The pathophysiologic explanation of pain in GBS is diverse. The acute phase is predominantly nociceptive pain, caused by inflammation of the nerve roots and peripheral nerves. Later pain is nonnociceptive but results from degeneration and/or regeneration of nerves such as is encountered in patients with chronic neuropathies. In contrast, the complaint of myalgias voiced by patients with GBS[52] and recovering from myositis seems related to mechanical factors from altered physical activity.

A pain treatment strategy begins with inquiring about the presence and severity of pain as a symptom. Opiates have a reliable analgesic effect, but sedation and ileus can limit their use. Data on nonopiate pharmacologic interventions are limited, but gabapentin or carbamazepine may reduce pain and opioid requirements in some patients. Methylprednisolone as part of pain management strategies has been studied but proved unsuccessful.[52]

Thromboembolism

Deep-vein thrombosis and subsequent pulmonary embolism are well-recognized complications of immobility for any hospitalized patient. The incidence of this complication specifically in acute neuromuscular disorders is uncertain; however, the aggregate risk in patients in neurointensive care units is high.[53] Studies have not addressed specific antithrombotic prophylaxis for GBS, but it is recommended that all minimally ambulant or nonambulant patients receive thromboembolism prophylaxis according to the American Society of Hematology.[54] Prophylaxis should be tailored to the patient's comorbidities, including bleeding risk, renal function, and recent procedures at noncompressible sites. The optimum duration of prophylaxis is unclear, but it should extend until ambulation is routine. Even with these measures, thromboembolism can still occur. Therefore, deep-vein thrombosis and pulmonary embolism should be on the short differential diagnosis of asymmetric leg edema, chest pain, shortness of breath, or hemodynamic instability.

Prevention of Complications

The prolonged immobility of patients with severe neuromuscular weakness places them at risk for hospital-acquired pneumonia and urinary tract infections, position-related nerve compression, skin and pressure ulceration, and contractures. Standard-of-practice preventive measures and treatment are strongly recommended.[28] Attention to body positioning, use of bracing and orthotics, pressure point padding, and frequent position changes constitute part of optimal care. Patients with incomplete eye closure from facial weakness can develop exposure keratitis. Corneal protection with artificial tears, lubricants, careful lid taping, or protective eye domes is essential. Multidisciplinary physical therapy should be initiated as soon as possible. Exercise programs for patients with neuromuscular weakness include passive range-of-motion stretching, stationary cycling, walking, and strength training have been shown to improve physical fitness and independence in activities of daily living. Management of complications is best handled by a multidisciplinary team consisting of nurses; physical, occupational, and speech therapists; physical medicine and rehabilitation specialists; and dieticians.[28]

SUMMARY

Specifically treatable neuromuscular disorders are a common group of conditions that are encountered by inpatient neurologists. The disorders discussed in this article present with acute to subacute progression of motor dysfunction affecting bulbar, respiratory, and limb function. Collecting the patient history and using first principles of neurologic examination aid in the localization and allow diagnosis and institution of proven treatments that can reduce morbidity and mortality. Close communication with intensive care colleagues allows neurologists to contribute to optimizing the outcome for this group of patients.

CLINICS CARE POINTS

- Plasma exchange and IVIg are equally efficacious in improving recovery from GBS. However, there is no evidence that offering repeated plasma exchange sessions or additional IVIg after the acute disease phase over is useful.

- Immunomodulatory regimens for treatment of inflammatory myopathies are based upon expert opinion.

- Reliance on pulse oximetry to judge respiratory stability in neuromuscular patients can be misleading. Measurement/estimates of force vital capacity are good indicators of impending respiratory failure.

- Electrodiagnostics can be especially useful when deciding upon which muscle to target for biopsy. The ideal muscle for selection is moderately weak.
- Suggested guidelines for nerve biopsy include when vasculitic neuropathy is suspected and when there is a clear treatment or prognostic implication.

DISCLOSURES

Research funding and consulting fees from Biogen, research funding and consulting fees from Epirium, research funding from Capricor, author has received medicolegal consulting fees for case reviews and expert witness testimony.

REFERENCES

1. Kamel H, Dhaliwal G, Navi BB, et al. A randomized trial of hypothesis-driven vs screening neurologic examination. Neurology 2011;77(14):1395–400.
2. Chimowitz MI, Logigian EL, Caplan LR. The accuracy of bedside neurological diagnoses. Ann Neurol 1990;28(1):78–85.
3. Nance JR, Mammen AL. Diagnostic evaluation of rhabdomyolysis. Muscle Nerve 2015;51(6):793–810.
4. Pestronk A. Available at: https://neuromuscular.wustl.edu/index.html. Accessed April 30, 2021.
5. Coco TJ, Klasner AE. Drug-induced rhabdomyolysis. Curr Opin Pediatr 2004; 16(2):206–10.
6. Tarnopolsky MA. Myopathies related to glycogen metabolism disorders. Neurotherapeutics 2018;15(4):915–27.
7. Selva-O'Callaghan A, Pinal-Fernandez I, Trallero-Araguás E, et al. Classification and management of adult inflammatory myopathies. Lancet Neurol 2018;17(9): 816–28.
8. Mammen AL, Allenbach Y, Stenzel W, et al. 239th ENMC International Workshop: Classification of dermatomyositis, Amsterdam, the Netherlands, 14-16 December 2018. Neuromuscul Disord 2020;30(1):70–92.
9. Pestronk A. Acquired immune and inflammatory myopathies: pathologic classification. Curr Opin Rheumatol 2011;23(6):595–604.
10. Rider LG, Ruperto N, Pistorio A, et al. 2016 ACR-EULAR adult dermatomyositis and polymyositis and juvenile dermatomyositis response criteria-methodological aspects. Rheumatology (Oxford) 2017;56(11):1884–93.
11. Callen JP. Relationship of cancer to inflammatory muscle diseases. Dermatomyositis, polymyositis, and inclusion body myositis. Rheum Dis Clin North Am 1994; 20(4):943–53.
12. Li X, Tan H. Value of (18)F-FDG PET/CT in the detection of occult malignancy in patients with dermatomyositis. Heliyon 2020;6(4):e03707.
13. Naddaf E, Milone M, Mauermann ML, et al. Muscle biopsy and electromyography correlation. Front Neurol 2018;9:839.
14. Preston DC, Shapiro BE. Electromyography and neuromuscular disorders: clinical-electrophysiologic correlations. 3rd edition. London; New York: Elsevier Saunders; 2013. p. xvii, 643.
15. Lai CH, Melli G, Chang YJ, et al. Open muscle biopsy in suspected myopathy: diagnostic yield and clinical utility. Eur J Neurol 2010;17(1):136–42.
16. Nix JS, Moore SA. What every neuropathologist needs to know: the muscle biopsy. J Neuropathol Exp Neurol 2020;79(7):719–33.

17. Gallo A, Abraham A, Katzberg HD, et al. Muscle biopsy technical safety and quality using a self-contained, vacuum-assisted biopsy technique. Neuromuscul Disord 2018;28(5):450–3.
18. Van De Vlekkert J, Maas M, Hoogendijk JE, et al. Combining MRI and muscle biopsy improves diagnostic accuracy in subacute-onset idiopathic inflammatory myopathy. Muscle Nerve 2015;51(2):253–8.
19. Wang LH, Friedman SD, Shaw D, et al. MRI-informed muscle biopsies correlate MRI with pathology and DUX4 target gene expression in FSHD. Hum Mol Genet 2019;28(3):476–86.
20. Kalia V, Leung DG, Sneag DB, et al. Advanced MRI techniques for muscle imaging. Semin Musculoskelet Radiol 2017;21(4):459–69.
21. Dalakas MC. Inflammatory muscle diseases. N Engl J Med 2015;373(4):393–4.
22. Aggarwal R, Rider LG, Ruperto N, et al. 2016 American College of Rheumatology/European League Against Rheumatism criteria for minimal, moderate, and major clinical response in adult dermatomyositis and polymyositis: an International Myositis Assessment and Clinical Studies Group/Paediatric Rheumatology International Trials Organisation Collaborative Initiative. Ann Rheum Dis 2017;76(5):792–801.
23. Dalakas MC, Illa I, Dambrosia JM, et al. A controlled trial of high-dose intravenous immune globulin infusions as treatment for dermatomyositis. N Engl J Med 1993; 329(27):1993–2000.
24. Aggarwal R, Charles-Schoeman C, Schessl J, et al. Prospective, double-blind, randomized, placebo-controlled phase III study evaluating efficacy and safety of octagam 10% in patients with dermatomyositis ("ProDERM Study"). Medicine (Baltimore) 2021;100(1):e23677.
25. Oddis CV, Reed AM, Aggarwal R, et al. Rituximab in the treatment of refractory adult and juvenile dermatomyositis and adult polymyositis: a randomized, placebo-phase trial. Arthritis Rheum 2013;65(2):314–24.
26. Saunders P, Tsipouri V, Keir GJ, et al. Rituximab versus cyclophosphamide for the treatment of connective tissue disease-associated interstitial lung disease (RECITAL): study protocol for a randomised controlled trial. Trials 2017;18(1):275.
27. So YT. Immune-mediated neuropathies. Continuum (Minneap Minn) 2012;18(1): 85–105.
28. Leonhard SE, Mandarakas MR, Gondim FAA, et al. Diagnosis and management of Guillain-Barre syndrome in ten steps. Nat Rev Neurol 2019;15(11):671–83.
29. Janssen JBE, Leow TYS, Herbschleb KH, et al. Immune checkpoint inhibitor-related guillain-barre syndrome: a case series and review of the literature. J Immunother 2021;44(7):276–82.
30. Haugh AM, Probasco JC, Johnson DB. Neurologic complications of immune checkpoint inhibitors. Expert Opin Drug Saf 2020;19(4):479–88.
31. Capasso A, Ompad DC, Vieira DL, et al. Incidence of Guillain-Barre Syndrome (GBS) in Latin America and the Caribbean before and during the 2015-2016 Zika virus epidemic: a systematic review and meta-analysis. PLoS Negl Trop Dis 2019;13(8):e0007622.
32. van Koningsveld R, Steyerberg EW, Hughes RA, et al. A clinical prognostic scoring system for Guillain-Barre syndrome. Lancet Neurol 2007;6(7):589–94.
33. Hughes RA, Swan AV, van Doorn PA. Intravenous immunoglobulin for Guillain-Barre syndrome. Cochrane Database Syst Rev 2014;9:CD002063.
34. Chevret S, Hughes RA, Annane D. Plasma exchange for Guillain-Barre syndrome. Cochrane Database Syst Rev 2017;2:CD001798.

35. Verboon C, van den Berg B, Cornblath DR, et al. Original research: second IVIg course in Guillain-Barre syndrome with poor prognosis: the non-randomised ISID study. J Neurol Neurosurg Psychiatry 2020;91(2):113–21.

36. Misawa S, Kuwabara S, Sato Y, et al. Safety and efficacy of eculizumab in Guillain-Barre syndrome: a multicentre, double-blind, randomised phase 2 trial. Lancet Neurol 2018;17(6):519–29.

37. Shimizu T, Morita T, Kumanogoh A. The therapeutic efficacy of intravenous immunoglobulin in anti-neutrophilic cytoplasmic antibody-associated vasculitis: a meta-analysis. Rheumatology (Oxford) 2020;59(5):959–67.

38. Stone JH, Merkel PA, Spiera R, et al. Rituximab versus cyclophosphamide for ANCA-associated vasculitis. N Engl J Med 2010;363(3):221–32.

39. de Groot K, Harper L, Jayne DR, et al. Pulse versus daily oral cyclophosphamide for induction of remission in antineutrophil cytoplasmic antibody-associated vasculitis: a randomized trial. Ann Intern Med 2009;150(10):670–80.

40. Almaani S, Fussner LA, Brodsky S, et al. ANCA-associated vasculitis: an update. J Clin Med 2021;10(7):1446.

41. Alshekhlee A, Miles JD, Katirji B, et al. Incidence and mortality rates of myasthenia gravis and myasthenic crisis in US hospitals. Neurology 2009;72(18):1548–54.

42. Hehir MK, Hobson-Webb LD, Benatar M, et al. Rituximab as treatment for anti-MuSK myasthenia gravis: multicenter blinded prospective review. Neurology 2017;89(10):1069–77.

43. Tandan R, Hehir MK 2nd, Waheed W, et al. Rituximab treatment of myasthenia gravis: a systematic review. Muscle Nerve 2017;56(2):185–96.

44. Muppidi S, Utsugisawa K, Benatar M, et al. Long-term safety and efficacy of eculizumab in generalized myasthenia gravis. Muscle Nerve 2019;60(1):14–24.

45. Yoon CH, Owusu-Guha J, Smith A, et al. Amifampridine for the management of lambert-eaton myasthenic syndrome: a new take on an old drug. Ann Pharmacother 2020;54(1):56–63.

46. Chevrolet JC, Deleamont P. Repeated vital capacity measurements as predictive parameters for mechanical ventilation need and weaning success in the Guillain-Barre syndrome. Am Rev Respir Dis 1991;144(4):814–8.

47. Lawn ND, Fletcher DD, Henderson RD, et al. Anticipating mechanical ventilation in Guillain-Barre syndrome. Arch Neurol 2001;58(6):893–8.

48. Nguyen TN, Badjatia N, Malhotra A, et al. Factors predicting extubation success in patients with Guillain-Barre syndrome. Neurocrit Care 2006;5(3):230–4.

49. Yonezawa N, Jo T, Matsui H, et al. Effect of early tracheostomy on mortality of mechanically ventilated patients with guillain-barre syndrome: a nationwide observational study. Neurocrit Care 2020;33(3):759–68.

50. Ali MI, Fernandez-Perez ER, Pendem S, et al. Mechanical ventilation in patients with Guillain-Barre syndrome. Respir Care 2006;51(12):1403–7.

51. Forsberg A, Press R, Holmqvist LW. Residual disability 10 years after falling ill in Guillain-Barre syndrome: a prospective follow-up study. J Neurol Sci 2012;317(1–2):74–9.

52. Ruts L, van Koningsveld R, Jacobs BC, et al. Determination of pain and response to methylprednisolone in Guillain-Barre syndrome. J Neurol 2007;254(10):1318–22.

53. Zhang P, Bian Y, Xu F, et al. The incidence and characteristics of venous thromboembolism in neurocritical care patients: a prospective observational study. Clin Appl Thromb Hemost 2020;26. 1076029620907954.

54. Ortel TL, Neumann I, Ageno W, et al. American Society of Hematology 2020 guidelines for management of venous thromboembolism: treatment of deep vein thrombosis and pulmonary embolism. Blood Adv 2020;4(19):4693–738.

Common Focal Neuropathies in the Hospitalized Patient

Mark Terrelonge Jr, MD, MPH*, Laura Rosow, MD

KEYWORDS

- Peripheral nerve injury • Focal neuropathy • Hospital Neurology

KEY POINTS

- Nerve injury may occur secondary to compression, stretch, and direct trauma, among other causes; understanding the cause of a patient's nerve injury is critical to understanding the injury's prognosis.
- Common focal neuropathies in the hospitalized patient include the ulnar, median, and radial nerves in the upper extremities, and the sciatic, peroneal, and femoral nerves in the lower extremity.
- Surgical and obstetric risk factors are important considerations in evaluation of patients with focal neuropathies.

INTRODUCTION

Focal neuropathies in the hospitalized patient are a common reason for neurologic consultation. A focal neuropathy may be discovered as part of a patient's intake examination or may develop during their hospital stay, either due to iatrogenic injury or as a complication of their underlying condition. Prompt recognition of these neuropathies can help reduce unnecessary testing, allow for timely intervention (if appropriate), and assist the neurologist in counseling, prognostication, and discharge and rehabilitation planning. Furthermore, identification of focal neuropathies may assist in the diagnosis of other comorbid conditions, including thyroid disease, diabetes, or even hereditary polyneuropathy.

In this article, the authors review common mechanisms of nerve injury in the hospitalized patient, history and physical examination findings associated with the most common focal neuropathies, and risk factors and surgeries that may predispose hospitalized patients to these neuropathies. Focal neuropathies that are attributable to chronic medical conditions or injuries sustained outside of the hospital (eg, fractures secondary to trauma) are touched on but are not the focus of this article.

University of California San Francisco, 400 Parnassus Avenue, 8th Floor, San Francisco, CA 94143, USA
* Corresponding author.
E-mail address: Mark.Terrelonge@ucsf.edu

Neurol Clin 40 (2022) 175–190
https://doi.org/10.1016/j.ncl.2021.08.013
0733-8619/22/© 2021 Elsevier Inc. All rights reserved.

CAUSES AND MECHANISMS OF NERVE FIBER INJURY

Nerves may be injured through various mechanisms, including: direct trauma, hypoperfusion, exposure to a neurotoxic substance, and inflammatory and thermal effects. Iatrogenic peripheral nerve injury in the hospitalized patient most frequently occurs due to stretch or compression.

Compressive injuries may present acutely or can develop gradually over time, typically due to prolonged or repeated excessive force from a hard surface (eg, surgical table or lithotomy stirrups) or a mass (eg, lipoma, cyst, metastasis). Traction injuries may happen secondary to surgical positioning and manipulation, expansile hematomas, or tourniquet use. Direct trauma may occur due to nerve laceration during surgery.

Beyond understanding the mechanisms of injury, the type and extent of nerve fiber damage predict the overall prognosis for recovery. The 3 primary types of nerve fiber damage described by the 1942 Seddon's classification are neuropraxia, axonotmesis, and neurotmesis (**Fig. 1**).[1]

Neuropraxia describes a nerve injury that is secondary to demyelination or ischemia and has no associated axonal damage. The biggest risk factor for this type of injury is nerve compression or entrapment. Because of focal demyelination or ischemia, the nerve will have decreased conduction velocity or conduction block across the site of injury.[2] With more motor nerve fibers being myelinated than sensory fibers, weakness usually predominates.[3] Injuries of this type have the best prognosis and can recover completely over weeks to months if the underlying cause is corrected.[4]

Axonotmesis describes an axonal nerve injury with preserved continuity of the epineurium, perineurium, and endoneurium.[2] It is caused most frequently by stretch, traction, and crush injuries. Distal to the injury, Wallerian degeneration occurs over the subsequent 7 to 10 days.[5] Sprouting occurs thereafter, and given the preserved endoneurium, axons are often able to reach denervated tissues, although a full

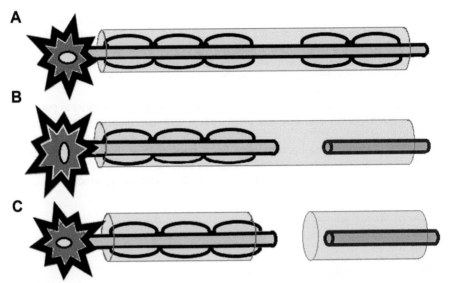

Fig. 1. Nerve injuries. (*A*) Neurapraxia: injury to the myelin, sparing the axon and the epineurium. (*B*) Axonotmesis: injury to the myelin and axon, sparing the epineurium. (*C*) Neurotmesis: injury to the myelin, axon, and epineurium.

recovery is not always seen. Regrowth occurs at 1 mm per day, and full recovery can take months to years.[6] If spontaneous recovery does not occur within a few months, surgery may be required to help promote and guide nerve regrowth at the site of injury.[7]

Neurotmesis describes an axonal nerve injury without continuity of the epineurium, perineurium, and endoneurium, that is, complete transection of the peripheral nerve. Risk factors include high-velocity trauma, lacerations, and penetrating injuries.[4] Endoneurium disruption along with scar tissue from surrounding tissue may impair nerve regrowth and reinnervation. Surgical nerve repair is the mainstay of treatment.[8]

COMMON FOCAL NEUROPATHIES

A summary of the presentations of common focal neuropathies can be found in **Table 1**.

ULNAR NEUROPATHY

Ulnar neuropathy is one of the most common focal neuropathies seen perioperatively in the hospital setting.[9,10] The ulnar nerve is formed from the C8 and T1 spinal nerve roots, which then travel into the lower trunk and medial cord of the brachial plexus before becoming a terminal nerve in the arm. The nerve travels posteriorly, close to the humerus, then traverses the retrocondylar groove of the elbow before continuing into the forearm. The shape and small size of this retrocondylar groove make the ulnar nerve especially prone to compressive injury. Prolonged flexion of the elbow may also

Table 1
Common focal neuropathies

Nerve	Roots	Motor Function	Sensory Function
Upper Extremity			
Ulnar	C8-T1	Wrist flexion, ulnar aspect; flexion of the fifth digit; abduction of the index and fifth digit; adduction of the thumb	Dorsum of the medial aspect of the hand and digits 4 and 5 (medial fourth finger)
Median	C6-T1	Thumb opposition; flexion of the thumb, second and third digit; forearm pronation; wrist flexion, radial aspect	Lateral palm; volar aspects of the thumb, index, middle, and lateral fourth finger; dorsal tips of aforementioned fingers
Radial	C5-C8	Elbow extension; Wrist extension; finger extension; forearm supination	Posterolateral arm and dorsal aspect of the hand and lateral three and a half fingers (sparing the fingertips)
Lower Extremity			
Sciatic	L4-S3	Flexion at the knee; all movements of the foot and toes	Entire foot and posterolateral leg below the knee
Peroneal	L4-S2	Dorsiflexion and eversion of the foot	Lateral calf and dorsum of foot
Femoral	L2-L4	Hip flexion; knee extension	Anterior thigh and medial calf (through the saphenous nerve)
Lateral femoral cutaneous	L2-L3	None	Anterolateral thigh

lead to mild stretch injury in the nerve.[11] Ulnar neuropathies are more common in men than women.[12]

There are several potential mechanisms of ulnar neuropathy in the hospitalized patient. In the perioperative setting, improper positioning or padding of the upper extremity may lead to nerve traction or compression. Ulnar neuropathy can happen with proper positioning as well, leading many to postulate that alternate, as yet unknown, factors may contribute to this entity.[9,13] In fact, approximately 0.5% of patients will develop an ulnar neuropathy after surgery, usually 2 to 7 days after their procedure. Additional mechanisms of ulnar neuropathy in hospitalized patients include subluxation, more proximal compression at the arcade of Struthers (a musculoaponeurotic structure between the medial humeral epicondyle and the medial head of the triceps brachii muscle), or infiltration by a mass.[14,15]

Classic signs of an ulnar neuropathy at the elbow include numbness or paresthesia in the fourth and fifth digits of the hand. Frank weakness is less common but can include the hand intrinsic muscles and occasionally grip weakness due to involvement of the flexor digitorum profundus (FDP) to digits 4 and 5. Occasionally, a Tinel sign at the elbow and/or medial elbow pain or paresthesia in the forearm may be present.

Differential for an ulnar neuropathy at the elbow also includes brachial plexus injury involving the medial cord or lower trunk or a C8 radiculopathy; these can sometimes be distinguished by noting associated weakness of muscles innervated by the median nerve, which is partly supplied by the medial cord, or by sensory loss extending into the medial forearm, which is supplied by the medial antebrachial cutaneous branch off the medial cord and supplied by C8 and T1. The presence of cervical or radicular pain can also provide a clue to an alternate localization.

Because iatrogenic ulnar neuropathy is typically associated with minimal axonal involvement, patients can usually expect to make a full or nearly full recovery; however, those with anatomic causes of continued nerve compression or stretch may require operative intervention and can have more variable improvement in symptoms.[16]

MEDIAN NEUROPATHY

Median neuropathy at the wrist is the most common focal neuropathy and is frequently encountered in the hospital setting, although it is unlikely to present acutely or as an iatrogenic/perioperative complication. However, there are mechanisms of median nerve injury more proximal to the wrist that may be seen acutely in the hospitalized patient. The median nerve consists of contributions from the medial and lateral cords of the brachial plexus and descends down the arm initially lateral then medial to the brachial artery. It enters the forearm through the cubital fossa and produces the anterior interosseous nerve (AION) and palmar cutaneous nerve before entering the hand through the carpal tunnel.

Humeral fractures, elbow dislocation, and radial fractures may injure the median nerve in the upper arm and forearm. Iatrogenic injury may occur during injection or cannulation of the arteries and veins near the antecubital fossa.[17] Stretch of inferior brachial plexus fibers contributing to the median nerve may occur near the axilla due to perioperative positioning or use of crutches (crutch paralysis).[18] Ischemia related to fistulas or a vasculitic process can affect the median nerve anywhere along its course.[19] Brachial neuritis, which can be idiopathic or secondary to viral infections or surgical interventions, may present preferentially with weakness of muscles innervated by the AION.[20]

A median neuropathy at the wrist, although most frequently idiopathic or related to hypertrophy of the flexor tendons across the carpal tunnel, can also be attributable to several medical conditions, including[21] hypothyroidism, acromegaly, amyloidosis, sarcoidosis, leprosy, wrist trauma, pregnancy, and masses (ie, lipomas, ganglion cysts).[22–25] This neuropathy typically present with nocturnal pain and paresthesia in the first three and a half fingers of the hand. Depending on the degree of injury, there may be sensory loss in the first three and a half fingers, sparing the thenar eminence, or even weakness of thumb abduction and opposition. An AION syndrome will spare the muscles typically involved in a median neuropathy at the wrist and is characterized by difficulty with making an "OK" sign due to weakness of the FDP to digit 1 and the flexor pollicis longus; other involved muscles include the pronator quadratus and FDP to digit 2.[26] More proximal injuries may further involve the pronator teres and flexor digitorum superficialis muscles.

Crutch compression, stretch neuropathies, and brachial neuritis–related injuries have the best chance for spontaneous recovery,[18] whereas injuries related to ongoing compression or medical conditions may require surgical intervention or treatment of the underlying cause.

RADIAL NEUROPATHY

The radial nerve originates from the posterior cord of the brachial plexus and travels down the arm through the radial groove, innervating the triceps proximally and the brachialis and brachioradialis muscles in the forearm. In the elbow, the nerve splits into 2 components—the posterior interosseous nerve (PIN), which is purely motor, and the superficial radial nerve, which is purely sensory.

The most common causes of injury to the radial nerve are fracture of the proximal humerus, dislocation at the shoulder joint, or pressure within the axilla as can be seen with improper crutch use or from direct pressure on the nerve against a firm object ("Saturday night palsy").[27,28] Other mechanisms of injury include ischemia, stretch injury (ie, improper arm positioning during surgery), intramuscular injection, masses, and immune-mediated brachial plexopathy, especially when the PIN is involved.[28–31]

Weakness and sensory deficits in a radial neuropathy depend on the location and extent of the injury. Proximally in the arm, radial nerve injury may lead to weakness of the triceps, wrist extensors, and finger extensors, along with sensory changes down the posterior aspect of the arm and in the lateral three and a half fingers in the dorsum of the hand. Injuries in the forearm may cause an incomplete syndrome with injuries to the superficial sensory branch or PIN only.

Given the strong association with humeral injuries, radiographs are frequently indicated to rule out a fracture.[32]

SCIATIC NEUROPATHY

Sciatic neuropathy is one of the more common focal neuropathies seen in the inpatient setting due to the frequency of nerve injury with hip and femur fractures and surgical repairs. The sciatic nerve is made up of fibers from the L4-S3 nerve roots, which descend from the lumbosacral plexus into the gluteal region, through the sciatic notch, then down the posterior thigh. Just above the popliteal fossa, the nerve bifurcates into the common peroneal and tibial nerves. Of note, the sciatic nerve maintains a somatotopic map of peroneal and tibial fibers, with peroneal fibers running more laterally.

Injury to the sciatic nerve can happen anywhere along its course. One of the more frequent locations of injury is near the sciatic notch, and this can be seen after hip surgery in up to 33% of cases or after hip fracture or dislocation.[33] Given the anatomic relationship between the femur, sciatic notch, and sciatic nerve, selective injury of the peroneal fibers is often seen and can mimic a common peroneal neuropathy

(**Fig. 2**).[34] Other causes of traumatic injury to the sciatic nerve include laceration or intragluteal injection directly into the nerve, including vaccines or other drugs.[35] Compressive injuries may occur from a posterior thigh compartment syndrome, hematoma, fibrous bands, or tumors (compressive or infiltrative).[36–38] Stretch- and traction-based injuries have been seen due to lithotomy positioning during vaginal delivery or certain gynecologic procedures.[39,40]

A complete sciatic neuropathy will result in weakness of all muscles below the knee and knee flexion, as well as significant sensory loss below the knee on the posterior and anterolateral aspect of the leg and the entirety of the foot. The ankle jerk reflex will be diminished. Sciatic neuropathies are often painful and may lead to shooting pains down the leg. The differential for a sciatic neuropathy includes lumbosacral radiculopathy or plexus injury, which may require electromyography and nerve conduction studies (EMG/NCS) and/or magnetic resonance neurography to distinguish.

PERONEAL NEUROPATHY

The peroneal nerve is formed from one of the terminal branches of the sciatic nerve. Above the knee, the peroneal fibers run laterally around the fibular head before separating into the deep and superficial branches. The superficial fibers innervate the peroneus longus and brevis—ankle evertors—and supply sensory information to the lateral calf and top of the foot. The deep peroneal nerve fibers provide motor innervation to the tibialis anterior, the main foot dorsiflexor, and additional toe extensors in the foot.

The most common site of injury is at the fibular neck and frequently occurs due to traction, compression, or laceration. Causes in hospitalized patients include direct

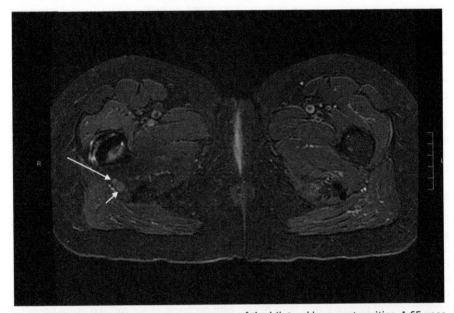

Fig. 2. Axial T2 magnetic resonance neurogram of the bilateral lower extremities. A 65-year-old woman who underwent a prolonged right hip arthroplasty with postoperative foot weakness and sensory deficits below the knee. The arrows point to the right sciatic nerve and show increased caliber due to intrafascicular edema at the level of the lesser trochanter. The nerve demonstrates a bifid morphology. The lateral branch (*long arrow*) gives rise to the peroneal fibers, whereas the medial branch (*short arrow*) gives rise to the tibial fibers.

manipulation during knee orthopedic surgery, prolonged bed rest, surgical positioning (particularly lateral hip rotation and knee flexion as is common in obstetric and gynecologic procedures), and compression from surgical positioning devices (ie, lithotomy knee stirrups).[41–46]

Weight loss is another risk factor for peroneal neuropathy, and patients with greater than 20 pounds of weight loss in 2 to 3 months are at particularly increased risk.[44] Bariatric surgery can be associated with development of bilateral peroneal neuropathies due to rapid weight loss.[45]

The most typical presentation of a common peroneal neuropathy is a foot drop, and this may be subtle and manifest with slight dragging of the toes while walking, whereas in more fulminant cases, the patient may have a frank steppage gait. Numbness, paresthesia, and pain in the lateral calf and top of the foot may be present, and the examiner may elicit a Tinel sign at the fibular head. Differential diagnosis includes L5 radiculopathy, lumbar plexopathy, or sciatic neuropathy. As described earlier, injury of the sciatic nerve more proximally may mimic a peroneal neuropathy due to the organization of nerve fibers and should always be on the differential of a common peroneal neuropathy; EMG/NCS of the leg and magnetic resonance neurography may be required to distinguish between these 2 possibilities.[46] An L5 radiculopathy can often be differentiated from a peroneal neuropathy by finding weakness of foot inversion, which reflects contribution of L5 to the tibial nerve.

In the case of compressive common peroneal neuropathies, avoidance of compression by adding cushioning near the fibular head may be helpful. An ankle foot orthotic may be used to help keep the foot dorsiflexed to aid in walking and prevent contractures until the patient is able to dorsiflex the foot.[47]

LATERAL FEMORAL CUTANEOUS NEUROPATHY

The lateral femoral cutaneous nerve of the thigh is a pure sensory nerve derived directly from the lumbar plexus. It provides sensory information from the anterolateral thigh. Because of its location near the inguinal ligament, it can easily be entrapped. When injured, it may lead to numbness and painful paresthesia over the anterior and lateral thigh without weakness, a syndrome known as "meralgia paresthetica."[48] Risk factors include obesity or rapid weight gain, diabetes mellitus, or direct compression (eg, by a belt or tight clothing).[49] Pregnant patients are at increased risk in general and may develop meralgia paresthetica during vaginal delivery due to prolonged hip flexion.[50]

Decreasing nerve compression is the mainstay of treatment, which may be achieved by weight loss and avoidance of tight/compressive garments. Management of diabetes may be helpful in the diabetic patient. Delivery of the fetus in pregnant patients often leads to complete reversal of symptoms.[50]

PREGNANCY, OBSTETRIC SURGERY, AND GYNECOLOGIC SURGERY

Peripheral nerve injury is a potential complication of childbirth, with obstetric neurologic injuries occurring in up to 2% of patients, although most are mild and resolve quickly.[51] Nerve compression in the pelvis by the fetal head and other external structures is the most common mechanism of injury, followed by ischemia and transection.[52] Anesthesia related to pregnancy and obstetric procedures is a risk factor, given that neuraxial blockade leads to less patient-initiated repositioning, decreased awareness of paresthesia or weakness that signal nerve injury, and more prolonged lithotomy position.[53] Other risk factors include prolonged second stage of labor and instrumented delivery.[51]

The femoral nerve may be injured in childbirth due to stretching or compression across the inguinal ligament, particularly during the lithotomy position.[54] Femoral neuropathies typically present with weakness of knee extension and depending on how proximal the lesion is, hip flexion as well. Sensory symptoms are seen over the anterior thigh and medial calf. The patellar reflex will be diminished or absent. The differential includes L2/3/4 radiculopathy or lumbar plexopathy and if symptoms are bilateral, the cauda equina, conus medullaris, or spinal cord. In bilateral cases, an MRI should be completed to rule out a central lesion. Prognosis is excellent, and patients generally experience a full or near-full recovery.[51,54]

The lithotomy position may lead to other neuropathies in the pregnant patient, such as common peroneal nerve compression from use of lithotomy supports.[40] In addition, this position predisposes the obturator nerve to stretch near the obturator foramen.[52] Patients with obturator neuropathy will often present with pain in the groin, anterior, or medial thigh, and there may be weakness of hip adduction on the side of the injury as well. The obturator nerve may also be injured during birth by compression from the fetal head against the pelvis.

Gynecologic surgery has among the highest rates of perioperative nerve complications, affecting approximately 2% of patients.[55] The most common mechanisms of injury are compression, stretch, or transection of nerve fibers. Transection injuries are most frequently related to incorrect surgical incision site.

Iatrogenic femoral nerve injury most commonly occurs after gynecologic surgery largely due to retractor use in abdominal hysterectomy or lithotomy position.[56,57] It is also important to consider the possibility of a plexopathy due to retroperitoneal hematoma or abscess, and computed tomography imaging of the pelvis may be necessary.[58]

The ilioinguinal and iliohypogastric nerves may also be injured, most commonly by suture entrapment at the lateral borders of the rectus abdominus muscle, particular after a Pfannenstiel incision.[59,60] Ilioinguinal injuries are more common than iliohypogastric injuries. Injury to the ilioinguinal nerve is characterized by sensory changes and pain in the mons pubis, labia majora, and proximal anterolateral thigh. The Tinel sign, elicited by tapping at the location of the nerve, may aid in diagnoses. Treatment usually involves neuropathic pain agents, local nerve blocks, or repeat surgery for decompression.[60]

Other less commonly injured nerves associated with gynecologic surgery include the obturator, pudendal, and genitofemoral nerves.[61]

A summary of injuries associated with pregnancy and obstetric and gynecologic surgery can be found in **Table 2**.

ORTHOPEDIC SURGERY

Sciatic neuropathies, which can occur as a complication of hip and femur surgery, have already been reviewed. Shoulder surgeries may cause focal injuries to the brachial plexus, cervical roots, or terminal nerve branches, particularly those nerves originating from the posterior and lateral cords (ie, axillary, radial, and median).[62] Traction is the most common mechanism of injury to these nerves, particularly following prosthetic arthroplasty or open surgery for treatment of shoulder instability.[63] Other causes of nerve injury include suture entrapment or nerve laceration.

CARDIOTHORACIC SURGERY

Phrenic nerve injury is commonly seen after cardiac surgery. The nerve originates from the third, fourth, and fifth cervical nerve roots and descends in the thorax to the

Table 2
Common nerve injuries associated with hospital procedures

Procedure	Nerve/Plexus Injuries	Common Risk Factors
Gynecologic/obstetric surgery & pregnancy	Femoral nerve Ilioinguinal/iliohypogastric nerve Obturator nerve Pudendal nerve Genitofemoral nerve Peroneal Nerve	• Stretching secondary to lithotomy positioning • Compression against inguinal ligament • Pfannenstiel incision • Suture entrapment • Stretch secondary to lithotomy positioning • Entrapment in sacrospinous ligament fixation • Compression/laceration during pelvic sidewall surgery • Compression against hard external surface
Orthopedic surgery	Sciatic nerve Brachial plexopathy	• Trauma/compression near the sciatic notch • Laceration • Traction injury after surgeries for shoulder instability • Suture entrapment
Cardiothoracic surgery	Phrenic nerve Long thoracic nerve	• "Ice-Slush" injury • Improper incision site • Sternal retraction
General anesthesia	Ulnar nerve Brachial plexus	• Compression/stretch against coronoid process • Traction injury secondary to arm positioning compression • Inflammatory reaction

diaphragm. The principle cause of injury is topical hypothermia due to the "ice-slush" used for myocardial protection during these procedures, with the left phrenic nerve being most susceptible due to its course near the heart.[64] The phrenic nerve may also be injured in internal mammary artery dissection.[64] Injury of the phrenic nerve leads to hemidiaphragm weakness, which can be evaluated with chest radiography, fluoroscopy, and ultrasonography, as well as delayed nerve conduction studies and electromyography.[65] Many patients with unilateral injury do not experience symptoms due to accessory muscle recruitment, but dyspnea with moderate physical activity or nocturnal orthopnea may be noted. Most of the phrenic neuropathies after coronary artery bypass grafting recover by 3 to 6 months.[66] Cardiac insulation pads may help decrease the risk of cold-induced phrenic neuropathies.[67]

The long thoracic nerve is also susceptible to injury during cardiac surgery, as well as during mastectomies and thoracotomies. It originates from the C5-C7 roots and innervates the serratus anterior muscle. In cardiac surgery, injury can occur due to improper incision site, sternal retraction, and positioning of the limbs in relation to the head and neck, thereby placing traction on the brachial plexus.[68,69] The serratus anterior muscle helps stabilize the scapula against the ribcage. Weakness can lead to a "winged scapula" (**Fig. 3**), wherein the shoulder blade protrudes abnormally from the back with shoulder flexion, limiting the ability to raise the arm above the head.[70] In some cases, nerve transfer or thoracic fixation surgery may be required.[71]

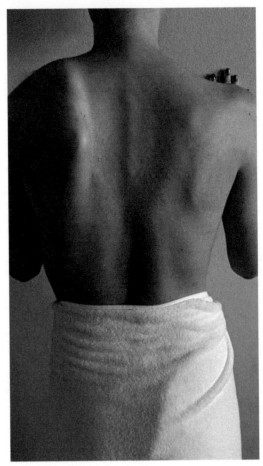

Fig. 3. A 30-year-old woman with a left-winged scapula due to injury of the left long thoracic nerve.

MULTIPLE MONONEUROPATHIES

In patients with multiple mononeuropathies occurring simultaneously or in rapid succession, it is important to maintain a high index of suspicion for inflammatory and vasculitic causes of neuropathy, particularly when pain is prominent.[72] A broad workup for primary and secondary causes of vasculitis should ensue accompanied by 4 limb EMG and NCS to fully characterize the neuropathy and rule out mimics (other inflammatory or demyelinating neuropathies). Nerve biopsy may be necessary before initiating treatment with immunosuppressive agents.[73]

In patients with recurrent mononeuropathies in locations susceptible to compression, an important diagnostic consideration is hereditary neuropathy with liability to pressure palsy.[74] Nerves in the brachial plexus and cranial nerves may even be involved. Avoidance of compression (eg, with situational awareness and protective equipment) is the mainstay of treatment.[74]

EVALUATION

Electrodiagnostic studies (with nerve conduction studies and electromyography) can help localize and characterize the severity of a focal neuropathy, allow for monitoring of nerve regrowth, and help assess prognosis and whether a patient may benefit from nerve repair surgery.

If axonal injury occurs, nerve conduction studies may show reduced compound muscle action potential amplitude in muscles distal to the site of nerve injury as early as a few days following the insult, depending on the rate of Wallerian degeneration. Alternatively, conduction block or focal slowing along a nerve segment may point to a primarily demyelinating injury. Sensory nerve action potentials (SNAPs) will usually be decreased 8 to 10 days after a nerve injury and often help with the differential of a nerve injury versus radicular injury, as the latter will be associated with normal SNAPs due to the preganglionic site of injury. Electromyography can detect active denervation in muscles supplied by an affected nerve. However, these changes may not be seen until up to 3 to 4 weeks after injury, and electrodiagnostic studies are most informative after this period. Repeat studies completed serially over months may help with prognostication by determining whether sprouting nerve fibers are able to find their target tissue.

Ultrasound may be helpful in the rapid assessment of peripheral nerve injury, granted the site of injury is within the ultrasound's field of view.[75] The use of magnetic resonance neurography has increased in recent years, including evaluation for T2 signal change in the nerves at the site of injury. The addition of diffusion-weighted imaging and diffusion tensor imaging provides valuable information about axon integrity,[76] and this may allow experienced neuroradiologists to describe the injury using Seddon's classification system, which assists with surgical determination and prognosis.[77]

TREATMENT

Treatment and prognosis generally depend on the mechanism and extent of neuropathy. A careful physical examination including detailed testing of strength, sensation, and reflexes is critical to localize the neuropathy and monitor recovery.[4] Sharp transecting nerve injuries may require urgent operative intervention within 72 hours to avoid nerve stump retraction.[78] A large percentage of iatrogenic injuries are neuropraxic in nature; most neuropathies with primarily sensory deficits may resolve in approximately 1 week, whereas those with motor deficits generally take 3 months or longer.[4]

Pain is a prominent component of many focal neuropathies and may require treatment with neuropathic pain agents.[79] Physical and occupational therapy has a role in helping patients regain strength and maintain flexibility and range of motion.[80] Depending on the limb injured, bracing and orthotics may be provided. In patients with sensory deficits, situational awareness and regular skin checks should be encouraged to avoid further injury.

In select cases, the nerve may not be able to heal without surgical intervention. The gold-standard treatment is direct end-to-end microsurgical epineural nerve repair, but other techniques including nerve grafting or nerve transfers have been associated with significant functional improvement in certain patients.[81] Research into further use of nerve conduits, stem cells, and gene therapy is currently underway.[82]

SUMMARY

Neurologists may encounter focal neuropathies in the hospital setting either related to the patient's presenting condition or due to events occurring during hospitalization. Common mechanisms of nerve injury include compression, stretch/traction, or direct trauma (eg, during surgical procedures). A careful history and physical examination are critical for prompt, accurate diagnosis and to monitor recovery. EMG/NCS and neuroimaging may play a role in select cases to help localize the neuropathy and determine prognosis but are usually most helpful 3 to 4 weeks after the injury. Treatment usually includes physical and occupational therapy and pain management. Most patients experience spontaneous and almost complete recovery, although nerve surgery may be required in select patients. For more severe neuropathies, posthospitalization follow-up with a neurologist, neuromuscular specialist, and/or neurosurgeon is recommended to monitor recovery and determine if additional interventions are necessary.

CLINICS CARE POINTS

- Iatrogenic peripheral nerve injury in the hospitalized patient most frequently occurs due to stretch or compression.
- The type and extent of nerve fiber damage predict the overall prognosis for recovery. Axon regrowth occurs at 1 mm per day.
- Nerve repair surgery is indicated in complete transection injuries or if no spontaneous recovery is detected within a few months of injury.
- EMG/NCS can help localize and characterize a focal neuropathy and is most informative when obtained at least 3 weeks following neuropathy onset.
- Magnetic resonance neurography is increasingly being used to diagnose focal neuropathies and to determine prognosis and appropriateness for nerve repair surgery.

DISCLOSURE

The authors have nothing to disclose.

REFERENCES

1. Seddon RJ. Surgical experiences with peripheral nerve injuries. Q Bull Northwest Univ Med Sch 1947;21(3):201–10.
2. Sunderland S. The anatomy and physiology of nerve injury. Muscle Nerve 1990; 13(9):771–84.
3. Lolis AM, Falsone S, Beric A. Common peripheral nerve injuries in sport: diagnosis and management. Handb Clin Neurol 2018;158:401–19.
4. Ferrante MA. The Assessment and Management of Peripheral Nerve Trauma. Curr Treat Options Neurol 2018;20(7):25.
5. Eder M, Schulte-Mattler W, Pöschl P. Neurographic course Of Wallerian degeneration after human peripheral nerve injury. Muscle Nerve 2017;56(2):247–52.
6. Smith BW, Sakamuri S, Spain DA, et al. An update on the management of adult traumatic nerve injuries-replacing old paradigms: A review. J Trauma Acute Care Surg 2019;86(2):299–306.
7. Bhandari PS. Management of peripheral nerve injury. J Clin Orthop Trauma 2019; 10(5):862–6.
8. Kaya Y, Sarikcioglu L. Sir Herbert Seddon (1903-1977) and his classification scheme for peripheral nerve injury. Childs Nerv Syst 2015;31(2):177–80.
9. Warner MA, Warner DO, Matsumoto JY, et al. Ulnar neuropathy in surgical patients. Anesthesiology 1999;90(1):54–9.
10. Chui J, Murkin JM, Posner KL, et al. Perioperative Peripheral Nerve Injury After General Anesthesia: A Qualitative Systematic Review. Anesth Analg 2018; 127(1):134–43.

11. Matev B. Cubital Tunnel Syndrome. Hand Surg 2003;08(01):127–31.

12. Contreras MG, Warner MA, Charboneau WJ, et al. Anatomy of the ulnar nerve at the elbow: potential relationship of acute ulnar neuropathy to gender differences. Clin Anat 1998;11(6):372–8.

13. Perreault L, Drolet P, Farny J. Ulnar nerve palsy at the elbow after general anaesthesia. Can J Anaesth 1992;39(5 Pt 1):499–503.

14. Dy CJ, Mackinnon SE. Ulnar neuropathy: evaluation and management. Curr Rev Musculoskelet Med 2016;9(2):178–84.

15. Caetano EB, Sabongi Neto JJ, Vieira LA, et al. The arcade of Struthers: an anatomical study and clinical implications. Rev Bras Ortop 2017;52(3):331–6.

16. Caliandro P, La Torre G, Padua R, et al. Treatment for ulnar neuropathy at the elbow. Cochrane Database Syst Rev 2016;11:CD006839.

17. Cheney FW, Domino KB, Caplan RA, et al. Nerve Injury Associated with Anesthesia : A Closed Claims Analysis. Anesthesiology 1999;90(4):1062–9.

18. Gross PT, Tolomeo EA. PROXIMAL MEDIAN NEUROPATHIES. Neurol Clin 1999; 17(3):425–45.

19. Sheetal S, Byju P, Manoj P. Ischemic monomelic neuropathy. J Postgrad Med 2017;63(1):42–3.

20. Wong L, Dellon AL. Brachial neuritis presenting as anterior interosseous nerve compression—Implications for diagnosis and treatment: A case report. J Hand Surg 1997;22(3):536–9.

21. Bland JDP. Carpal tunnel syndrome. Curr Opin Neurol 2005;18(5):581–5.

22. Ezzat S, Forster MJ, Berchtold P, et al. Acromegaly. Clinical and biochemical features in 500 patients. Medicine (Baltimore) 1994;73(5):233–40.

23. Padua L, Di Pasquale A, Pazzaglia C, et al. Systematic review of pregnancy-related carpal tunnel syndrome. Muscle Nerve 2010;42(5):697–702.

24. van Dijk MAJ, Reitsma JB, Fischer JC, et al. Indications for requesting laboratory tests for concurrent diseases in patients with carpal tunnel syndrome: a systematic review. Clin Chem 2003;49(9):1437–44.

25. Tenosynovial and Cardiac Amyloidosis in Patients Undergoing Carpal Tunnel Release | Journal of the American College of Cardiology. Available at: https://www.jacc.org/doi/full/10.1016/j.jacc.2018.07.092. Accessed April 20, 2021.

26. ANTERIOR INTEROSSEOUS NERVE LESIONS | The Bone & Joint Journal. Available at: https://online.boneandjoint.org.uk/doi/abs/10.1302/0301-620X.78B2.0780238. Accessed April 20, 2021.

27. Floranda EE, Jacobs BC. Evaluation and treatment of upper extremity nerve entrapment syndromes. Prim Care 2013;40(4):925–943, ix.

28. Bumbasirevic M, Palibrk T, Lesic A, et al. Radial nerve palsy. EFORT Open Rev 2016;1(8):286–94.

29. Midroni G, Moulton R. Radial entrapment neuropathy due to chronic injection-induced triceps fibrosis. Muscle Nerve 2001;24(1):134–7.

30. Nelson G. Radial nerve compression due to lipoma. J Vis Commun Med 2007; 30(2):84–5.

31. Yang JS, Cho YJ, Kang SH, et al. Neuralgic Amyotrophy Manifesting as Mimicking Posterior Interosseous Nerve Palsy. J Korean Neurosurg Soc 2015; 58(5):491–3.

32. Entrapment Neuropathies in the Upper and Lower Limbs: Anatomy and MRI Features. Available at: https://www.hindawi.com/journals/rrp/2012/230679/. Accessed April 20, 2021.

33. Plewnia C, Wallace C, Zochodne D. Traumatic sciatic neuropathy: a novel cause, local experience, and a review of the literature. J Trauma 1999;47(5):986–91.

34. Sunderland S. The relative susceptibility to injury of the medial and lateral popliteal divisions of the sciatic nerve. Br J Surg 1953;41(167):300–2.

35. Mishra P, Stringer MD. Sciatic nerve injury from intramuscular injection: a persistent and global problem. Int J Clin Pract 2010;64(11):1573–9.

36. Feinberg J, Sethi S. Sciatic Neuropathy: Case Report and Discussion of the Literature on Postoperative Sciatic Neuropathy and Sciatic Nerve Tumors. HSS J 2006;2(2):181–7.

37. Tani JC. Fibrous band compression of the tibial nerve branch of the sciatic nerve. Am J Orthop (Belle Mead Nj) 1995;24(12):910–2.

38. Distad BJ, Weiss MD. Clinical and Electrodiagnostic Features of Sciatic Neuropathies. Phys Med Rehabil Clin N Am 2013;24(1):107–20.

39. Romfh JH, Currier RD. Sciatic neuropathy induced by the lithotomy position. Arch Neurol 1983;40(2):127.

40. Burkhart FL, Daly JW. Sciatic and peroneal nerve injury: a complication of vaginal operations. Obstet Gynecol 1966;28(1):99–102.

41. Baima J, Krivickas L. Evaluation and treatment of peroneal neuropathy. Curr Rev Musculoskelet Med 2008;1(2):147–53.

42. Feinberg JH, Nadler SF, Krivickas LS. Peripheral nerve injuries in the athlete. Sports Med 1997;24(6):385–408.

43. Nercessian OA, Ugwonali OFC, Park S. Peroneal Nerve Palsy After Total Knee Arthroplasty. J Arthroplasty 2005;20(8):1068–73.

44. Sotaniemi KA. Slimmer's paralysis–peroneal neuropathy during weight reduction. J Neurol Neurosurg Psychiatry 1984;47(5):564–6.

45. Fares MY, Dimassi Z, Fares J, et al. Peroneal neuropathy and bariatric surgery: untying the knot. Int J Neurosci 2020;130(4):417–23.

46. Van Langenhove M, Pollefliet A, Vanderstraeten G. A retrospective electrodiagnostic evaluation of footdrop in 303 patients. Electromyogr Clin Neurophysiol 1989;29(3):145–52.

47. Garozzo D, Ferraresi S, Buffatti P. Surgical treatment of common peroneal nerve injuries: indications and results. A series of 62 cases. J Neurosurg Sci 2004;48(3):105–12.

48. Harney D, Patijn J. Meralgia paresthetica: diagnosis and management strategies. Pain Med 2007;8(8):669–77.

49. Parisi TJ, Mandrekar J, Dyck PJB, et al. Meralgia paresthetica: relation to obesity, advanced age, and diabetes mellitus. Neurology 2011;77(16):1538–42.

50. Sax TW, Rosenbaum RB. Neuromuscular disorders in pregnancy. Muscle Nerve 2006;34(5):559–71.

51. Richards A, McLaren T, Paech MJ, et al. Immediate postpartum neurological deficits in the lower extremity: a prospective observational study. Int J Obstet Anesth 2017;31:5–12.

52. Harper RL, Eckford SD, Williams H, et al. Obstetric neurological injuries. Obstetrician & Gynaecologist 2020;22(4):305–12.

53. Moen V, Dahlgren N, Irestedt L. Severe neurological complications after central neuraxial blockades in Sweden 1990-1999. Anesthesiology 2004;101(4):950–9.

54. O'Neal MA. Lower Extremity Weakness and Numbness in the Postpartum Period: A Case-Based Review. Neurol Clin 2019;37(1):103–11.

55. Cardosi RJ, Cox CS, Hoffman MS. Postoperative neuropathies after major pelvic surgery. Obstet Gynecol 2002;100(2):240–4.

56. Chan JK, Manetta A. Prevention of femoral nerve injuries in gynecologic surgery. Am J Obstet Gynecol 2002;186(1):1–7.

57. Goldman JA, Feldberg D, Dicker D, et al. Femoral neuropathy subsequent to abdominal hysterectomy. A comparative study. Eur J Obstet Gynecol Reprod Biol 1985;20(6):385–92.

58. Parmer SS, Carpenter JP, Fairman RM, et al. Femoral neuropathy following retroperitoneal hemorrhage: case series and review of the literature. Ann Vasc Surg 2006;20(4):536–40.

59. Loos MJ, Scheltinga MR, Mulders LG, et al. The Pfannenstiel incision as a source of chronic pain. Obstet Gynecol 2008;111(4):839–46.

60. Whiteside JL, Barber MD, Walters MD, et al. Anatomy of ilioinguinal and iliohypogastric nerves in relation to trocar placement and low transverse incisions. Am J Obstet Gynecol 2003;189(6):1574–8 ; discussion 1578.

61. Kuponiyi O, Alleemudder DI, Latunde-Dada A, et al. Nerve injuries associated with gynaecological surgery. The Obstetrician & Gynaecologist 2014;16(1): 29–36.

62. Ball CM. Neurologic complications of shoulder joint replacement. J Shoulder Elbow Surg 2017;26(12):2125–32.

63. Richards RR, Hudson AR, Bertoia JT, et al. Injury to the brachial plexus during Putti-Platt and Bristow procedures. A report of eight cases. Am J Sports Med 1987;15(4):374–80.

64. O'Brien JW, Johnson SH, VanSteyn SJ, et al. Effects of internal mammary artery dissection on phrenic nerve perfusion and function. Ann Thorac Surg 1991;52(2): 182–8.

65. Nason LK, Walker CM, McNeeley MF, et al. Imaging of the diaphragm: anatomy and function. Radiographics 2012;32(2):E51–70.

66. Tripp HF, Bolton JW. Phrenic nerve injury following cardiac surgery: a review. J Card Surg 1998;13(3):218–23.

67. Esposito RA, Spencer FC. The effect of pericardial insulation on hypothermic phrenic nerve injury during open-heart surgery. Ann Thorac Surg 1987;43(3): 303–8.

68. Gozna ER, Harris WR. Traumatic winging of the scapula. J Bone Joint Surg Am 1979;61(8):1230–3.

69. Vahl CF, Carl I, Müller-Vahl H, et al. Brachial plexus injury after cardiac surgery. The role of internal mammary artery preparation: a prospective study on 1000 consecutive patients. J Thorac Cardiovasc Surg 1991;102(5):724–9.

70. Warner JJ, Navarro RA. Serratus anterior dysfunction. Recognition and treatment. Clin Orthop Relat Res 1998;349:139–48.

71. Vetter M, Charran O, Yilmaz E, et al. Winged Scapula: A Comprehensive Review of Surgical Treatment. Cureus. 9(12). doi:10.7759/cureus.1923

72. Collins MP, Hadden RD. The nonsystemic vasculitic neuropathies. Nat Rev Neurol 2017;13(5):302–16.

73. Mathew L, Talbot K, Love S, et al. Treatment of vasculitic peripheral neuropathy: a retrospective analysis of outcome. QJM 2007;100(1):41–51.

74. Potulska-Chromik A, Sinkiewicz-Darol E, Ryniewicz B, et al. Clinical, electrophysiological, and molecular findings in early onset hereditary neuropathy with liability to pressure palsy. Muscle Nerve 2014;50(6):914–8.

75. Pham M, Bäumer T, Bendszus M. Peripheral nerves and plexus: imaging by MR-neurography and high-resolution ultrasound. Curr Opin Neurol 2014;27(4):370–9.

76. Martín Noguerol T, Barousse R, Gómez Cabrera M, et al. Functional MR Neurography in Evaluation of Peripheral Nerve Trauma and Postsurgical Assessment. RadioGraphics 2019;39(2):427–46.

77. Martín Noguerol T, Barousse R, Socolovsky M, et al. Quantitative magnetic resonance (MR) neurography for evaluation of peripheral nerves and plexus injuries. Quant Imaging Med Surg 2017;7(4):398–421.

78. Campbell WW. Evaluation and management of peripheral nerve injury. Clin Neurophysiol 2008;119(9):1951–65.

79. Brooks KG, Brooks TLK, author KG. Treatments for neuropathic pain. Pharm J. Available at: https://pharmaceutical-journal.com/article/research/treatments-for-neuropathic-pain. Accessed April 20, 2021.

80. Suszyński K, Marcol W, Górka D. Physiotherapeutic techniques used in the management of patients with peripheral nerve injuries. Neural Regen Res 2015; 10(11):1770–2.

81. Griffin JW, Hogan MV, Chhabra AB, et al. Peripheral Nerve Repair and Reconstruction. JBJS 2013;95(23):2144–51.

82. Panagopoulos Georgios N, Megaloikonomos Panayiotis D, Mavrogenis Andreas F. The Present and Future for Peripheral Nerve Regeneration. Orthopedics 2017;40(1):e141–56.

Neurologic Complications of Surgery and Anesthesia

Daniel Talmasov, MD[a], Joshua P. Klein, MD, PhD[b],*

KEYWORDS

- Surgery • Anesthesia • Complication • Stroke • Myasthenia • Antiplatelet
- Anticoagulation

KEY POINTS

- The most common cause of early postoperative stroke after cardiac or aortic vascular surgery is a thromboembolism resulting from a new cardiac arrythmia, typically postoperative atrial fibrillation.
- Factors to be considered when deciding if and how to interrupt antithrombotic therapy for surgery include the types of antithrombotic medicines a patient is taking, the bleeding risk of the surgery itself, and the degree of underlying vascular risk.
- For patients taking antiplatelet medications for a neurovascular indication, it is generally advised to hold antiplatelet therapy before elective surgery, for a period of time equivalent to the average platelet lifespan (7–10 days).
- Patients who remain somnolent or hypoactive for a prolonged period of time following surgery or those who awaken but seem confused, inattentive, disoriented, or agitated should be evaluated for common causes of encephalopathy, including reversible and treatable infections and metabolic abnormalities.

INTRODUCTION

Surgery and anesthesia carry risks of ischemic, hemorrhagic, hypoxic, and metabolic complications, all of which can result in neurologic symptoms and deficits. Patients with underlying cardiovascular and cerebrovascular risk factors are particularly vulnerable. The authors review here the neurologic complications of surgery and anesthesia, with a focus on the role of the neurologic consultant in preoperative evaluation and risk stratification and diagnosis and management of postoperative complications.

[a] Department of Neurology, New York University School of Medicine, 222 East 41st Street, 14th Floor, New York, NY 10017, USA; [b] Department of Neurology, Brigham and Women's Hospital, Harvard Medical School, Room 4018, 60 Fenwood Road, Boston 02115, MA, USA
* Corresponding author.
E-mail address: jpklein@bwh.harvard.edu

Neurol Clin 40 (2022) 191–209
https://doi.org/10.1016/j.ncl.2021.08.014
0733-8619/22/© 2021 Elsevier Inc. All rights reserved.

PREOPERATIVE NEUROLOGIC EVALUATION
The Role of Neurologists in the Preoperative Evaluation: Risk Stratification, Antithrombotic Management, and Establishment of a Neurologic Baseline

Neurologists are often called by surgical or anesthesia teams to consult on patients anticipating surgery. Most commonly, the goal of such a consultation is to assess the risk of periprocedural neurologic complications, principally stroke, and to aid in preventing these outcomes. Neurologists play an important role in the preoperative evaluation by stratifying patients according to their degree of underlying neurovascular risk factors including any preexisting burden of neurovascular disease, by guiding the periprocedural management of antithrombotic medications, and by establishing a preoperative neurologic baseline for comparison, should concern for an acute stroke arise during or after the surgery.

Preoperative evaluation: establishing a preoperative neurologic baseline—correlating the examination and neuroimaging

When consulting on a preoperative patient, neurohospitalists should perform a careful and meticulous neurologic examination to establish and document a preoperative baseline; this will be an important standard for comparison should concern for a new neurologic deficit arise postoperatively. If the evaluation raises concern for preexisting neurologic disease, either by history or via some abnormality on neurologic examination, available studies pertinent to the localization should be reviewed or obtained if not previously evaluated. Any abnormal findings revealed on imaging should be correlated to the preoperative neurologic examination.

Preoperative evaluation: neurovascular risk stratification

Average lifespan has increased in recent years, in part due to improvements in living conditions and disease prevention but also as a consequence of advances in treatments aimed at reducing complications of otherwise highly morbid medical conditions. As a result, the medical complexity of the average surgical patient has increased.[1] Patients undergoing surgery, especially cardiac or vascular surgery, are thus more likely to have significant underlying risk factors for stroke—including hypertension, hyperlipidemia, diabetes mellitus, or a history of prior stroke or transient ischemic attack (TIA). Part of the role of a neurologist can be to assist surgical teams in weighing the risk of surgery—for example, patients with a history of recent ischemic stroke (within 3 months) were found to have a much higher risk of major cardiovascular complications (odds ratio 14.23; 95% confidence interval 11.61–17.45), with risk plateauing at about 9 months after ischemic stroke.[2] It is therefore recommended that elective surgery be deferred for at least 9 months after an ischemic stroke.[1]

Many surgical patients will already be on antithrombotic therapy for stroke prevention, via antiplatelet therapies (eg, aspirin or clopidogrel) and/or anticoagulants (eg, warfarin, direct oral anticoagulants). Because continuation of antiplatelet or antithrombotic agents through surgery can carry a risk of catastrophic intraoperative or postoperative bleeding, surgical teams will often consult neurologists to assist in stratifying the risk of ischemic stroke when interrupting these therapies.

Preoperative evaluation: types of antithrombotic medicines in use

Secondary stroke prevention is a rapidly evolving landscape, with several innovations in recent years affecting standard of care. Among these is the use of short-term dual antiplatelet therapy (DAPT, a combination of aspirin and clopidogrel most commonly) in patients following a TIA or minor stroke and the use of direct oral anticoagulants (DOACs) rather than warfarin for stroke prevention in patients with nonvalvular chronic atrial fibrillation.[3] Furthermore, reversal agents for DOACs have been developed; their availability increases the safety profile of DOACs.[1] Consulting neurologists should be familiar with common neurologic indications and the typical course of therapy for all of the aforementioned medicines. This, together with a knowledge of their pharmacokinetics, will guide the neurohospitalist in navigating the interruption and resumption of antiplatelet and antithrombotic therapy perioperatively.

Certain conditions call for anticoagulation over antiplatelet therapy for more effective long-term cardioembolic stroke prevention. These conditions include nonvalvular atrial fibrillation, heart failure with a left ventricular ejection fraction under 35%, a known atrial thrombus, an acute anterior ST-elevation myocardial infarction with apical wall-motion abnormalities, the presence of a left ventricular assistance device (LVAD), rheumatic valvular heart disease, and the presence of a mechanical valve.[3] Of these, the most common is atrial fibrillation, the prevalence of which is increasing with aging of the population.[3] For patients with atrial fibrillation, scoring systems such as CHA_2DS_2-VASc have been developed to estimate the annual risk of stroke and guide decision-making regarding initiation of anticoagulation.[4] More recently, the DOACs are replacing warfarin as standard therapy, with the key advantage of DOACs being a simpler pharmacokinetic profile, leading to simpler dosing strategies without need for frequent laboratory monitoring, a faster onset and offset of action, fewer drug interactions, and studies showing both noninferiority to warfarin and a superior safety profile.

Perioperative management—interrupting and resuming antithrombotic medicines

Approximately 10% to 15% of patients on long-term anticoagulation for atrial fibrillation will require interruption of anticoagulant treatment of an elective surgical procedure.[5–7] Factors to be considered when deciding if and how to interrupt antithrombotic therapy include the types of antithrombotic medicines a patient is taking, the bleeding risk of the surgery/procedure itself, and the degree of underlying vascular risk in a patient. In some cases, antithrombotic medicines need not be interrupted before surgery at all, in others they will need to be discontinued preoperatively and later resumed. Finally, in some cases, it may be wiser to postpone a procedure (ie, in the case of elective surgery) until a patient's vascular risk profile has become more favorable, such as in patients who experienced an ischemic stroke less than 9 months ago.[1,2]

The timing of when to interrupt and resume the dosing of anticoagulants depends on pharmacokinetic properties of the specific agent being used (**Table 1**). Additional considerations include bleeding risk associated with the surgery (a surgical consideration that in some cases may extend the window of time postoperatively for which anticoagulation remains interrupted) and the urgency of surgery.

Whether to bridge anticoagulant therapy

Two major trials have assessed the risks and benefits of providing an anticoagulant "bridging" therapy, which is done via dosing a shorter-acting anticoagulant while a patient's primary anticoagulant (warfarin or a DOAC) was held preprocedurally. Both the BRIDGE (in which patients were taking warfarin) and PAUSE (in which patients were taking apixaban or rivaroxaban) trials found no benefit to providing bridging anticoagulation preoperatively, as anticoagulants were held before elective surgery.[9,10] It is important to note, however, that the studies apply most directly to patients with nonvalvular atrial fibrillation undergoing elective surgery. Special considerations need to be made for individual cases based on both a patient's degree of vascular risk factors and the relative urgency of the surgery. Conditions such as the presence of a mechanical heart valve, underlying hypercoagulable state, or recent history of cardioembolic events all significantly increase the daily risk of a cerebrovascular event and must be considered when stratifying a patient's overall level of risk in temporarily suspending anticoagulation.

Table 1
Perioperative interruption, resumption, and reversal of common antithrombotic agents

Antithrombotic Medications	Mechanism	When to Interrupt Therapy Before Elective surgery[1,7]	When to Resume Therapy Following Elective surgery[1,7]	Reversal Agents (for Emergency Surgery)
Antiplatelet Agents				
Aspirin	Cyclooxygenase (COX) inhibitor	7–10 d before surgery	Resume when periprocedural bleeding risk has diminished[1]	No specific reversal agent
Clopidogrel	P2Y12 inhibitor	7–10 d before surgery	Resume when periprocedural bleeding risk has diminished[1]	No specific reversal agent
Anticoagulants				
Warfarin	Vitamin K antagonist	5 d before surgery	12–24 h postoperatively	Prothrombin complex concentrate • replacement of vitamin K–dependent coagulation factors) + IV vitamin K[8]
Dabigatran	Direct thrombin inhibitor	*Patient with normal renal function:* 1 d before low bleeding risk procedure 2 d before high bleeding risk procedure[1,7] *Patient with impaired renal function (CrCl < 50mLmin):* 2 d before low bleeding risk procedure 4 d before high bleeding risk procedure	*All patients:* 1 d following low bleeding risk procedure 2–3 d following high bleeding risk procedure	Idarucizumab • monoclonal antibody, binds dabigatran

Apixaban	Factor Xa inhibitor	1 d before low bleeding risk procedure 2 d before high bleeding risk procedure	1 d following low bleeding risk procedure 2–3 d following high bleeding risk procedure	Andexanet alfa • Recombinant protein, factor Xa mimic
Rivaroxaban	Factor Xa inhibitor	1 d before low bleeding risk procedure 2 d before high bleeding risk procedure	1 d following low bleeding risk procedure 2–3 d following high bleeding risk procedure	Andexanet alfa • Recombinant protein, factor Xa mimic
Edoxaban	Factor Xa inhibitor	1 d before low bleeding risk procedure 2 d before high bleeding risk procedure	1 d following low bleeding risk procedure 2–3 d following high bleeding risk procedure	Andexanet alfa • Recombinant protein, factor Xa mimic

If bridging is indicated for patients taking warfarin, after the drug is held 5 days before surgery, therapeutic-dose low-molecular-weight heparin (LMWH) is dosed every 12 hours starting 3 days before surgery, with the last preoperative dose given 24 hours before surgery (and no dose given 12 hours before surgery).[1,7] LMWH is resumed 48 to 72 hours after surgery and continued until warfarin is again therapeutic.[1,7] An infusion of intravenous unfractionated heparin may be used as well. The DOACs generally do not require bridging therapy for perioperative interruptions due to their short half-lives (see **Table 1**).

Direct oral anticoagulant reversal agents—a resource for emergency surgery

One concern around DOACs has been a lack of effective reversal agents. The safety profile of DOACs continues to evolve, however, and reversal agents are becoming increasingly available. This becomes pertinent for perioperative management of anticoagulated patients when rapid reversal of anticoagulation is necessary for emergency surgery. DOAC reversal agents also can have a role in cases where anticoagulation with a DOAC is resumed postoperatively but the patient suffers a bleeding complication.

Dabigatran was the first DoAC for which a specific reversal agent, idarucizumab, was approved by the US Food and Drug Administration (FDA) and became commercially available. Idarucizumab, a monoclonal antibody, has been demonstrated to be effective in reversing the anticoagulant effects of dabigatran in clinical situations requiring a rapidly acting antidote (ie, gastrointestinal bleeding, intracerebral hemorrhage, and emergency surgery).[11]

Reversal agents for antifactor Xa drugs are under development, promising to further enhance their safety profile. Andexanet alfa, a recombinant protein engineered to structurally mimic human factor Xa, has been approved by the FDA for use as a reversal agent for the factor Xa inhibitors rivaroxaban, apixaban, and edoxaban, following success in clinical trials.[12,13] Prothrombin complex concentrate (PCC), which is available in 3-factor and 4-factor varieties, can also be used to reverse the anticoagulant effects in patients receiving active factor Xa inhibition. Four-factor PCC was found to be effective in treating about 70% of hemorrhages associated with apixaban or rivaroxaban. Failure of treatment, however, was more common in intracranial hemorrhage.[14]

Understanding indications for antiplatelet therapy

Patients may be on a variety of antiplatelet regimens for different indications, and it is always helpful to ascertain the specific indications for antiplatelet therapy in a patient before deciding whether (and for how long) to interrupt usage of these medicines. Some patients may be on antiplatelet monotherapy for stroke prevention based on a history of a prior stroke or TIA. Others will be on DAPT (ie, both aspirin and clopidogrel daily) for 3 weeks following a minor stroke or TIA,[15,16] followed by antiplatelet monotherapy. The same regimen (DAPT for 90 days followed by monotherapy) is recommended for ischemic stroke due to intracranial atherosclerotic disease.[17] In these cases, it may be advisable to delay surgery due to the recency of the stroke or TIA, rather than to interrupt DAPT. Neurologists should remain aware that patients may be on antiplatelet regimens for reasons other than stroke prevention, such as recent coronary artery stent placement.

Interrupting antiplatelet therapy

Both aspirin and P2Y12 inhibitors (eg, clopidogrel, ticlopidine, prasugrel) irreversibly inhibit platelet function for the entire lifetime of the exposed platelets; thus, for patients taking these agents for a neurovascular indication (ie, secondary stroke prevention), it is generally advised to hold antiplatelet therapy before elective surgery, for a period of time equivalent to the average platelet lifespan, or 7 to 10 days.[7,18] Patients who have had a percutaneous coronary intervention should have their cardiologist consulted before interrupting aspirin periprocedurally.[1] In contrast to aspirin being used for stroke prevention, aspirin used for secondary cardiovascular prevention is often continued through surgery, with the exception of several conditions that confer unacceptable risk of perioperative bleeding in patients taking aspirin, including intracranial and intramedullary spine operations.[19]

Of note, ticagrelor, a reversible P2Y12 inhibitor, can be interrupted with a shorter lead time before surgery, and a time interval of 2 to 3 days may be sufficient, as was the case in a study of patients on ticagrelor before coronary artery bypass graft surgery.[20]

MANAGEMENT OF POSTOPERATIVE NEUROLOGIC COMPLICATIONS
Perioperative Stroke—Assessment and Management

Perioperative stroke refers to strokes that occur both during surgical procedures (intraoperative stroke) and postoperatively. Distinguishing these entities by comparing the time of onset of stroke-related deficits or imaging findings to the time of surgery can help identify the cause of stroke. Intraoperative stroke is commonly associated with proximal embolic events or intraoperative cerebral hypoperfusion; postoperative stroke is often due to new-onset arrythmias (eg, atrial fibrillation).[21] Cardiac and aortic surgeries carry an increased risk of perioperative stroke and thus deserve special attention—rates of permanent neurologic deficits following cardiac surgery have been reported as high as 6%.[22,23]

Intraoperative stroke
The most common causes of intraoperative ischemic stroke are thromboembolism, comprising 70% to 80% of cases, and hypoperfusion, which makes up 20% to 30% of intraoperative strokes.[21,24,25] Causes of embolic intraoperative stroke are myriad; they can result from paradoxic venous thromboembolism through a patent foramen ovale, atrial fibrillation and other sources of intracardiac thrombus, aortic and carotid atherosclerosis, or more rarely can result from embolization of air (discussed later).[21] Hypoperfusion may result from intraoperative hypotension, a particular problem in the setting of severe extracranial or intracranial arterial stenosis.

Postoperative stroke
Postoperative strokes can be divided into early postoperative stroke (within 7 days of surgery) and late postoperative stroke (7–30 days following surgery).[21] The most common cause of early postoperative stroke after cardiac or aortic vascular surgery is a thromboembolism resulting from a new cardiac arrythmia, typically postoperative atrial fibrillation.[21,26,27] Other important causes of early postoperative stroke include a variety of causes of cerebral hypoperfusion, such as bleeding, distributive shock (eg, sepsis), and cardiogenic shock (particularly following cardiac surgery).[21]

Perioperative stroke evaluation and management
If concern emerges for acute neurologic deficits in a patient following surgery, the patient should be immediately evaluated by a neurologist for the possibility of an acute stroke. The goal of this evaluation is to establish a diagnosis (hemorrhagic stroke, ischemic stroke, or neither) and for ischemic strokes, to assess the patient's candidacy for time-sensitive interventions—namely intravenous thrombolysis and/or endovascular thrombectomy. Guidelines from the American Heart Association specify that recent (within 3 months) intracranial or intraspinal surgery is an absolute

contraindication to the use of intravenous thrombolysis, and other recent surgery is a relative contraindication[28]; there is actually little clinical evidence to support these and other specific contraindications; some are thought to be overly restrictive.[29] Thrombolysis may be feasible in select patients after discussion of the ability to control potential bleeding into the surgical site with the patient's surgeon. Patients with perioperative strokes may still be candidates for endovascular thrombectomy, which has been shown to be safe in this patient population.[30]

Patients with perioperative stroke should be evaluated in the same manner as those with nonperioperative stroke. In addition, the surgical procedure should be reviewed with the surgeon to determine whether thrombus formed at any venous or arterial anastomosis could have reached the cerebral circulation, and the intraoperative anesthesia record should be reviewed as well for periods of hypotension or other hemodynamic events. Perioperative or postoperative atrial fibrillation in a patient with no history of atrial fibrillation lasting for more than 48 hours should be treated with a minimum of 4 weeks of anticoagulation, and continuation of anticoagulation beyond that time point is based on an analysis of other cardiovascular and cerebrovascular risk factors.

There is currently no strong evidence that preoperative screening for carotid artery stenosis reduces the risk of perioperative or postoperative stroke in otherwise neurologically asymptomatic patients. A tailored approach to screening based on patient risk factors and other high-risk features is recommended by most experts.

Acute and Chronic Encephalopathy After Surgery

Postoperative encephalopathy is very common and is underdiagnosed.[31] Incidence varies based on demographic factors (elderly patients are at highest risk) and the existence of relevant risk factors (including underlying cognitive impairment[32] or a history of substance/alcohol use). Risk also varies among different procedures, with contributions from factors such as invasiveness of the surgery and length of time spent under general anesthesia. Encephalopathy is also more likely to occur with, or be prolonged by, the presence other complications of hospitalization, such as nosocomial infection[31,33,34] and medication toxicity (eg, from anticholinergic agents, opioid-based pain medications causing impairment of consciousness). Because encephalopathy is addressed at length in another chapter in this volume, it will only be briefly discussed here.

Acute postsurgical encephalopathy

Patients who remain somnolent or hypoactive for a prolonged period of time following surgery or those who awaken but seem confused, inattentive, disoriented, and/or agitated should be evaluated for common causes of encephalopathy, including reversible and treatable infections and metabolic abnormalities. If a basic infectious, metabolic, and toxic screen (including review of the patient's inpatient medication regimen for potential iatrogenic contributions to encephalopathy) does not yield an answer, other workup for additional causes may be considered (**Table 2**), especially if the encephalopathy is not improving.

Prolonged/chronic postsurgical encephalopathy

Some patients will remain encephalopathic for a prolonged period of time following surgery. In such cases, consulting neurologists should first ensure that a thorough workup for toxic, metabolic, and infectious causes of encephalopathy has been performed, and this should include an exhaustive evaluation for iatrogenic or nosocomial complications, including excessive dosing of deliriogenic or sedating medications, kidney or liver injury, and hospital-borne infections. Often, careful investigation will

Table 2 Common causes of postoperative encephalopathy		
Toxic Encephalopathy • Prolonged effects of anesthesia/analgesia • Perioperative drugs (benzodiazepines, opioids, serotonergic agents, anticholinergic agents) Increased risk from: advanced age, impaired drug metabolism and/or clearance	**Metabolic Encephalopathy** • Renal failure • Liver failure • Hypercapnia • Hypoxia • Hyponatremia • Hypernatremia • Hyperosmolarity • Metabolic acidosis	**Septic Encephalopathy** • Triggered by underlying infection (bacterial, viral, fungal, and so forth) • Encephalopathy from combined effects of direct pathogenic factors (eg, bacterial endotoxin), and host response (eg, inflammatory internal milieu/cytokine release, oxidative stress, immune mobilization)[35]
Seizure • Generalized (bilateral tonic-clonic) seizures followed by postictal encephalopathy • Nonconvulsive status epilepticus (focal status epilepticus with loss of awareness or with altered awareness)	**Stroke** • Hemorrhagic • Ischemic: thromboembolism (most common); hypoxic injury due to hemodynamic hypoperfusion (ie, watershed infarctions); fat embolism; air embolism	Global anoxic/ischemic brain injury • Follows profound hypoperfusion and/or cardiac arrest

Data from Refs.[41–43]

yield an actionable diagnosis, and the reversible inciting factor may be addressed. If this evaluation fails to yield a likely cause for prolonged encephalopathy, other causes should be considered, including seizure, stroke, nosocomial meningitis or encephalitis, or in some cases, global hypoxic-ischemic brain injury.

The role of electroencephalogram in evaluating prolonged encephalopathy
Nonconvulsive status epilepticus can be a cause of prolonged unresponsiveness and can be ruled out with routine electroencephalogram (EEG). However, seizures, especially when brief and focal, may also be incidental to an underlying, often more ominous, cause of the encephalopathy, such as global hypoxic-ischemic injury or encephalitis. If the EEG reveals seizure activity, treatment with nonsedating antiseizure medications may improve mental status to the degree that a conclusion can be drawn that epileptic activity was responsible for its alteration. If the mental status does not improve, an alternative cause should be sought. Even when not revealing any epileptic phenomena, the EEG can be helpful in assessing encephalopathic patients—a globally slow EEG with poor background organization supports the clinical assessment; the presence of diffuse triphasic waves suggests a toxic-metabolic encephalopathy; and an extremely attenuated record with little spontaneous activity or reactivity elevates concern for potential global anoxic-ischemic brain injury—perhaps from a cardiac arrest or prolonged hypoperfusional state.

The role of MRI in evaluating prolonged encephalopathy
Brain MRI is helpful in evaluating for occult perioperative stroke in encephalopathic or unresponsive patients, as well as in evaluating for global injury associated with

hypoperfusion, as may occur in the setting of cardiac arrest, intraoperative blood loss resulting in hemorrhagic shock, or other causes of shock overwhelming a patient's capacity for maintaining cerebral perfusion. Patterns of signal abnormality on MRI, if present, may offer clues as to the cause of a patient's prolonged impaired arousal.

Multifocal ischemic infarcts in different arterial distributions (especially bilaterally) strongly suggest emboli arising from a proximal source. Infarcts in arterial border zone regions (those areas bordering 2 major arterial perfusion territories) elevate suspicion that the patient experienced clinically significant hypoperfusion, and MRI can also reveal evidence of global hypoxic-ischemic brain injury. Because MRI is not completely sensitive for diffuse anoxic injury, a scan can potentially seem normal despite the presence of severe and irreversible injury.

NEUROLOGIC COMPLICATIONS OF ADVANCED CIRCULATORY SUPPORT
Neurologic Complications of Extracorporeal Membrane Oxygenation and Cardiopulmonary Bypass

Cardiopulmonary bypass and extracorporeal membrane oxygenation (ECMO) are remarkable means of mechanically providing external cardiopulmonary support. Cardiopulmonary bypass is the term applied to extrinsic cardiopulmonary support used intraoperatively for patients undergoing invasive cardiac surgery. The term ECMO is applied for such extracorporeal support outside of the operative setting, most often due to severe cardiac shock and respiratory failure in adults.[36] Patients requiring treatment with ECMO suffer from severe refractory cardiac failure and thus are among the sickest patients in the hospital. This makes it difficult to attribute the cause of subsequent neurologic complications to any one factor, whether a consequence of underlying illness or iatrogenic, but data on neurologic complications in this population are available.

In a retrospective study of 8398 adult patients receiving ECMO drawn from a national inpatient cohort, neurologic complications occurred in 9.6%.[36] Cardiac arrest, shock, and sepsis all independently predicted an increased chance of neurologic complications, the most common of which were ischemic stroke, intracranial hemorrhage (ICH), and seizure. Among ECMO patients with neurologic complications, ICH was the only one that increased the odds ratio of mortality (and survivors had higher rates of disability and thus discharge to long-term care); acute ischemic stroke was also associated with increased need for discharge to a long-term care facility but not increased mortality, whereas clinical outcomes of patients with seizures did not differ significantly from ECMO patients without neurologic complications.[36] Of these complications, acute ischemic stroke was the most common, occurring in 4.62% of adult patients in the study.[36] Other important complications of ECMO include limb ischemia, arterial dissection, pseudoaneurysm formation, groin infection, retroperitoneal bleeding, and peripheral plexus or nerve injury (in the groin due to mechanical trauma and elsewhere due to ischemia).

Neurologists should be aware that brain injury in a patient whose hospital course involved ECMO may not become apparent until later in their clinical course—this is first because clinical deficits may not be initially apparent because of sedation, neuromuscular blockade, or critical illness polyneuropathy/myopathy. Second, as the ECMO circuit itself is MRI incompatible, neuroimaging in patients actively receiving ECMO is limited to computed tomography (CT), a less sensitive modality, particularly for acute ischemic and hypoxic complications, and thus one less likely to detect brain injury. An observational neuropathological study demonstrated that brain injury following ECMO is more common and varied than radiologically observed, occurring in 35 of 43 patients, although only deceased patients were included in this study.[37] Of note, 9 patients in this study had negative antemortem neuroimaging with no abnormalities noted, but 6 of 9 of those had brain injuries on pathologic examination.

Neurologic Complications in Patients with Left Ventricular Assist Devices

Patients with end-stage heart failure who await cardiac transplantation are increasingly being managed with LVAD, as these carry marked survival advantages (52% as compared with 25% survival at 1 year) for such patients over optimal medical therapy alone, based on the 2001 Randomized Evaluation of Mechanical Assistance for the Treatment of Heart Failure (REMATCH) trial.[38] LVAD therapy in the era of REMATCH, while conferring marked survival advantages, also carries a significantly increased rate of neurologic complications; this risk was 4.35 times higher in patients on an LVAD than in patients on optimal medical therapy alone. Stroke risk is especially high, with an incidence of 8% to 25%.[39,40]

Physicians taking care of patients on an LVAD, and especially neurohospitalists based in centers caring for such populations, should be aware that changes in hematologic physiology in patients with LVADs confer an increased risk of both ischemic and hemorrhagic stroke. In these patients, interactions between blood and the surface of the LVAD device confer an increased risk of bleeding as well as thromboembolic events.[41] Research has shown that this results from a combination of hematologic changes following LVAD implantation, including acquired von Willebrand disease, hemolysis, and platelet activation.[39] Acquired von Willebrand disease seems to result in part from shear stress imposed by the LVAD,[42] causing increased proteolysis of von Willebrand factor by the enzyme ADAMTS-13, resulting in both hemorrhagic and ischemic stroke as complications[39]; this is compounded by both an increase in platelet activation by mechanical stress on platelets leading to platelet aggregation and adherence to the foreign surface of the device and is further compounded by LVAD-associated hemolysis, which indirectly triggers the accumulation of active von Willebrand factor multimers and predisposes to clot formation.[39] Taken together, the altered hematologic milieu, with increased hemolysis and platelet activation superimposed on an acquired deficiency of von Willebrand factor, disrupts the homeostatic balance of bleeding and clotting in LVAD patients, leading to increased stroke risk. As a result, patients on an LVAD are treated with anticoagulant medications.

NEUROLOGIC COMPLICATIONS IN SPECIFIC SURGICAL POPULATIONS
Spinal Cord Ischemia in Thoracoabdominal Vascular Surgery

Spinal cord infarction is a complication of vascular surgery involving the thoracic and abdominal aorta (**Fig. 1**). Although rare, reliable prevention of this complication has proved elusive in part because spinal cord blood supply is complex and highly variable.[43] The great anterior radiculomedullary artery (artery of Adamkiewicz), a dominant source of the inferior spinal cord's blood supply, has a variable origin and can arise from posterior intercostal, subcostal, or lumbar branches of the descending aorta, on either the left (most commonly) or the right side.[43,44] In a series of 18 patients with paraplegia or paraparesis due to spinal cord ischemia following an abdominal aortic surgery, review of preoperative CT, MRI, and aortographic data failed to visualize the artery of Adamkiewicz,[45] likely due to its variable location and appearance. Patients who experience spinal cord ischemia as a result of abdominal aortic surgery often manifest an anterior spinal arterylike syndrome, with paraparesis or paraplegia and a sensory level affecting spinothalamic tract function; dorsal column sensory function can be preserved in many cases but not uniformly.

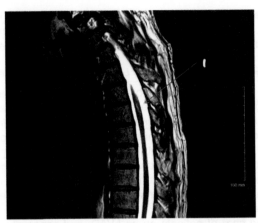

Fig. 1. Thoracic spinal cord ischemia and myelomalacia following aortobifemoral bypass. Sagittal T2-weighted MRI of the thoracic spine 5 months after development of sudden post-operative paraparesis, showing a focal area of abnormal T2 hyperintensity (*arrow*) in the central spinal cord, consistent with myelomalacia related to spinal cord infarction.

Cerebrospinal fluid drainage via placement of a lumbar drain has long been used preoperatively and prophylactically for patients undergoing thoracoabdominal aneurysm repair as a means of reducing intraspinal pressure, increasing blood flow to the spinal cord, and preventing ischemic cord complications. The same procedure has been advocated as a treatment strategy in cases of acute spinal cord ischemic infarction as a means of reducing the damage to the cord. Given the rarity and multiple causes of spinal cord infarction, no definitive clinical trial data exist to guide usage of lumbar drains in this setting. Complications of lumbar drains, including symptoms related to intracranial hypertension or hypotension, subdural hematoma formation, and infection, should be considered. Beyond cerebrospinal fluid shunting, blood pressure augmentation, avoidance of hypotension, and maintenance of oxygenation are recommended.

Neurologic Complications of Nutritional Deficiencies After Bariatric Surgery

Bariatric surgery as a means of managing obesity is increasingly common. The Roux-en-Y gastric bypass is one of the most common and effective methods of bariatric surgery and involves a surgical anastomosis between a pouch fashioned from the superior aspect of the stomach directly to the jejunum, thereby bypassing most of the stomach and the entire duodenum. A complication of this bypass is impaired absorption of several vitamins and minerals, including the vitamins folate, B_1, B_{12}, D, and E, and the minerals iron, calcium, magnesium, and phosphate.[46] Of these, iron, folate, and vitamin B_{12} deficiencies seem to occur most commonly following gastric bypass surgery.[47,48]

A range of neurologic complications has been reported following bariatric surgery, including encephalopathy, behavioral abnormalities, seizures, cranial nerve palsies, myelopathy, plexopathies, peripheral neuropathy, mononeuropathies including carpal tunnel syndrome and meralgia paresthetica, myopathy, and ataxia.[46]

In a series of 435 patients who underwent bariatric surgery at the Mayo Clinic, as many as 71 (16%) developed peripheral neuropathy.[49] The most common patterns of neuropathy among these patients were polyneuropathy (n = 27), mononeuropathy (n = 39, of which 31 developed carpal tunnel syndrome), and radiculoplexus neuropathy (n = 5). Risk factors for developing neuropathy included both the rate and absolute amount of weight loss and loss to follow-up by a nutritional clinic following the bariatric surgery.[49]

Other less common but important neurologic complications of bariatric surgeries are illustrated in **Table 3**.

Fat and Air Embolism

Uncommonly, neurologists will encounter patients with neurologic complications of nonthrombotic emboli—most commonly fat, air, or amniotic fluid emboli. Fat emboli can arise as a result of orthopedic trauma (ie, a fat embolus in the setting of a traumatic femoral neck fracture) but also occur iatrogenically in surgical patients undergoing arthroplasty.[52] Air embolism can occur as a result of any procedure that introduces air intravascularly, and neurologic complications of cerebral air embolism have been reported in association with a multitude of procedures including central venous catheter instrumentation,[53] cardiac ablation,[54] esophagogastroduodenoscopy,[55] and cerebral angiography.[56] In both cases, emboli become trapped in pulmonary capillaries, causing an increase in right heart pressure and potential direct embolization of fat or air into the left heart circulation, particularly if a patent foramen ovale or other interatrial connection is present. Once the emboli have reached the left heart circulation, direct occlusion of cerebral and other arteries may occur. Air and fat emboli can cause diffuse cerebral infarctions, producing focal or nonfocal clinical deficits that range in severity from mild symptoms to coma and MRI findings of scattered foci of restricted diffusion (**Figs. 2** and **3**). Unlike thromboembolic infarctions, neurologic symptoms usually develop gradually and progressively over the course of a day or two. Symptoms related to damage of other organ systems may be present as well; respiratory compromise and a petechial rash have both been described. Treatment is primarily supportive, although in the case of air embolism, hyperbaric oxygen may be considered.[57]

Clinical case—fat embolism following total hip arthroplasty

An 84-year-old man underwent a total hip arthroplasty. He was stable immediately following the procedure, but the following morning was found to be dysarthric, weak, somnolent, and hypoxemic. A CT of the head showed no abnormalities. A CT of the chest showed 2 small subsegmental pulmonary emboli in the left upper lobe. An MRI of the brain showed numerous foci of restricted diffusion involving the cerebral cortex and subcortical white matter (see **Fig. 2**). The cervical and intracranial arteries were patent, echocardiogram showed evidence of pulmonary hypertension and no patent foramen ovale, heart rhythm was normal sinus, and no other source of emboli was identified. The presumed stroke (and pulmonary embolism) mechanism was fat iatrogenically introduced into the venous system during the arthroplasty procedure and a presumed intracardiac or extracardiac shunt.

Perioperative Management of Patients with Myasthenia Gravis

Patients with myasthenia gravis (MG), a chronic autoimmune disease in which antibodies against acetylcholine receptors result in impaired neurotransmission and neuromuscular weakness, and in some cases, respiratory compromise, warrant special perioperative consideration. Neurologists evaluating patients with MG preoperatively should focus on ascertaining which muscle groups are affected in the patient during disease exacerbations (with special attention to any history of respiratory compromise and bulbar symptoms), understanding the patient's recent course of illness and assessing whether the patient is currently optimized on medical therapy.[58]

Table 3
Neurologic complications of nutritional deficiencies after bariatric surgery

Nutrient Deficiency	Complications
Vitamin B$_1$ (thiamine)	Wernicke encephalopathy • Confusion or mild memory impairment • Oculomotor abnormalities • Cerebellar dysfunction Peripheral neuropathy
Vitamin B$_{12}$ (cobalamin)	Subacute combined degeneration • loss of vibration and joint position sense • pyramidal weakness, hyperreflexia, extensor plantar response • peripheral neuropathy • neuropsychiatric disturbances (psychosis, mood disorder, dementia)
Vitamin D	Myopathy
Vitamin E	Axonal peripheral neuropathy, spinocerebellar ataxia, myopathy
Folate deficiency	Peripheral neuropathy
Iron deficiency	Restless leg syndrome[50,51]
Copper deficiency	Myelopathy Peripheral neuropathy
Hypocalcemia	Muscle spasms, ophthalmoplegia • occurs secondary to vitamin D deficiency

Medications that patients may take at home include acetylcholinesterase inhibitors (eg, pyridostigmine), oral corticosteroids, or other immunosuppressive drugs (eg, azathioprine).[58,59] Patients with a severe exacerbation of their disease requiring hospitalization may be treated with intravenous immunoglobulin (IVIg)[60] or plasmapheresis.[59] Elective surgery should take place during a stable phase of illness in a patient with MG, with the patient optimized on medical therapy. The definition of optimization will vary with the patient, but a common goal is a patient requiring no or minimal corticosteroids with stable symptoms on pyridostigmine monotherapy.[58] If urgent

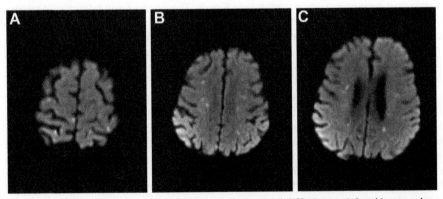

Fig. 2. Fat embolism following total hip arthroplasty. Axial diffusion-weighted images show numerous small bihemispheric cortical and subcortical acute infarctions. There were no infratentorial lesions.

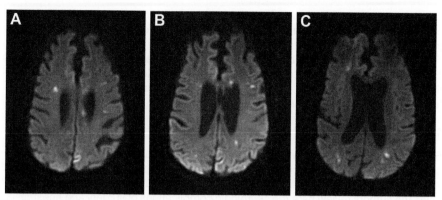

Fig. 3. Air embolism following esophagogastroduodenoscopy (EGD). Axial diffusion-weighted images show numerous small bihemispheric cortical and subcortical acute infarctions after air embolism in a 52-year-old man undergoing dilation of esophageal strictures. There were no infratentorial lesions.

or emergent surgery is necessary for a patient with MG in an active phase of their illness, IVIg or plasmapheresis can be used to optimize them in preparation for surgery.[58]

Neurologists should be aware that there are special considerations for anesthesia in patients with MG, particularly with the use of medications such as depolarizing neuromuscular blockers that can significantly worsen myasthenic symptoms. The greatest risk to myasthenic patients in this setting is perioperative myasthenic crisis, or respiratory compromise due to weakness of the respiratory muscles, combined with aspiration risk from impaired clearance of secretions that comes with bulbar myasthenia. Postoperatively, it is important that myasthenic patients receive sufficient pulmonary hygiene and pain control to facilitate successful tracheal extubation.[58] Drugs that interfere with neuromuscular transmission, such as aminoglycosides,[61] should be avoided, as should drugs such as benzodiazepines whenever possible, as these reduce respiratory drive and patients with MG can be especially sensitive to them.[61] Factors predictive of a postoperative need for mechanical ventilation in myasthenic patients include duration of myasthenia, respiratory disease, pyridostigmine dosage, and vital capacity.[62] If a patient with MG has experienced a postoperative myasthenic crisis, they should continue to receive ventilatory support until the underlying cause of crisis can be diagnosed and treated.[58] Intravenous immunoglobulin should be administered or plasmapheresis performed in cases where the patient requires ongoing ventilatory support past 24 hours.[58,63]

Identification and Treatment of Malignant Hyperthermia, a Severe Response to Anesthesia

Malignant hyperthermia is a severe hypermetabolic reaction of skeletal muscle to anesthetic agents that occurs in genetically susceptible patients.[64] Mutations in the RYR1, CACNA1S, and STAC3 genes are known to increase the risk of malignant hyperthermia and are inherited in an autosomal dominant manner. Patients with inherited muscle diseases including central core myopathy are at increased risk as well. However, up to half of those with a susceptibility to malignant hyperthermia have neither a gene mutation in RYR1, CACNA1S, or STAC3 nor a myopathy.

Patients experience hyperthermia, tachycardia, muscle rigidity, and rhabdomyolysis; become acidotic and hyperkalemic; and exhibit increased end-tidal CO_2 despite an increase in minute ventilation.[64] It is known to occur in response to the depolarizing neuromuscular blocker succinylcholine, as well as to inhaled anesthetics such as halothane, isoflurane, sevoflurane, and desflurane.[64]

Malignant hyperthermia is rare with an incidence between 1:10,0000 and 1:250,000.[65,66] Dantrolene sodium, a postsynaptic muscle relaxant that serves effectively as an antidote in cases of malignant hyperthermia, should be promptly administered and titrated to tachycardia and hypercarbia.[64]

SUMMARY

Surgery and anesthesia carry risks of ischemic, hemorrhagic, hypoxic, and metabolic complications, all of which can result in neurologic symptoms and deficits. Patients with underlying cardiovascular and cerebrovascular risk factors are particularly vulnerable. The authors review here the neurologic complications of surgery and anesthesia, with a focus on the role of the neurohospitalist in preoperative evaluation and risk stratification and diagnosis and management of postoperative complications.

CLINICS CARE POINTS

- Patients with a history of ischemic stroke within 3 months before a surgery have a much higher risk of major cardiovascular complications, with risk plateauing at about 9 months.
- There is no strong evidence that preoperative screening for carotid artery stenosis reduces the risk of perioperative or postoperative stroke in otherwise neurologically asymptomatic patients.
- Postoperative encephalopathy is very common and is underdiagnosed.

DISCLOSURE

The authors have nothing to disclose.

REFERENCES

1. Hornor MA, Duane TM, Ehlers AP, et al. American College of Surgeons' Guidelines for the perioperative management of antithrombotic medication. J Am Coll Surg 2018;227(5):521–36.e1.
2. Jørgensen ME, Torp-Pedersen C, Gislason GH, et al. Time elapsed after ischemic stroke and risk of adverse cardiovascular events and mortality following elective noncardiac surgery. JAMA 2014;312(3):269–77.
3. Kim AS. Medical management for secondary stroke prevention. Continuum (Minneap Minn) 2020;26(2):435–56.
4. Lip GY, Nieuwlaat R, Pisters R, et al. Refining clinical risk stratification for predicting stroke and thromboembolism in atrial fibrillation using a novel risk factor-based approach: the euro heart survey on atrial fibrillation. Chest 2010;137(2):263–72.
5. Douketis JD, Healey JS, Brueckmann M, et al. Perioperative bridging anticoagulation during dabigatran or warfarin interruption among patients who had an elective surgery or procedure. Substudy of the RE-LY trial. Thromb Haemost Mar 2015;113(3):625–32.
6. Sherwood MW, Douketis JD, Patel MR, et al. Outcomes of temporary interruption of rivaroxaban compared with warfarin in patients with nonvalvular atrial

fibrillation: results from the rivaroxaban once daily, oral, direct factor Xa inhibition compared with vitamin K antagonism for prevention of stroke and embolism trial in atrial fibrillation (ROCKET AF). Circulation 2014;129(18):1850–9.

7. Tafur A, Douketis J. Perioperative management of anticoagulant and antiplatelet therapy. Heart 2018;104(17):1461–7.

8. Hanley JP. Warfarin reversal. J Clin Pathol 2004;57(11):1132–9.

9. Douketis JD, Spyropoulos AC, Duncan J, et al. Perioperative management of patients with atrial fibrillation receiving a direct oral anticoagulant. JAMA Intern Med 2019;179(11):1469–78.

10. Douketis JD, Spyropoulos AC, Kaatz S, et al. Perioperative bridging anticoagulation in patients with atrial fibrillation. N Engl J Med 2015;373(9):823–33.

11. Pollack CV, Reilly PA, van Ryn J, et al. Idarucizumab for dabigatran reversal — full cohort analysis. New Engl J Med 2017;377(5):431–41.

12. Connolly SJ, Milling TJ, Eikelboom JW, et al. Andexanet alfa for acute major bleeding associated with factor xa inhibitors. New Engl J Med 2016;375(12): 1131–41.

13. Connolly SJ, Crowther M, Eikelboom JW, et al. Full study report of andexanet alfa for bleeding associated with factor xa inhibitors. New Engl J Med 2019;380(14): 1326–35.

14. Majeed A, Ågren A, Holmström M, et al. Management of rivaroxaban- or apixaban-associated major bleeding with prothrombin complex concentrates: a cohort study. Blood 2017;130(15):1706–12.

15. Johnston SC, Easton JD, Farrant M, et al. Clopidogrel and aspirin in acute ischemic stroke and high-risk TIA. New Engl J Med 2018;379(3):215–25.

16. Wang Y, Wang Y, Zhao X, et al. Clopidogrel with aspirin in acute minor stroke or transient ischemic attack. New Engl J Med 2013;369(1):11–9.

17. Chimowitz MI, Lynn MJ, Derdeyn CP, et al. Stenting versus aggressive medical therapy for intracranial arterial stenosis. New Engl J Med 2011;365(11):993–1003.

18. Bell AD, Roussin A, Cartier R, et al. The use of antiplatelet therapy in the outpatient setting: Canadian cardiovascular society guidelines. Can J Cardiol 2011; 27(Suppl A):S1–59.

19. Gerstein NS, Schulman PM, Gerstein WH, et al. Should more patients continue aspirin therapy perioperatively?: clinical impact of aspirin withdrawal syndrome. Ann Surg 2012;255(5):811–9.

20. Gherli R, Mariscalco G, Dalén M, et al. Safety of preoperative use of ticagrelor with or without aspirin compared with aspirin alone in patients with acute coronary syndromes undergoing coronary artery bypass grafting. JAMA Cardiol 2016;1(8): 921–8.

21. Gaudino M, Benesch C, Bakaeen F, et al. Considerations for reduction of risk of perioperative stroke in adult patients undergoing cardiac and thoracic aortic operations: a scientific statement from the american heart association. Circulation 2020;142(14):e193–209.

22. Bucerius J, Gummert JF, Borger MA, et al. Stroke after cardiac surgery: a risk factor analysis of 16,184 consecutive adult patients. Ann Thorac Surg 2003;75(2): 472–8.

23. Roach GW, Kanchuger M, Mangano CM, et al. Adverse cerebral outcomes after coronary bypass surgery. Multicenter study of perioperative ischemia research group and the ischemia research and education foundation investigators. N Engl J Med 1996;335(25):1857–63.

24. Gottesman Rebecca F, Sherman Paul M, Grega Maura A, et al. Watershed strokes after cardiac surgery. Stroke 2006;37(9):2306–11.

25. Hori D, Brown C, Ono M, et al. Arterial pressure above the upper cerebral autoregulation limit during cardiopulmonary bypass is associated with postoperative delirium. Br J Anaesth 2014;113(6):1009–17.

26. Gaudino M, Rahouma M, Di Mauro M, et al. Early versus delayed stroke after cardiac surgery: a systematic review and meta-analysis. J Am Heart Assoc 2019; 8(13):e012447.

27. Kotoh K, Fukahara K, Doi T, et al. Predictors of early postoperative cerebral infarction after isolated off-pump coronary artery bypass grafting. Ann Thorac Surg 2007;83(5):1679–83.

28. Jauch EC, Saver JL, Adams HP Jr, et al. Guidelines for the early management of patients with acute ischemic stroke: a guideline for healthcare professionals from the American Heart Association/American Stroke Association. Stroke 2013;44(3): 870–947.

29. Fugate JE, Rabinstein AA. Absolute and relative contraindications to IV rt-PA for acute ischemic stroke. Neurohospitalist 2015;5(3):110–21.

30. Premat K, Clovet O, Frasca Polara G, et al. Mechanical thrombectomy in perioperative strokes. Stroke 2017;48(11):3149–51.

31. Robinson TN, Eiseman B. Postoperative delirium in the elderly: diagnosis and management. Clin Interv Aging 2008;3(2):351–5.

32. Robinson TN, Raeburn CD, Tran ZV, et al. Postoperative delirium in the elderly: risk factors and outcomes. Ann Surg 2009;249(1):173–8.

33. Talmasov D, Klein JP. Neuroimaging, electroencephalography, and lumbar puncture in medical psychiatry. In: Summergrad P, Silbersweig DA, Muskin PR, et al, editors. Textbook of medical psychiatry. American Psychiatric Association Publishing; 2020. p. 51–83.

34. Rabinstein AA, Keegan MT. Neurologic complications of anesthesia: a practical approach. Neurol Clin Pract 2013;3(4):295–304.

35. Ziaja M. Septic encephalopathy. Curr Neurol Neurosci Rep 2013;13(10):383.

36. Nasr DM, Rabinstein AA. Neurologic complications of extracorporeal membrane oxygenation. J Clin Neurol 2015;11(4):383–9.

37. Khan IR, Gu Y, George BP, et al. Brain histopathology of adult decedents after extracorporeal membrane oxygenation. Neurology 2021;96(9):e1278–89.

38. Rose EA, Gelijns AC, Moskowitz AJ, et al. Long-term use of a left ventricular assist device for end-stage heart failure. New Engl J Med 2001;345(20):1435–43.

39. Goodwin K, Kluis A, Alexy T, et al. Neurological complications associated with left ventricular assist device therapy. Expert Rev Cardiovasc Ther 2018;16(12): 909–17.

40. Slaughter MS, Rogers JG, Milano CA, et al. Advanced heart failure treated with continuous-flow left ventricular assist device. New Engl J Med 2009;361(23): 2241–51.

41. Himmelreich G, Ullmann H, Riess H, et al. Pathophysiologic role of contact activation in bleeding followed by thromboembolic complications after implantation of a ventricular assist device. Asaio J 1995;41(3):M790–4.

42. Crow S, Chen D, Milano C, et al. Acquired von Willebrand syndrome in continuous-flow ventricular assist device recipients. Ann Thorac Surg 2010; 90(4):1263–9.

43. Melissano G, Civilini E, Bertoglio L, et al. Angio-CT imaging of the spinal cord vascularisation: a pictorial essay. Eur J Vasc Endovascular Surg 2010;39(4): 436–40.

44. Koshino T, Murakami G, Morishita K, et al. Does the adamkiewicz artery originate from the larger segmental arteries? J Thorac Cardiovasc Surg 1999;117(5):898–905.

45. Rosenthal D. Spinal cord ischemia after abdominal aortic operation: is it preventable? J Vasc Surg 1999;30(3):391–7.
46. Berger JR. The neurological complications of bariatric surgery. Arch Neurol 2004; 61(8):1185–9.
47. Halverson JD. Metabolic risk of obesity surgery and long-term follow-up. Am J Clin Nutr 1992;55(2 Suppl):602s–5s.
48. Skroubis G, Sakellaropoulos G, Pouggouras K, et al. Comparison of nutritional deficiencies after Roux-en-Y gastric bypass and after biliopancreatic diversion with Roux-en-Y gastric bypass. Obes Surg 2002;12(4):551–8.
49. Thaisetthawatkul P, Collazo-Clavell ML, Sarr MG, et al. A controlled study of peripheral neuropathy after bariatric surgery. Neurology Oct 26 2004;63(8): 1462–70.
50. Connor JR, Boyer PJ, Menzies SL, et al. Neuropathological examination suggests impaired brain iron acquisition in restless legs syndrome. Neurology 2003; 61(3):304.
51. Krieger J, Schroeder C. Iron, brain and restless legs syndrome. Sleep Med Rev 2001;5(4):277–86.
52. Morales-Vidal SG. Neurologic complications of fat embolism syndrome. Curr Neurol Neurosci Rep 2019;19(3):14.
53. Heckmann JG, Lang CJG, Kindler K, et al. Neurologic manifestations of cerebral air embolism as a complication of central venous catheterization. Crit Care Med 2000;28(5):1621–5.
54. Ionel D, Odago F, Pettigrew L, et al. An unusual case of cerebral air embolism (5349). Neurology 2020;94(15 Supplement):5349.
55. Farouji I, Chan KH, Abed H, et al. Cerebral air embolism after gastrointestinal procedure: a case report and literature review. J Med Cases 2021;12(3):119–25.
56. Rand MV, Richard ARF. Cerebral air embolism occurring at angiography and diagnosed by computerized tomography. J Neurosurg 1984;60(1):177–8.
57. Murphy BP, Harford FJ, Cramer FS. Cerebral air embolism resulting from invasive medical procedures. Treatment with hyperbaric oxygen. Ann Surg 1985;201(2): 242–5.
58. Jamal BT, Herb K. Perioperative management of patients with myasthenia gravis: prevention, recognition, and treatment. Oral Surg Oral Med Oral Pathol Oral Radiol Endod 2009;107(5):612–5.
59. Dau PC, Lindstrom JM, Cassel CK, et al. Plasmapheresis and immunosuppressive drug therapy in myasthenia gravis. New Engl J Med 1977;297(21):1134–40.
60. Dalakas MC. Intravenous immunoglobulin in autoimmune neuromuscular diseases. Jama 2004;291(19):2367–75.
61. Pittinger CB, Eryasa Y, Adamson R. Antibiotic-induced paralysis. Anesth Analg 1970;49(3):487–501.
62. Leventhal SR, Orkin FK, Hirsh RA. Prediction of the need for postoperative mechanical ventilation in myasthenia gravis. Anesthesiology 1980;53(1):26–30.
63. Hetherington KA, Losek JD. Myasthenia gravis: myasthenia vs. cholinergic crisis. Pediatr Emerg Care 2005;21(8):546–8.
64. Rosenberg H, Pollock N, Schiemann A, et al. Malignant hyperthermia: a review. Orphanet J Rare Dis 2015;10:93.
65. Halliday NJ. Malignant hyperthermia. J Craniofac Surg Sep 2003;14(5):800–2.
66. Ording H. Incidence of malignant hyperthermia in Denmark. Anesth Analg 1985; 64(7):700–4.

Quality Improvement Metrics and Methods for Neurohospitalists

Kathryn A. Kvam, MD[a,*], Eric Bernier, MSN, RN[b],
Carl A. Gold, MD, MS[a]

KEYWORDS

- Quality improvement • Quality measures • Core measures
- Performance improvement • Hospital rankings • Neurohospitalist • Neurology
- Hospital medicine

KEY POINTS

- Quality improvement is a systematic approach to solving problems in health care to improve how neurohospitalists care for patients, typically through continuous or iterative interventions.
- Nationally, performance measures are largely driven by the requirements of the Centers for Medicare and Medicaid Services and large accrediting bodies such as The Joint Commission.
- Common measures include length of stay, readmissions, mortality, hospital-acquired complications, and stroke core measures.
- Hospital rankings also depend heavily on performance on quality and patient safety measures.
- A structured A3-based quality improvement method can help define the problem in clinical care, systematically analyze it, and iterate solutions to drive improvement.

INTRODUCTION

At the heart of the movement away from fee-for-service care toward pay-for-performance programs is an effort to better align reimbursement with the quality of care being provided for patients.[1,2] How to best measure the quality of care being provided continues to be a ripe area for research,[3,4] particularly for neurohospitalists who care for complex patients with rare diseases.[5,6] Effectively implementing changes to improve care is an even greater challenge, but one neurohospitalists are uniquely

[a] Neurohospitalist Program, Department of Neurology and Neurological Sciences, Stanford University School of Medicine, 453 Quarry Road, Stanford, CA 94305-5235, USA; [b] Stanford Health Care, 300 Pasteur Drive, MC 5255, Stanford, CA 94305, USA
* Corresponding author.
E-mail address: kkvam@stanford.edu

Neurol Clin 40 (2022) 211–230
https://doi.org/10.1016/j.ncl.2021.08.011
0733-8619/22/© 2021 Elsevier Inc. All rights reserved.

poised to meet given our skill as multidisciplinary team leaders and our insights from a clinical practice that is deeply influenced by gaps in our systems of care.

BACKGROUND
What Is Quality Improvement?

Quality improvement (QI) is a systematic approach to solving problems in health care to improve how we care for patients, typically through continuous or iterative interventions.[7–9] Where research primarily aims to generate new generalizable knowledge, QI primarily aims to improve a process or performance on an outcome, often by implementing existing knowledge in a specific setting.[8,10] The Institute of Medicine's 6 aims for improvement[11] define the dimensions of optimal patient care as *safe* (reducing errors and avoiding preventable harm), *effective* (providing care that is based on current evidence and guidelines), *patient-centered, efficient* (avoiding wasted time and resources), *timely,* and *equitable.*

Clinical audit and performance in practice initiatives like that in the Maintenance of Certification program[12] also focus on iterative improvement and yet differ in that their primary intent is to provide quality assurance[8,13] rather than enable physicians and their multidisciplinary teams to effect change. Improving quality is a key strategy for improving value in health care, where value is defined as the quality of care divided by the cost of care.

Why Should Neurohospitalists Engage in Quality Improvement?

The common program requirements for all Accreditation Council for Graduate Medical Education fellowships including vascular neurology, epilepsy, neuromuscular medicine, clinical neurophysiology, and sleep medicine dictate that "fellows must…play an active role in system improvement processes…and apply these skills to effect quality improvement measures."[14] Similarly, QI has been proposed as a core competency for both internal medicine and pediatric hospitalists.[15,16] Neurohospitalists are similarly uniquely poised to lead QI initiatives and are in fact often tapped for these roles. Neurohospitalists possess advanced systems-based practice skills, can advocate for the distinct needs of neurology patients, and provide value to the local and regional health care system by developing pathways for cost-effective, evidence-based care and helping health systems avoid penalties.[17–19] Becoming facile in understanding how neurohospitalist care is measured can aid neurohospitalists in understanding their value and garnering resources to support both improving how we care for patients with neurologic disease as well as institutional priorities.

QUALITY IMPROVEMENT METRICS
How is Neurohospitalist Care Measured?

Centers for Medicare and Medicaid Services programs and measures
Nationally, measurement of clinical performance is largely driven by the requirements of the Centers for Medicare and Medicaid Services (CMS) and large accrediting bodies such as The Joint Commission. The details of these programs are ever-changing but fundamentally the concepts remain similar: payment and certification systems that emphasize quality and safety outcomes with an increasing emphasis on cost containment over time.

CMS's Quality Payment Program (QPP) determines physician reimbursements under Medicare part B. The QPP was set up as part of the Medicare Access and Children's Health Insurance Program Reauthorization Act of 2015. The QPP has 2 tracks[20,21]:

- the Merit-based Incentive Payment System (MIPS)
- participation in an approved Advanced Alternative Payment Model (APM)

For neurohospitalists affiliated with a large academic institution or healthcare center, participation is likely through the APM track. MIPS replaces the preexisting Physician Quality Reporting System (PQRS), Value-based Payment Modifier Program, and Meaningful Use Programs. Previous studies suggest that the most common PQRS measures used by neurologists were adoption/use of electronic health record (EHR), inquiry regarding tobacco use, verification of current medications, advising smokers to quit, and deep venous thrombosis prophylaxis for ischemic stroke or intracranial hemorrhage.[22]

MIPS includes 4 categories: quality, improvement activities, promoting interoperability, and cost. Quality is based on reporting of a set number of quality measures. Improvement activities include an array of options.[23] Promoting interoperability focuses on EHR meaningful use. Cost includes Medicare spending per beneficiary, total per capita cost, and a growing number of episode-based cost measures. Performance in 2021 in these categories is calculated into a score that determines payment adjustments in 2023, which can be as much as −9% to +9%.[20,24]

Under MIPS, physicians and physician groups who are facility-based (>75% of billed Medicare Part B services occur inpatient, hospital outpatient [ie, patients in observation units], or emergency department) can be scored in the quality and cost categories based on their hospital's performance in the Hospital Value-Based Purchasing Program.[25]

A new reporting option intended for implementation in 2021, MIPS Value Pathways (MVPs), was delayed due to the COVID-19 pandemic. MVPs is centered on specialty-specific and condition-specific outcome measures that CMS intends to develop in partnership with specialty societies, including the American Academy of Neurology (AAN).[21]

CMS has 3 additional value-based programs for hospital reimbursement[25]:

- Hospital Value-Based Purchasing Program, in which hospitals are financially awarded or incur payment reduction (up to 2%) based on mortality, complications, safety, patient experience, efficiency, and cost reduction measure performance.
- Hospital Readmission Reduction Program, in which hospitals with excess readmissions within 30 days for select conditions are subject to reduced payments, capped at 3%. Neurologic conditions are currently not included.
- Hospital-Acquired Conditions Reduction Program, in which the worst-performing hospitals on central line–associated bloodstream infection, catheter-associated urinary tract infection, surgical site infection, methicillin-resistant *Staphylococcus aureus* bacteremia, *Clostridioides difficile* infection, and the CMS Recalibrated Patient Safety Indicator Composite score (PSI 90) receive reduced payments (1% for the hospitals performing in the lowest quartile).

Hospitals submit performance measures electronically, including core measures originally developed by The Joint Commission[3] and hospital-acquired conditions. For cases in which a hospital-acquired condition (HAC) was not present on admission, Medicare payment for the acquired condition may be withheld.[26]

Disease-specific stroke measures
In addition to hospital and program accreditation, The Joint Commission provides disease-specific certification programs. Those most encountered by neurology

include Acute Stroke Ready, Primary Stroke Center, Thrombectomy-Capable Stroke Center, and Comprehensive Stroke Center.[27] Each level of certification requires measure reporting, with the set increasing in volume and complexity along with the certification level. Relevant stroke measures are listed in **Table 1**.

Hospital rankings

Hospital rankings also depend heavily on performance on quality and patient safety measures. Perhaps the most widely known, US News & World Report (USNWR) Best Hospital Honor Roll, annually ranks the best hospitals for neurology in combination with neurosurgery,[28] All hospitals in the United States are eligible to be ranked, but many are excluded based on low clinical volume. The rankings are intended to be data-driven evaluations of hospital resources related to patient care, the process of delivering care, and patient outcome measures.[29] Specialties, such as neurology and neurosurgery, are defined by the Medicare Severity Diagnosis Related Group (MS-DRG) classification system, not by the specialty of the discharging physicians.

The specific methodology for the 2020 to 2021 USNWR specialty rankings is explained extensively in a 167-page document.[29] Patient outcomes relevant to neurohospitalists include risk-adjusted 30-day mortality rate and discharge to home rate for Medicare patients for calendar years 2016 to 2018, the last 3 years for which full data sets were available. Since 2019 to 2020, the rankings have also evaluated patient experience using linear mean overall scores from Hospital Consumer Assessment of Healthcare Providers and Systems (HCAHPS). A transparency measure was newly added to the neurology and neurosurgery ranking for the 2020 to 2021 rankings. A hospital received credit for this measure if it had voluntarily reported stroke care measures to the public through the Get With The Guidelines stroke QI program of the American Heart Association.

Vizient is a health care performance improvement company that includes a member consortium of voluntarily contracted academic medical centers and community hospitals.[30] Vizient ranks hospitals annually based on performance on the Quality and Accountability Scorecard. The elements of this scorecard and their relative weighting vary from year to year, but typically include the ratio of observed to expected mortality rate, 30-day readmissions, the ratio of observed to expected length of stay, patient safety indicators, and patient experience based on specific items from HCAHPS survey. Unlike USNWR, which only includes data from Medicare patients, Vizient includes data from all patients discharged from a given hospital. Specialty-specific rankings are not publicly reported by Vizient in the same manner as USNWR, but Vizient data can be filtered by specialty so individual institutions can benchmark their performance against peer institutions. Similar to USNWR, specialties such as neurology are defined by MS-DRG. Other hospital rankings include the Leapfrog Hospital Safety Grade[31] and the Lown Institute Hospitals Index.[32]

American Academy of Neurology quality measures

In 2008, the AAN began developing neurology-specific quality measures in an effort to ensure that meaningful, valid, and reliable metrics are available for neurology practices for both reporting and improvement purposes. Starting with the Parkinson's quality measures published in 2010,[33] the AAN has developed 16 quality measurement sets for epilepsy, headache, essential tremor, multiple sclerosis, stroke, amyotrophic lateral sclerosis, muscular dystrophy, distal symmetric polyneuropathy, child neurology, neuro-oncology, neurotology, inpatient and emergency neurology, universal neurology, and neurology outcomes.[34] The Axon Registry was developed to provide participating neurologists with feedback on the quality of care provided to

Table 1
Stroke measures by The Joint Commission certification type

The Joint Commission Stroke Measures	Acute Stroke Ready Center	Primary Stroke Center	Thrombectomy-Capable Stroke Center	Comprehensive Stroke Center
ASR-IP-1: Thrombolytic therapy initiated in the emergency department (followed by inpatient admission to the ASRH)	X			
ASR-IP-2: Antithrombotic therapy by end of hospital day 2	X			
ASR-IP-3: Discharged on antithrombotic therapy	X			
ASR-OP-1: Thrombolytic therapy (drip and ship)	X			
CSTK-01: NIHSS for patients with ischemic stroke		X	X	X
CSTK-02: Modified Rankin score at 90 days			X	X
CSTK-04: Procoagulant reversal agent initiation for ICH				X
CSTK-03: Severity measurement performed for SAH and ICH (overall rate)				X
CSTK-05a and b: Patients with hemorrhagic transformation treated with IV or IA t-PA or MER			X	X
CSTK-06: Nimodipine treatment administered for SAH				X
CSTK-08: TICI reperfusion grade after thrombolysis			X	X
CSTK-09a and b: Time (in minutes) from hospital arrival to skin puncture			X	X
CSTK-10: Favorable outcome at 90 d (mRS≤2)				X
CSTK-11: Rate of rapid effective reperfusion from hospital arrival				X
CSTK-12: Rate of rapid effective reperfusion from skin puncture				X
STK-1: Venous thromboembolism (VTE prophylaxis)		X	X	X
STK-10: Assessed for rehabilitation		X	X	X
STK-2: Discharged on antithrombotic therapy		X	X	X
STK-3: Anticoagulation therapy for atrial fibrillation/flutter		X	X	X
STK-4: Thrombolytic therapy		X	X	X

(continued on next page)

Table 1
(continued)

The Joint Commission Stroke Measures	Acute Stroke Ready Center	Primary Stroke Center	Thrombectomy-Capable Stroke Center	Comprehensive Stroke Center
STK-5: Antithrombotic therapy by end of hospital day 2		X	X	X
STK-6: Discharged on statin medication		X	X	X
STK-8: Stroke education		X	X	X
STK-OP-1: Door to transfer to another hospital (time in minutes-ischemic and hemorrhagic stroke)		X		

Where X indicates the presence of a particular measure within each level of stroke certification.

Abbreviations: ASR, acute stroke ready; ASRH, acute stroke ready hospital; CSTK, comprehensive stroke center; IA, intra-arterial; CH, intracerebral hemorrhage; IP, inpatient; IV, intravenous; LVO, large vessel occlusion; MER, mechanical endovascular revascularization; NIHSS, National Institutes of Health stroke scale; OP, outpatient; SAH, subarachnoid hemorrhage; STK, stroke; t-PA, tissue plasminogen activator; TICI, thrombolysis in cerebral infarction; mRS, modified Rankin score; TICI 2B, thrombolysis in cerebral infarction Grade 2B—complete filling of all of the expected vascular territory is visualized, but the filling is slower than normal; VTE, venous thromboembolism.

patients.[35] Participating practices can also use the registry to report performance measures to the MIPS program. The AAN has studied the data accuracy of the Axon Registry and has now seated a workgroup with the intent of serially revising and/or retiring quality measures after incorporation of data from the Axon Registry regarding performance of the measure (validity and reliability measurements, including whether measures have "topped off" at near perfect performance indicating there is no longer a gap in care).[36,37] It is important to note that at present the Axon Registry does not include data from hospital admissions or emergency department visits, severely limiting its usefulness for neurohospitalists.

Which Existing Metrics Should Neurohospitalists Know About?

Mortality

Mortality is defined by CMS as risk-standardized mortality within 30 days of index hospital admission date. It is easily measured and understood and meaningful to patients and physicians. However, crude mortality rates fail to capture preexisting risk and there are varying risk-adjustment models that can produce disparate results.[38] Patients on hospice at the time of death but physically in the hospital are included, which critics argue undervalues patient-centered palliative care in favor of aggressive disease-directed treatment.[39] Unlike CMS, Vizient measures only risk-adjusted deaths that occur within the hospital and none that occur after hospital discharge, which may incentivize some hospitals to "discharge" dying patients to hospice services within the hospital setting. In current neurologic practice, mortality rates are typically low,[40] limiting the reliability of mortality as an indicator for the quality of care provided by neurohospitalists.[41,42]

Length of stay

Length of stay is discharge date minus admission date, but notably does not include nights spent on observation level of care. More commonly thought of as a measure of hospital efficiency and cost, at least one previous study found a correlation between a patient's risk-adjusted length of stay and a quality of care judgment (good care vs poor care) from physician peer reviewers.[43]

Readmission rate

Under the CMS definition, any unplanned readmission that happens within 30 days of discharge from the index admission, whether the patient is readmitted to the same or different hospital, is counted as a readmission. Some readmissions may be avoidable; however, studies have found widely varying rates ranging from 5% to 79% likely due to the subjectivity of this term.[44] The CMS definition of "planned" readmission is very limited. One study of neurology readmissions found that 16% of readmissions were planned by clinicians, but only 2% were considered planned by CMS definitions.[45]

Patient experience

HCAHPS surveys are distributed to a random sample of patients (except those discharged to hospice or who died while inpatient) and measure patient experience across a variety of domains. These include communication with nurses, communication with doctors, responsiveness of hospital staff, communication about medicines, discharge information, care transitions, and an overall rating and a likelihood to recommend measure. Challenges in using patient satisfaction as a measure of care include low response rate, difficulty attributing responses to a single physician or even group (rather than a patient's experiences with doctors globally during the hospital stay), potential age bias,[46] and delayed reporting.

Hospital-acquired complications

Starting in 2008, CMS began reducing reimbursements for hospitalizations in which one of a selected set of HACs occurred that was not documented to be "present on admission." These HACs were selected based on being high cost or high volume and considered to be preventable through evidence-based guidelines.[26] A recent review highlighted hospital-acquired complications of particular relevance to neurohospitalists.[47]

1. *Falls.* Falls are a common hospital-acquired complication. Up to 30% of falls result in injury and 4% to 6% result in severe injury.[48] Neurology patients are at high risk of falls due to gait, balance, strength, visual, and cognitive impairments, as well as medications they may be receiving. A fall is defined as unintentionally coming to rest on the ground, floor, or other lower level surface, including an episode in which a patient loses balance and would have fallen if not for staff intervention.[34]
2. *Venous thromboembolism* (VTE). Patients with neurologic disease are at high risk of VTE due to immobility.[49] Incidence of potentially preventable VTE is defined as the number of patients diagnosed with confirmed VTE during hospitalization (not present on admission) who did not receive VTE prophylaxis between admission and the day before the VTE diagnostic test order date.[50]
3. *Catheter-associated urinary tract infection* (CAUTI). Patients with neurologic disease are at higher risk of urinary tract infection due to neurogenic bladder dysfunction. Per the Centers for Disease Control and Prevention definition, a CAUTI is defined as a symptomatic urinary tract infection diagnosis in the setting of an indwelling urinary catheter in place more than 2 days (note this excludes intermittent straight catheters, suprapubic catheters, and external devices) or within 1 day of its discontinuation.[51]
4. *Catheter-associated blood stream infection* (CLABSI). Patients with a central line for plasmapheresis or antibiotics are at risk of intravascular device–related bacteremia. A CLABSI is defined as bacteremia that occurs in the setting of an eligible central line in place more than 2 days following first access of the central line in the inpatient location or within 1 day of its removal.[52]
5. *Stroke measures*[27] (**Table 1**)
6. *Proposed AAN inpatient and emergency quality measures.* In 2017, a workgroup with representatives from the AAN, Neurocritical Care Society, and Neurohospitalist Society published a set of proposed inpatient and emergency quality measures.[53] Measures included documenting advance directives and goals of care, delirium screening, prevention and treatment, reducing urinary catheter utilization, and treatment of status epilepticus, Guillain-Barre, myasthenic crisis, and bacterial meningitis. Of note, performance on these measures has not been benchmarked and no data registry exists to support comparison among peer institutions. Using Vizient and manual chart review, one study found that a measure regarding dexamethasone for bacterial meningitis measure was not a reliable indicator of quality of care provided by neurohospitalists because this treatment decision is rarely made by neurohospitalists.[54]

QUALITY IMPROVEMENT TOOLS AND THEIR APPLICATION

Awareness of this national landscape and your institution's reporting requirements and performance serves several purposes for neurohospitalists:

1. to identify and prioritize QI opportunities
2. to incorporate existing validated quality measures into QI project design

3. to understand the ways in which neurohospitalists can add tangible value to their hospital or health care system and help advocate for additional resources

A variety of QI methods exist, including Lean and Six Sigma,[55,56] Model for Improvement (Institute for Healthcare Improvement),[57] and Failure Modes and Effects Analysis.[58] At many institutions, an A3-based approach is the common language and structure for improvement efforts. An example A3 is included in **Fig. 1**, and the relevant steps in its completion are outlined in **Table 2**.

What Are Some Examples of Published Quality Improvement Studies in Neurology?

"Learning from the Best" is a core concept in QI. Understanding what other groups or organizations have done to solve a problem in health care, including how they measured their performance, key drivers they identified, and interventions that were impactful can all be valuable in designing and implementing a local QI initiative. Published reports regarding quality of care in neurology span a wide range of topics from improving clinic access[68,69] to reducing length of stay,[70] readmissions,[45,71] and hospital-acquired complications.[72] Most focus on understanding the current state and/or predictors, whereas others prospectively evaluate the effect of an intervention (**Table 3**). Neurohospitalists may also benefit from reviewing QI reports published by hospital medicine physicians. For those interested in publishing their own QI reports, helpful guides exist that are relevant across specialties.[82] As in other fields, many neurology-specific journals require QI reports to adhere to SQUIRE 2.0 guidelines.[83]

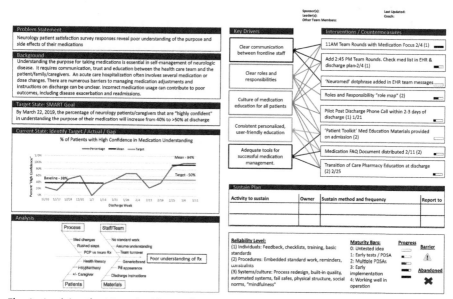

Fig. 1. Applying the A3 method for quality improvement: improving patients' understanding of their medications. FAQ, frequently asked questions; PCP, primary care physician; PDSA, plan, do, study, act; Rx, prescription; SMART, Specific, Measurable, Achievable, Relevant, Time-Bound. (*Courtesy* of David B. Larson. From Larson DB, Mickelsen LJ, Garcia K. Realizing Improvement through Team Empowerment (RITE): A Team-based, Project-based Multidisciplinary Improvement Program. Radiographics. 2016;36(7):2170–2183. doi:10.1148/rg.2016160136.

Table 2
Steps of an A3 approach to clinical problem solving

Step	Comments on Application
Identify the stakeholders, project team, and sponsors	• Stakeholders may include patients, caregivers, physicians, nurses, case managers, pharmacists, and others hospital staff. • Representatives from each stakeholder group may be represented on the project team. • The sponsor is often an executive who can provide resources and back the project if obstacles occur.[59]
Identify available resources	• Resources may include expertise, time, tools, or funding.
Define the problem statement	• Clearly state the problem you are trying to solve. • Be careful to state "what" but not "why."
Describe the background	• How does this problem affect patients, providers, and/or health care systems? • Are there tangible ways that it is important to the mission of the organization? Note: Making links here can help you get support from your hospital administration to effect change and to garner resources.
Understand and define current state	• What is the current level of performance? • Carefully think through the best measures of success. • Consider process measures, outcome measures, and balancing measures.[60]
Create a process map	• Go and see the process as it is currently occurring.[61] • Map the process.[62] • Identify any waste, such as wasted time or redundant steps.[63]
Create a run chart (**Fig. 1**)	• Refine what you will measure and how often. In a run chart, this is often a process measure to enable real-time data collection. • Note current average performance and target performance. • As the project processes, annotate the chart with interventions and dates.
Decide on a SMART goal	• Specific, Measurable, Achievable, Relevant, and Time-bound.
Analyze the problem	• Transition from "what" to understanding "why" a problem is occurring. • Perform a fishbone analysis[64] and/or Pareto chart[65] to understand the key contributing factors. • "5 Whys" can be a useful tool to understand root causes.[66]

(continued on next page)

Step	Comments on Application
Table 2 **(continued)**	
Develop the key drivers	• These are the things that must happen consistently for interventions to be successful—the "road map to success." (Examples: Order sets, electronic medical record alert systems, protocols). • Key drivers should be directly drawn from the analysis (fishbone, 5 whys, and/or Pareto).
Brainstorm, prioritize, and test interventions	• Brainstorm interventions that enable your key drivers to occur. Each intervention should be linked to at least one key driver. • Prioritize based on effort and impact, ideally aiming for high impact, low effort interventions. • Aim for high reliability interventions that are embedded in systems (EHR, physical structure), rather than depend on individuals. • Each intervention should have an owner and the maturity of the intervention should be specified. • Test interventions, at small scale to start, and use your run chart to visualize whether the desired change in your outcomes is occurring. Perform plan, do, study, act (PDSA) cycles to iterate interventions.[67] • If an intervention is successful, consider expanding its scope or scale.
Create a sustain plan	• Identify who owns each intervention and at what frequency they will report ongoing progress. • Embed the changes and tracking in existing institutional structures to maximize ongoing success. • Use your run chart to visualize whether success is maintained or further advanced. • Continue to refine and iterate.

Abbreviation: EHR, electronic health record.

(Data from Larson DB, Mickelsen LJ, Garcia K. Realizing Improvement through Team Empowerment (RITE): A Team-based, Project-based Multidisciplinary Improvement Program. Radiographics. 2016;36(7):2170–2183. https://doi.org/10.1148/rg.2016160136)

RESOURCES AND ADDITIONAL TRAINING OPPORTUNITIES IN QUALITY IMPROVEMENT

The Institute for Healthcare Improvement Open School has a wide array of online courses for learning and teaching QI.[57] The Society of Hospital Medicine offers additional online training and resources.[84] The AAN Quality Improvement page provides links to basic QI tools.[85]

Training neurology residents and fellows in QI is a gap. There are only a handful of published QI curricula for neurology residents,[86,87] one for medical students on a neurology clerkship,[88] and none to our knowledge for neurology fellows. A

Table 3
Representative published prospective quality improvement studies in neurology

Study	Population	Measure	Study Design	Interventions	Study Duration	Results
Patel, *Epilepsia* 2020[73]	Patients with pediatric epilepsy	Seizure rescue medication dosing compliance	Single-center quality improvement study[a]	Prefilled midazolam syringes; electronic chart tools; monthly pharmacy review; physician and RN education	4 y	Substantial decrease in underdosed rescue medications, from 3.5% noncompliance to 0.4%
Ostendorf,[74] *Pediatric Neurology* 2018	Admitted pediatric patients with status epilepticus on the floor	Percentage of patients treated with a BZD within 10 min and ICU transfer rate	Single-center quality improvement study	Seizure simulations with floor staff; emphasizing IN midazolam over IV lorazepam; relocating medications	2 y	Proportion of patients who received a benzodiazepine within 10 min improved from 39% to 79% and there were significantly fewer ICU transfers (39% down to 9%)
Machline-Carrion, *JAMA Neurology* 2019[75]	Patients with stroke or TIA	Composite adherence to evidence-based performance measures	Multicenter, cluster-randomized controlled trial	Case management; reminders; checklist; educational materials; periodic audit and feedback	22 mo	Trend toward better adherence in intervention group that was not significant
Kassardjian,[76] *Neurology* 2015	Patients undergoing muscle biopsy	Percentage of delayed or canceled muscle biopsies	Single-center quality improvement study	Move informed consent visit to the afternoon; create patient education brochures detailing preoperative restrictions	21 mo	Reduced delayed muscle biopsies from 21% of all cases to 7%

Source	Population	Metric	Study design	Intervention	Duration	Results
Nance,[77] *Journal of Parkinson's Disease* 2020	Hospitalized patients with Parkinson disease	On-time administration of levodopa	Single-center quality improvement study	EHR alert; stocking on unit dispensaries; medication reconciliation and education	3 y	Significantly improved on-time medication administration (from 42% to 71% within 15 min of scheduled time)
Busby,[78] *Journal of Neurointervention Surgery* 2015	Patients with stroke	Door-to-needle time	Single-center quality improvement study	Implementation of "CODE FAST" workflow including prehospital notification; standard work for 2 RNs in parallel with neurology MD evaluation	1 y	Significant reduction in door-to-needle time from a median of 62–25 min
Coughlin,[79] *Neurocritical Care* 2018	Patients transferring out of neurointensive care to the floor	Percentage of "Bouncebacks" to the ICU	Single-center quality improvement study	Implementation of an enhanced handoff process for "high-risk" patients	2 y retrospective + 15 mo prospective	Bounceback rate improved from 6.7% pre-intervention to 2.8% post
Duncan,[80] *Circulation: Cardiovascular Quality and Outcomes* 2020	Patients with stroke or TIA discharged from the hospital	Functional status	Multicenter cluster-randomized controlled trial	Comprehensive postdischarge transitional care	2 y	No significant difference in functional status between intervention and controls

(continued on next page)

Table 3
(continued)

Study	Population	Measure	Study Design	Interventions	Study Duration	Results
Bravata,[81] *JAMA Network Open* 2020	VA patients with transient neurologic symptoms	Percentage of patients who received all 7 guideline recommended processes of care they were eligible for	Multicenter nonrandomized cluster controlled trial	Clinical program; data feedback; education; EHR tools	4 y	Significantly improved mean "without-fail" rate following the intervention compared with controls

Abbreviations: BZD, benzodiazepine; EHR, electronic health record; ICU, intensive care unit; IN, intranasal; IV, intravenous; MD, medical doctor; RN, registered nurse; TIA, transient ischemic attack; VA, Department of Veterans Affairs.

[a] Quality improvement studies: those that used traditional single-center, nonrandomized, iterative Plan-Do-Study-Act cycles ± statistical process control for analysis.

standardized national curriculum is needed to ensure this core competency is met. Finding faculty qualified to teach this curriculum when most neurologists lack formal training is an unmet professional development need.

SUMMARY

Equipped with a basic understanding of QI tools and metrics, neurohospitalists can be prepared to lead multidisciplinary teams in improving how we care for our patients. Knowledge of how the care we provide is measured can facilitate identifying readily available data for measuring project success and help neurohospitalists prioritize improvement efforts that will add value.

CLINICS CARE POINTS

- QI is a systematic approach to solving problems in how we care for patients.
- Common clinical performance measures for hospitalized neurology patients include length of stay, readmissions, mortality, hospital-acquired complications, and stroke core measures.
- A structured A3-based QI method can be used to translate a gap in care (a bad outcome or near miss) into an opportunity to design and lead a QI project that impacts how we care for future patients.
- Publishing QI projects can be both an opportunity for scholarship and disseminating best practices.

DISCLOSURE

The authors have nothing to disclose.

ACKNOWLEDGMENTS

The authors thank Drs Frank Longo, Yuen So, and Greg Albers and Alison Kerr for their support of QI in the Stanford Department of Neurology and Neurologic Sciences. The authors thank Dr David Larson for his mentorship and his direction of the Stanford Realizing Improvement through Team Empowerment and Clinical Effectiveness Leadership Training programs. The authors thank Mark Ramirez for his additional contributions and Dr Brian Scott for allowing inclusion of example QI tools used in his multidisciplinary project on medication education.

REFERENCES

1. Porter ME, Teisberg EO. How physicians can change the future of health care. JAMA 2007;297(10):1103.
2. Stevens JC. Pay for performance and the physicians quality reporting initiative in neurologic practice. Neurol Clin 2010;28(2):505–16.
3. Chassin MR, Loeb JM, Schmaltz SP, et al. Accountability measures — using measurement to promote quality improvement. N Engl J Med 2010;363(7):683–8.
4. Pimentel MPT, Austin JM, Kachalia A. To improve quality, keep your eyes on the road. BMJ Qual Saf 2020;29(11):943–6.
5. Naessens JM, Van Such MB, Nesse RE, et al. Looking under the streetlight? A framework for differentiating performance measures by level of care in a value-based payment environment. Acad Med 2017;92(7):943–50.

6. Douglas VC, Josephson SA. A proposed roadmap for inpatient neurology quality indicators. Neurohospitalist 2011;1(1):8–15.
7. Does improving quality save money? | The Health Foundation. Available at: https://www.health.org.uk/publications/does-improving-quality-save-money. Accessed March 16, 2021.
8. Backhouse A, Ogunlayi F. Quality improvement into practice. BMJ 2020;368: m865.
9. Academy of Medical Royal Colleges. Quality improvement - training for better outcomes. Academy of Medical Royal Colleges. Available at https://www.aomrc.org.uk/reports-guidance/quality-improvement-training-better-outcomes/. Accessed April 23, 2021.
10. Finkelstein JA, Brickman AL, Capron A, et al. Oversight on the borderline: quality improvement and pragmatic research. Clin Trials 2015;12(5):457–66.
11. Institute of Medicine (US). Committee on quality of health care in America. Crossing the quality chasm: a new health system for the 21st century. National Academies Press (US); 2001. Available at: http://www.ncbi.nlm.nih.gov/books/NBK222274/. Accessed March 16, 2021.
12. Faulkner LR, Tivnan PW, Johnston MV, et al. Invited article: the ABPN maintenance of certification program for neurologists: past, present, and future. Neurology 2008;71(8):599–604.
13. Johnston G, Crombie I, Alder E, et al. Reviewing audit: barriers and facilitating factors for effective clinical audit. Qual Health Care 2000;9(1):23–36.
14. Accreditation Council for Graduate Medical Education. Neurology Program Requirements and FAQs. Available at: https://acgme.org/Specialties/Program-Requirements-and-FAQs-and-Applications/pfcatid/37/Neurology. Accessed April 23, 2021.
15. The core competencies in hospital medicine: a framework for curriculum development by the Society of Hospital Medicine. J Hosp Med 2006;1(S1):iii–iv.
16. Stucky ER, Ottolini MC, Maniscalco J. Pediatric hospital medicine core competencies: development and methodology. J Hosp Med 2010;5(S2):110–4.
17. Simpson JR, Rosenthal LD, Cumbler EU, et al. Inpatient falls: defining the problem and identifying possible solutions. Part II: application of quality improvement principles to hospital falls. Neurohospitalist 2013;3(4):203–8.
18. Cumbler EU, Simpson JR, Rosenthal LD, et al. Inpatient falls: defining the problem and identifying possible solutions. Part I: an evidence-based review. Neurohospitalist 2013;3(3):135–43.
19. Probasco JC, Greene J, Harrison A, et al. Neurohospitalist practice, perspectives, and burnout. Neurohospitalist 2019;9(2):85–92.
20. QPP Overview - QPP. Available at: https://qpp.cms.gov/about/qpp-overview. Accessed March 16, 2021.
21. MIPS Value Pathways - QPP. Available at: https://qpp.cms.gov/mips/mips-value-pathways. Accessed March 16, 2021.
22. Cohen AB, Sanders AE, Swain-Eng RJ, et al. Quality measures for neurologists. Neurol Clin Pract 2013;3(1):44–51.
23. Improvement activities. Available at: https://www.aan.com/siteassets/home-page/tools-and-resources/practicing-neurologist–administrators/quality-payment-program/merit-based-incentive-payment-system/17-updateiatipsheet.pdf. Accessed April 29, 2021.
24. Quality Payment Program (QPP). Available at: https://www.aan.com/tools-and-resources/practicing-neurologists-administrators/value-based-care/quality-payment-program/. Accessed March 16, 2021.

25. QPP | Quality Payment Program. Available at: https://www.hospitalmedicine.org/practice-management/qpp-quality-payment-program/. Accessed March 16, 2021.

26. Hospital-Acquired Conditions (Present on Admission Indicator) | CMS. Available at: https://www.cms.gov/Medicare/Medicare-Fee-for-Service-Payment/HospitalAcqCond?redirect=/hospitalacqcond/01_over-view.asp. Accessed March 16, 2021.

27. Stroke Fact Sheet. Available at: https://www.heart.org/-/media/files/professional/quality-improvement/get-with-the-guidelines/get-with-the-guidelines-stroke/stroke-fact-sheet_-comprehensive_-final_ucm_501843.pdf?la=en. Accessed April 23, 2021.

28. Best Hospitals for Neurology & Neurosurgery | Rankings & Ratings | US News Best Hospitals. Available at: https://health.usnews.com/best-hospitals/rankings/neurology-and-neurosurgery. Accessed April 23, 2021.

29. Olmsted M, Powell R, Murphy J. Methodology US News & World Report 2020-2021 best hospitals: specialty rankings. Available at: https://health.usnews.com/media/best-hospitals/BH_Methodology_2020-21. Accessed April 23, 2021.

30. Vizient Inc.| Member-driven healthcare performance improvement. Available at: https://www.vizientinc.com/. Accessed April 23, 2021.

31. Healthcare ratings and reports. Leapfrog. 2015. Available at: https://www.leapfroggroup.org/ratings-reports. Accessed April 23, 2021.

32. Rankings. Lown Institute Hospital Index. Available at: https://lownhospitalsindex.org/rankings/. Accessed April 23, 2021.

33. Cheng EM, Tonn S, Swain-Eng R, et al. Quality improvement in neurology: AAN Parkinson disease quality measures: report of the Quality Measurement and Reporting Subcommittee of the American Academy of Neurology. Neurology 2010; 75(22):2021–7.

34. Quality measures. Available at: https://www.aan.com/practice/quality-measures/. Accessed March 16, 2021.

35. Sigsbee B, Goldenberg JN, Bever CT, et al. Introducing the Axon Registry: an opportunity to improve quality of neurologic care. Neurology 2016;87(21):2254–8.

36. Baca CM, Benish S, Videnovic A, et al. Axon Registry® data validation: accuracy assessment of data extraction and measure specification. Neurology 2019; 92(18):847–58.

37. Victorio MCC, Lundgren K, Johnston-Gross M, et al. Implementation of a data accuracy plan to improve data extraction yield in the Axon Registry®. Neurology 2020;95(3):e310–9.

38. Shahian DM, Wolf RE, Iezzoni LI, et al. Variability in the measurement of hospital-wide mortality rates. N Engl J Med 2010;363(26):2530–9.

39. Holloway RG, Quill TE. Mortality as a measure of quality: implications for palliative and end-of-life care. JAMA 2007;298(7):802.

40. Douglas VC, Scott BJ, Berg G, et al. Effect of a neurohospitalist service on outcomes at an academic medical center. Neurology 2012;79(10):988–94.

41. Goldfarb. Risk-adjusted overall mortality as a quality measure in the cardiovascular intensive care unit | Ovid. Available at: https://oce-ovid-com.stanford.idm.oclc.org/article/00045415-201811000-00004/HTML. Accessed April 9, 2021.

42. Koennecke H-C, Belz W, Berfelde D, et al. Factors influencing in-hospital mortality and morbidity in patients treated on a stroke unit. Neurology 2011;77(10): 965–72.

43. Thomas JW, Guire KE, Horvat GG. Is patient length of stay related to quality of care? Hosp Health Serv Adm 1997;42(4):489–507.

44. van Walraven C, Bennett C, Jennings A, et al. Proportion of hospital readmissions deemed avoidable: a systematic review. CMAJ 2011;183(7):E391–402.

45. Le ST, Josephson SA, Puttgen HA, et al. Many neurology readmissions are non-preventable. Neurohospitalist 2017;7(2):61–9.

46. Chen JG, Zou B, Shuster J. Relationship between patient satisfaction and physician characteristics. J Patient Exp 2017;4(4):177–84.

47. Sand H, Owen M, Amin A. CMS' hospital-acquired conditions for the neurohospitalist. Neurohospitalist 2012;2(1):18–27.

48. Hitcho EB, Krauss MJ, Birge S, et al. Characteristics and circumstances of falls in a hospital setting. J Gen Intern Med 2004;19(7):732–9.

49. Schneck MJ. Venous thromboembolism in neurologic disease. Handb Clin Neurol 2014;119:289–304.

50. Specifications manual for joint commission national quality measures (v2020A. Available at: https://manual.jointcommission.org/releases/TJC2020A/MIF0163. html. Accessed April 23, 2021.

51. National Healthcare Safety Network. Urinary tract infection. 2021. Available at: https://www.cdc.gov/nhsn/PDFs/pscManual/7pscCAUTIcurrent.pdf. Accessed April 23, 2021.

52. National Healthcare Safety Network. Bloodstream infections. 2021. Available at: https://www.cdc.gov/nhsn/pdfs/pscmanual/4psc_clabscurrent.pdf. Accessed April 23, 2021.

53. Josephson SA, Ferro J, Cohen A, et al. Quality improvement in neurology: inpatient and emergency care quality measure set: executive summary. Neurology 2017;89(7):730–5.

54. Dujari S, Gummidipundi S, He Z, et al. Administration of dexamethasone for bacterial meningitis: an unreliable quality measure. Neurohospitalist 2021;11(2):101–6.

55. Lean Enterprise Institute. What is lean? Lean Enterprise Institute. 2018. Available at: https://www.lean.org/WhatsLean/. Accessed April 23, 2021..

56. Application of lean thinking to health care: issues and observations | International Journal for Quality in Health Care | Oxford Academic. Available at: https://academic.oup.com/intqhc/article/21/5/341/1831537. Accessed April 24, 2021.

57. Institute for Healthcare Improvement (IHI). IHI resources: how to improve. IHI; 2018. Available at: http://www.ihi.org/resources/Pages/HowtoImprove/default.aspx.

58. DeRosier J, Stalhandske E, Bagian JP, et al. Using health care failure mode and effect analysis: the VA national center for patient safety's prospective risk analysis system. Jt Comm J Qual Improv 2002;28(5):248–67, 209.

59. Kotter JP. Leading change: why transformation efforts fail. Harv Bus Rev 1995;73(2):59–67. Available at: https://hbr.org/1995/05/leading-change-why-transformation-efforts-fail-2. Accessed April 23, 2021.

60. Toma M, Dreischulte T, Gray NM, et al. Balancing measures or a balanced accounting of improvement impact: a qualitative analysis of individual and focus group interviews with improvement experts in Scotland. BMJ Qual Saf 2018;27(7):547–56.

61. McClam Liebengood S, Cooper M, Nagy P. Going to the gemba: identifying opportunities for improvement in radiology. J Am Coll Radiol 2013;10(12):977–9.

62. Antonacci G, Reed JE, Lennox L, et al. The use of process mapping in healthcare quality improvement projects. Health Serv Manage Res 2018;31(2):74–84.

63. Green CF, Crawford V, Bresnen G, et al. A waste walk through clinical pharmacy: how do the "seven wastes" of lean techniques apply to the practice of clinical pharmacists. Int J Pharm Pract 2015;23(1):21–6.

64. Phillips J, Simmonds L. Using fishbone analysis to investigate problems. Nurs Times 2013;109(15):18–20.

65. Harvey HB, Sotardi ST. The pareto principle. J Am Coll Radiol 2018;15(6):931.

66. Brook OR, Kruskal JB, Eisenberg RL, et al. Root cause analysis: learning from adverse safety events. Radiographics 2015;35(6):1655–67.

67. Taylor MJ, McNicholas C, Nicolay C, et al. Systematic review of the application of the plan–do–study–act method to improve quality in healthcare. BMJ Qual Saf 2014;23(4):290–8.

68. Ross SC. An option for improving access to outpatient general neurology. Neurol Clin Pract 2014;4(5):435–40.

69. Elrashidi MY, Philpot LM, Young NP, et al. Effect of integrated community neurology on utilization, diagnostic testing, and access. Neurol Clin Pract 2017; 7(4):306–15.

70. Probasco JC, Hawley G, Burnett M, et al. Facilitating early-in-day discharge for multiple sclerosis patients treated with intravenous methylprednisolone: a quality improvement project. Neurohospitalist 2015;5(4):197–204.

71. Condon C, Lycan S, Duncan P, et al. Reducing readmissions after stroke with a structured nurse practitioner/registered nurse transitional stroke program. Stroke 2016;47(6):1599–604.

72. Halperin JJ, Moran S, Prasek D, et al. Reducing hospital-acquired infections among the neurologically critically ill. Neurocrit Care 2016;25(2):170–7.

73. Using quality improvement to implement the CNS/AAN quality measure on rescue medication for seizures - Patel - 2020 - Epilepsia - Wiley Online Library. Available at: https://onlinelibrary-wiley-com.stanford.idm.oclc.org/doi/full/10.1111/epi.16713. Accessed April 6, 2021.

74. Ostendorf AP, Merison K, Wheeler TA, et al. Decreasing seizure treatment time through quality improvement reduces critical care utilization. Pediatr Neurol 2018;85:58–66.

75. Effect of a quality improvement intervention on adherence to therapies for patients with acute ischemic stroke and transient ischemic attack: a cluster randomized clinical trial | Cerebrovascular Disease | JAMA Neurology | JAMA Network. Available at: https://jamanetwork-com.stanford.idm.oclc.org/journals/jamaneurology/fullarticle/2732174. Accessed April 6, 2021.

76. Kassardjian CD, Williamson ML, van Buskirk DJ, et al. Residency training: quality improvement projects in neurology residency and fellowship: applying DMAIC methodology. Neurology 2015;85(2):e7–10.

77. Nance MA, Boettcher L, Edinger G, et al. Quality improvement in Parkinson's disease: a successful program to enhance timely administration of levodopa in the hospital. J Park Dis 2020;10(4):1551–9.

78. Busby L, Owada K, Dhungana S, et al. CODE FAST: a quality improvement initiative to reduce door-to-needle times. J Neurointerv Surg 2016;8(7):661–4.

79. Coughlin DG, Kumar MA, Patel NN, et al. Preventing early bouncebacks to the neurointensive care unit: a retrospective analysis and quality improvement pilot. Neurocrit Care 2018;28(2).175–83.

80. Duncan Pamela W, Bushnell Cheryl D, Jones Sara B, et al. Randomized pragmatic trial of stroke transitional care. Circ Cardiovasc Qual Outcomes 2020; 13(6):e006285.

81. Assessment of the protocol-guided rapid evaluation of veterans experiencing new transient neurological symptoms (PREVENT) program for improving quality of care for transient ischemic attack: a nonrandomized cluster trial | Cerebrovascular Disease | JAMA Network Open | JAMA Network. Available at: https://

jamanetwork-com.stanford.idm.oclc.org/journals/jamanetworkopen/fullarticle/ 2770248. Accessed April 6, 2021.

82. Larson DB, Duncan JR, Nagy PG, et al. Guide to effective quality improvement reporting in radiology. Radiology 2014;271(2):561–73.

83. SQUIRE | SQUIRE 2.0 guidelines. Available at: http://www.squire-statement.org/ index.cfm?fuseaction=Page.ViewPage&pageId=471. Accessed April 23, 2021.

84. SHM's center for quality improvement. Available at: https://www.hospitalmedicine. org/clinical-topics/clinical-topic-overview/. Accessed April 23, 2021.

85. Quality Improvement. AAN. Available at: https://www.aan.com/policy-and-quidelines/quality/quality-improvement/quality-toolkit-and-resources/. Accessed April 23, 2021.

86. Maski KP, Loddenkemper T, An S, et al. Development and implementation of a quality improvement curriculum for child neurology residents: lessons learned. Pediatr Neurol 2014;50(5):452–7.

87. Miller-Kuhlmann R, Kraler L, Bozinov N, et al. Education research: a novel resident-driven neurology quality improvement curriculum. Neurology 2020; 94(3):137–42.

88. McInnis RP, Lee AJ, Schwartz B, et al. A quality improvement curriculum for the neurology clerkship: a practice-based approach to discharge education. eNeurologicalSci 2019;16:100196.

Social Determinants of Health in Neurology

Nicole Rosendale, MD

KEYWORDS

- Social determinants of health • Structural determinants of health • Health equity
- Health disparity • Neurodisparity

KEY POINTS

- Social determinants of health are the conditions in which people are born, grow, and live that affect health access and outcomes.
- Social structures are stratified based on structural determinants of health, or the political and social policies that define individual positions within hierarchies of access to power and resources.
- Disparities in disease incidence, prevalence, and outcomes exist throughout neurology, including in stroke, epilepsy, headache, amyotrophic lateral sclerosis, multiple sclerosis, and dementia.
- Neurologic health equity requires multilevel interventions, including at the individual, interpersonal, organizational, community, and policy levels, to create sustained change.

INTRODUCTION

Social determinants of health (SDH) are the conditions in which people are born, live, and grow that affect health access and outcomes.[1] The US Department of Health and Human Services Healthy People 2030 recommendations outline 5 primary domains of SDH: health care access and quality, education access and quality, social and community context, economic stability, and neighborhood and built environment.[1] These conditions are stratified into social hierarchies that determine an individual's differential exposure and vulnerability to health conditions and access to available resources.[2] These social strata are created and sustained through *structural determinants of health*, that is, the political and social policies that define individual positions within hierarchies of power and access to resources.[2]

There are multiple frameworks available to conceptualize the interplay between structural determinants of health, social determinants of health, and health outcomes. In 2010, the World Health Organization published a framework that also names intermediate determinants of health: material circumstances, behavior and biological factors, and psychosocial factors (**Fig. 1**).[2] Another framework to conceptualize this

Neurohospitalist Division, Department of Neurology, University of California San Francisco, 1001 Potrero Avenue, Building 1, Room 101, Box 0870, San Francisco, CA 94110, USA
E-mail address: Nicole.Rosendale@ucsf.edu

Neurol Clin 40 (2022) 231–247
https://doi.org/10.1016/j.ncl.2021.08.012
0733-8619/22/© 2021 Elsevier Inc. All rights reserved.
neurologic.theclinics.com

Figure A. Final form of the CSDH conceptual framework

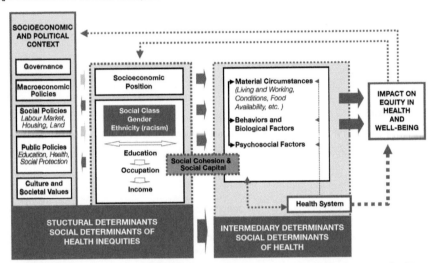

Fig. 1. The World Health Organization social determinants of health framework. (*From* World Health Organization. A Conceptual Framework for Action on the Social Determinants of Health: Debates, Policy & Practice, Case Studies.; 2010. Accessed March 26, 2021. http://apps.who.int/iris/bitstream/10665/44489/1/9789241500852_eng.pdf; with permission)

interplay between the individual and society is the social ecological model (**Fig. 2**).[3] These frameworks serve as the basis for the subsequent discussion of SDH in neurologic care presented in this article.

The connection between social structures and health gained increased attention in the late twentieth century, although references to the relationship between a person's social position and health can be found throughout medical history. In the 1700s, Johann Peter Frank argued for changing the economic, environmental, social, and occupational conditions of workers to promote public health and advocated for physicians' roles in that change.[4] In 1848, Rudolph Virchow said that "if medicine is to accomplish its great task, it must intervene in political and social life."[5] Following World War II, the World Health Organization was founded with a constitution that defined health as a "state of complete physical, mental and social well-being."[6]

During the late 1990s and early 2000s, there was renewed focus to tackle health inequities and address SDH worldwide.[6] In 2002, for example, Sweden launched a determinants-oriented national public health strategy in which health objectives were framed in terms of SDH, such as people's economic security and access to employment.[6] This recognition of the importance of social structures on individual health gained momentum in the United States as well. A 2011 meta-analysis highlighted that the number of deaths in the United States in 2000 attributable to low education, racial segregation, and limited social support was comparable to the deaths due to myocardial infarction, cerebrovascular disease, and lung cancer, respectively.[7] In 2014, Braveman and Gottlieb[8] wrote that a "large and compelling body of evidence…reveals a powerful role for social factors – apart from medical care – in shaping health."

The global novel coronavirus disease 2019 (COVID-19) pandemic in 2020 led to even further attention on structural and social determinants of health with particular focus on the role of structural racism leading to disproportionate COVID-19 morbidity

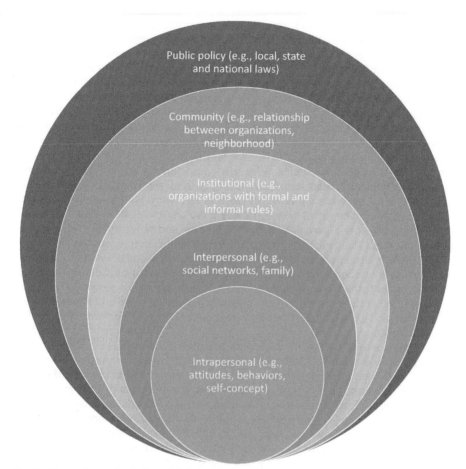

Fig. 2. The social ecological model. (*Data from* McLeroy KR, Bibeau D, Steckler A, Glanz K. An Ecological Perspective on Health Promotion Programs. Health Education Quarterly. 1988;15(4):351-377. https://doi.org/10.1177/109019818801500401)

and mortality in Black/African American, Indigenous/Native American, and Latinx communities. An analysis of COVID-19 mortality in Black individuals compared with White individuals, for example, found that after adjustment for age, sex, insurance status, comorbidities, neighborhood deprivation, and site of care, there was no statistically significant difference in risk of mortality between the 2 groups.[9] The investigators highlighted that it was therefore not race itself as a social construct that determined risk, but rather social determinants (access to hospital care),[9] a factor inextricably linked to structural racism.

Disparities in health due to systemic discrimination do not only affect Black, Indigenous, and people of color. Individuals who identify as lesbian, gay, bisexual, transgender, and queer (LGBTQ+), for example, experience disparate access to and outcomes in health as well. LGBTQ+ youth are at higher risk for substance use, depression, anxiety, and suicide.[10] LGBTQ+ adults are at higher risk for a number of conditions, including adverse mental health outcomes, substance use, cancer, and cardiovascular disease.[11] Individuals with disabilities report higher rates of obesity, smoking, adverse mental health, and cardiovascular disease.[12]

A full understanding of SDH also requires an understanding of intersectionality. Intersectionality refers to the interconnected nature of multiple identities in determining an individual's experiences with and exposure to discrimination. With ties to the advocacy of Sojourner Truth and Audre Lord, Kimberlé Crenshaw[13] formalized the term in relation to the experiences of Black women in 1989. Since that time, this framework has been used to understand the complex influence of an individual's social and personal identities on health access and outcomes. A 2021 study of structural oppression and Black sexual minority men's health, for example, found that structural racism (measured using the State Racism Index) was associated with symptoms of anxiety, perceived burdensomeness (a proximal cause of suicidal ideation), and heavy drinking.[14] Anti-LGBTQ+ policies were also associated with anxiety symptoms, perceived burdensomeness and heavy drinking, and were negatively associated with human immunodeficiency virus (HIV) testing frequency. Further analysis showed a significant interaction effect between these 2 factors: the positive association between structural racism, perceived burdensomeness, and heavy drinking were stronger for individuals living in states with high levels of anti-LGBTQ+ policies.[14]

More recently, research has begun to connect the experience of living in a discriminatory society to specific physiologic changes. The concept of allostatic load, for example, refers to the physiologic cost of chronic neuroendocrine responses induced by exposure to chronic or repeated psychosocial stressors.[15] Poverty, neighborhood segregation, and experiences of discrimination, whether due to race/ethnicity, weight, acculturation status, sexual orientation, or gender identity/expression, are all associated with higher allostatic load.[15] In turn, higher allostatic load is associated with risk for cardiovascular disease,[16] adverse mental health,[17] adverse maternal-fetal outcomes,[18] and even mortality.[16] Other studies have assessed the role of epigenetic changes in response to psychosocial stress. A study of sexual minority men living with HIV found that stress related to sexual minority identity was associated with differential expression in leukocyte genes in pathways that are implicated in inflammation, immune function, cancer, and cardiovascular function.[19] A combination of allostatic load and epigenetic changes may influence the function of biological pathways and ultimately some clinical outcomes associated with SDH.

SOCIAL DETERMINANTS OF HEALTH IN NEUROLOGY

Disparities exist throughout neurology. Examples can be found across all neurologic subspecialties and illnesses,[20] including stroke,[21] epilepsy,[22] headache,[23] dementia,[24] amyotrophic lateral sclerosis,[25] and multiple sclerosis.[26] A recent study found that Black individuals were nearly 30% less likely to see an outpatient neurologist and Hispanic individuals nearly 40% less likely compared with White counterparts, even after adjusting for demographic, insurance, and health status differences.[27] Not surprisingly, Black and Hispanic individuals in this study had higher emergency department use and more inpatient utilization compared with White participants.[27] These inequities have only been exacerbated in the setting of COVID-19.[28]

Although a description of the breadth of disparities in neurology is outside the scope of this article, disparities in stroke prevalence and outcomes serve as a representative example. The incidence of stroke is higher in Mexican American and American Indian/Alaska Native individuals compared with non-Hispanic White Americans.[29,30] Black individuals have higher risk of stroke at younger ages, higher risk of recurrent stroke, and higher stroke mortality compared with non-Hispanic White individuals.[30] Asian American individuals have similar prevalence of stroke to non-Hispanic White Americans and lower stroke mortality,[31] although a 2019 study using data from the Get with the Guidelines-Stroke program found that Asian American individuals with stroke presented with greater stroke severity, were less likely to receive intravenous thrombolysis (odds ratio [OR] 0.95, 95% confidence interval [CI] 0.91–0.98) and had worse functional outcomes (Modified Rankin Score of 0–1 OR 0.90, 95% CI 0.83–0.97) compared with White individuals, even after controlling for presenting National Institutes of Health stroke score (NIHSS).[32]

If we apply the social ecologic model to stroke disparities, we can understand how existing social and political structures perpetuate these disparities.

Intrapersonal Factors

On an *intrapersonal level*, for example, research suggests that stereotype threat plays an important role in perpetuating health disparities. Stereotype threat occurs when cues in an environment make negative stereotypes associated with a person's identity salient to that individual, triggering psychological and physiologic processes that can have a detrimental effect on the individual's cognitive and physical function.[33] This phenomenon can lead to difficulty with adherence to treatment recommendations, limited comprehension of patient education, and disengagement.[33]

Experiences of discrimination across the lifespan may directly influence vascular health as well. Research suggests a positive association between higher levels of internalized racism and stroke risk factors of obesity and hypertension.[34] In a 2007 study on cardiovascular recovery in Black and White men, both Black and White men who inhibited their anger during a debate had delayed total peripheral vascular recovery, whereas only Black men had delayed recovery when expressing their anger during debate.[35] As the title of the article suggests, this study demonstrates that whether Black men express or repress anger there are cardiovascular consequences.

Interpersonal Factors

At the *interpersonal level*, there are multiple potential contributors to disparities in stroke and stroke risk factors. Although data are limited, available studies suggest that Black individuals presenting with stroke are less likely to receive thrombolysis compared with White individuals.[30] In one of the available studies, this difference was significant even after accounting for delays in presentation.[36] The emergent nature of the decision to administer thrombolysis necessitates rapid decision making, which is often when the effect of implicit bias is greatest. Another potential contributor to this disparity is differential rates of refusal of intravenous tissue plasminogen activator (IV tPA). In a study using Get With the Guidelines-Stroke registry data, Black individuals had 2 times higher odds of not consenting to IV tPA even after adjusting for age, self-pay status, prior stroke, NIHSS, and hypertension (adjusted OR 2.5, 95% CI 1.3–4.6).[37] Although the reasons for refusal were not available, the investigators highlight that these consent conversations require effective communication between the clinician and the patient or surrogate, which may be influenced by interpersonal bias, health literacy, or trust in the clinician or health care system,[37] particularly if there is race discordance between the clinician and patient or surrogate.[38]

Other examples of the effects of interpersonal racism contributing to stroke disparities is the differential rate of urine toxicology screens in patients presenting with stroke or transient ischemic attack (TIA). In this study, younger age (<50 years) and Black race were the factors that significantly predicted the performance of a urine toxicology screen.[39] This finding is concerning for multiple reasons: the preferential performance of toxicology screening in Black patients may reinforce existing biases about the prevalence of drug use as the etiology of stroke and TIA in this population. In addition, the failure to test all individuals presenting with stroke or TIA means that other populations may not have the stroke risk factor of drug use identified, thereby missing an important opportunity for targeted intervention. Interpersonal racism is associated with other stroke risk factors as well, including higher ambulatory blood pressure,[40] smoking,[41] diabetes,[42] and sleep.[43]

Organizational Factors

At the *organizational level*, one study showed that Black individuals had longer wait times to see a physician after arriving to the emergency department with stroke symptoms compared with White individuals.[44] This study found that wait times for Hispanic individuals were similar to White individuals; however, another study found that Hispanic individuals with stroke symptoms also had longer wait times.[45] In both of these studies, arrival by ambulance was associated with being seen sooner by a physician and Black and Hispanic individuals may be less likely to use ambulance services.[30] Although the differential use of ambulance services may be an explanation for the difference in wait times, this finding then highlights other upstream structural barriers in need of intervention, such as economic disparities or barriers due to language. Among Hispanic adults who have immigrated to the United States, degree of acculturation (defined as a combination of citizenship status, birthplace, and length of stay in the United States) was associated with use of emergency services: the least acculturated adults were 14.4% less likely to use emergency services compared with US-born non-Hispanic White individuals.[46] A 2019 study found that statements about immigration made during President Trump's campaign (building a wall, deportation, and denying services to immigrants) was associated with fear in accessing emergency department services and led half of surveyed Latinx immigrants without documentation to delay presentation by a median of 2 to 3 days.[47] In the setting of stroke, these delays could lead to further disability and widen the existing gap in stroke outcomes.

After stroke, there are also racial difference in stroke education that influence an individuals' ability to respond to recurrent stroke or to a stroke in their social network. Hispanic, Asian, native Hawaiian/Pacific Islander, and American Indian/Alaska Native stroke survivors had lower odds of recognizing all 5 signs of stroke and calling 911 compared with non-Hispanic White stroke survivors (OR 0.42, 95% CI 0.25–0.71).[48] Although the reasons for this may be multifactorial, the nature of stroke education provided by organizations at the time of the initial stroke may play a large role and speaks to the idea of striving for equity (meeting the specific educational needs of the patient you are treating) rather than equality (providing the same education to all patients).

Community Factors

Neighborhood factors, part of the *community level* in the social ecologic model, have well-described connections to stroke and stroke risk factors. Higher neighborhood socioeconomic status (defined as median household income for the zip code) was associated with shorter onset-to-treatment times as well as reduced in-hospital mortality.[49] A study using data from the North Manhattan Study found that participants living less than 100 m from a major roadway had a 42% (95% CI 1.01–2.02) higher rate of ischemic stroke compared with those living more than 400 m away.[50] Neighborhood factors also influence stroke risk factors. Urban sprawl, limited access to healthy food, access to safe public space for exercise, and neighborhood social environment (defined as social capital, collective efficacy, and crime) have all been associated with risk of obesity.[51] Access to healthy food options, neighborhood safety, and social cohesion are also associated with lower rates of hypertension.[52] In stroke survivors, neighborhood also influences outcomes. Data from The Brain Attack Surveillance in Corpus Christi Project showed higher neighborhood socioeconomic status (defined as census-tract level income, wealth, education, and employment) was associated with better function, better psychosocial health, and fewer depressive symptoms after moderate to severe stroke, and better function in those with minor strokes.[53]

Differences in neighborhood characteristics are due to in part to structural discriminatory practices that created and perpetuate residential segregation, such as redlining, an example of a *policy level* determinant of health. In response to the Great Depression, the US government established the Federal Housing Administration (FHA) in 1934, which underwrote mortgages to incentivize home ownership. They formalized a process to exclude certain neighborhoods from this opportunity based on racial composition, a process that became known as redlining. Redlining led to White individuals purchasing homes with the benefit of this subsidy in particular neighborhoods. Individuals seeking to purchase a home in a redlined neighborhood were denied a mortgage, regardless of their financial stability. This practice limited opportunity for the development and maintenance of quality housing in redlined neighborhoods and set the stage for residential disparities and segregation that persist to this day. Data from the Multiethnic Study of Atherosclerosis (MESA), for example, show that higher neighborhood segregation scores were significantly associated with cardiovascular disease outcomes in Black individuals, and higher segregation scores were associated with lower cardiovascular disease outcomes for White individuals,[52] largely due to differential resources available in predominantly White neighborhoods compared with predominantly Black neighborhoods. The FHA did not discontinue mortgage restrictions based on race until the 1960s, and although redlining is one example of a public policy contributing to disparities in stroke prevalence and outcome, it is not the only one.

These connections between the individual and society also can be multidirectional. For example, scarcity leads to impairment in executive function, which can then directly influence decision making around health-related behaviors, such as substance use, as well as an individual's ability to plan, organize, and navigate a complex health care system.[54] This impairment can increase risk of outcomes like stroke that can result in disability and further exacerbate poverty. Experiencing racial discrimination may impair the function of the prefrontal cortex and alter the salience network, potentially contributing to disparities in mental health and chronic pain.[17] This influence of the social environment on cognitive networks can be seen throughout the lifespan. Brain development is influenced by environmental factors, including exposure to toxins such as pollution, poor nutrition, poverty, and psychosocial stress. This exposure has direct impact on the development of the prefrontal cortex and limbic system, which then leads to differences in impulse control, working memory, and cognitive flexibility.[54] Income volatility during young adulthood has been shown to affect cognition and microstructure integrity of the brain in midlife.[55]

The social ecological model also can be applied to other neurologic conditions. There are racial and ethnic disparities in epilepsy, for example, particularly with regard to treatment.[56] In a 2014 article, Szaflarski[57] discusses the various levels of structural and social determinants as they relate to epilepsy, highlighting the complexity of the relationship between society and the individual. Lower socioeconomic status, for example, has been associated with higher incidence and prevalence of epilepsy; however, epilepsy is also a risk factor for lower socioeconomic status.[57,58] People with epilepsy may experience discrimination or stigma related to epilepsy in addition to other social and personal identities they hold.[59] Institutional, community, and policy-level factors also influence access to care, quality of that care, and cost, all of which can perpetuate or exacerbate existing disparities in epilepsy treatment.[57,60]

This framework also can be used to understand neurologic disparities in other populations. Research suggests a number of neurologic disparities in LGBTQ+ individuals, for example, including higher risk of ischemic stroke in transgender women and sexual minority women[20] and higher risk of migraine in sexual minority men and women.[61,62] The drivers of these disparities can be conceptualized through the social ecologic framework. The absence of federal protection from discrimination in housing, education, and, until June 2020, employment leads to higher rates of poverty in LGBTQ+ individuals,[63] particularly LGBTQ+ people of color.[64] Poverty has been associated with higher migraine prevalence and migraine-related disability.[65] Serious psychological distress and hours of regular sleep accounted for a significant proportion of the disparity in headache between sexual minority and heterosexual adults in a study using data from the 2013 to 2018 National Health Interview Survey.[66] Mental health disparities have been associated with experiences of discrimination and stigma in sexual minority individuals.[67] Sleep outcomes are influenced by multiple levels of the framework, including experiences of discrimination[43] and neighborhood factors.[68]

An understanding of the influence of structural and social determinants of health on neurology necessitates an intersectional lens. In the National Health Interview Survey, Black lesbian and bisexual women reported higher prevalence of stroke compared with Black heterosexual women (adjusted prevalence ratio [aPR] 3.25, 95% CI 1.63–6.49).[69] The difference in stroke prevalence was even greater, however, compared with White heterosexual women (aPR 4.51%, 95% CI 2.16–9.39),[69] suggesting an effect of both sexual orientation and race in this disparity. Although this type of analysis requires larger populations to provide sufficient statistical power, it more accurately reflects our patients' experiences as they navigate the health care system and their daily lives.

SOCIAL DETERMINANTS OF HEALTH IN HOSPITAL MEDICINE

Social determinants of health influence hospitalization and hospital care. This influence may manifest in lack of access to preventive care that leads individuals to present to the hospital at a later stage of illness or may influence risk of readmission. A 2019 study of the effect of SDH on hospitalizations in the Veterans Health Administration found decreased odds of hospitalization associated with higher neighborhood socioeconomic status even after controlling for patient-level characteristics of race and Gagne comorbidity score.[70] Another study using survey data from Veterans Health Administration patients found that respondents with multiple SDH vulnerabilities, defined as loneliness, sleep quality, material needs, depression, social support, patient activation, food insecurity, medication insecurity and recent life stressors, had 50% higher odds of 180-day hospital admission compared with those with minimal SDH vulnerabilities (OR 1.53, 95% CI 1.09–2.14).[71] Individuals with more health-related social needs (defined in domains of employment, family, psychosocial, housing, and socioeconomic status) had higher risk of 30-day, 60-day, and 90-day readmission in a dose-response relationship: for example, 30-day readmission rate for those with 1 domain was 11.9% versus 63.5% for individuals with 5 domains.[72]

Social determinants may also influence the type of diagnoses with which individuals present. In a study using data from the 2006 to 2011 California State Inpatient Database, individuals experiencing homelessness were more likely to be admitted for seizure and traumatic brain injury compared with housed individuals.[73] In this study, homelessness was an independent risk factor for 30-day readmission after neurologic admission, even after adjusting for differential readmission rates inherent in particular neurologic diagnoses.[73]

INTERVENTIONS TO ADDRESS SOCIAL DETERMINANTS OF HEALTH

The framing of neurologic health disparities through the lens of structural and social determinants is gaining traction. This approach has already been recommended broadly by the National Academies of Sciences, Engineering, and Medicine in their 2019 report "Integrating Social Care into the Delivery of Health Care: Moving Upstream to Improve the Nation's Health."[74] Given the complex interaction between structural and social determinants of health with the individual, interventions to promote health equity must be multipronged (**Table 1**). In a Cochrane Review of interventions for secondary stroke prevention, for example, organizational interventions as opposed to educational or behavioral interventions improved blood pressure control, although did not affect other risk factors or incidence of recurrent stroke.[75] These findings suggest interventions that address each level of vulnerability, from the individual to national or international policy, are required to enact sustained change.

Table 1
Selection of suggested interventions to address structural and social determinants of health in neurology

Level of Intervention	Proposed Interventions
Policy	• Incorporate social determinant variables into value-based reimbursement algorithms • Fund research on best practices for collection and validation of social determinants variables in various care settings • Ensure appropriate reimbursement for clinicians and health systems to address social determinants • Address gaps in health care coverage to promote preventive rather than reactive health care
Community	• Create partnerships between community organizations and health care systems to identify the social needs of the local community and connect people to resources • Build coalitions between local organizations to promote collaboration and advocacy
Institutional	• Create a resource list to connect patients to local services depending on need identified • Incorporate social workers/case managers into clinical model to facilitate connection to available resources • Remove identity cues in a clinical environment to reduce triggering stereotype threat • Develop multimodal patient education materials, including written and visual communication, and provide necessary information in multiple languages
Interpersonal	• Focus on interventions and counseling to build resilience and self-efficacy of patients • Provide education to trainees and colleagues on the identification and intervention for social determinants
Individual	• Identify one's own implicit biases that may be affecting care decisions and counseling • Engage in critical self-reflection of one's own skills in identifying and intervening on social determinants of health • Seek ongoing education and training in the manifestations of social determinants in neurology and potential interventions • Advocate for interventions to address social issues on an institutional, community, and/or policy level

One of the first steps necessary to intervene on disparities due to SDH is to identify the SDH driving those disparities. Despite recognizing the importance of these data, however, there remains inconsistency on which variables are important and how to best capture them. There may also be a sense of futility in collecting SDH information if there are not clear procedures or referral processes to connect patients with needed resources. These concerns can be addressed through intentional organizational redesign, including the development of a referral list for the various types of social needs identified, integration of social service navigators or case managers into clinic models, and leveraging technology to automate referrals within the electronic health record once a need has been identified. On a policy level, it is essential that clinicians and health care systems are appropriately compensated for the time and expertise in addressing these issues as a part of health care. It is also important to be mindful around which variables are collected, how they are interpreted, and how they are used so as to not exacerbate current inequities. As Gottlieb and Alderwick[76] wrote in a 2019 article, "[i]f the potential for bias based on social data goes unchecked, the result could be an inequitable de-escalation of care for specific groups of patients." Best practices for the collection and use of SDH variables, therefore, must be guided by research and community engagement.

On a policy level, SDH variables need to be integrated into discussions of health care reimbursement. As health care reimbursement shifts from reimbursement based on number of services rendered to the value of services rendered, incorporating social risk factors into these algorithms is essential to ensure equitable reimbursement and resource allocation. In a study using 2012 to 2016 New York City hospital discharge data, including SDH scores into the model used in the Centers for Medicare and Medicaid Services Hospital Readmissions Reduction Program (HRRP) significantly affected projected penalties for hospitals caring for the highest proportion of patients with high SDH scores. They conclude that ongoing omission of these data from the HRRP model leads to inappropriate attribution of readmission to hospitals themselves and leads to inequitable penalties for hospitals caring for vulnerable patient populations.[77] Policy-level interventions are also important to address ongoing gaps in health care access for specific populations and to ensure appropriate funding for high-quality research into best practices for identifying and intervening on SDH.

At the institutional level, there is increasing focus on the need to train clinicians in structural competency: the idea that education and intervention on health disparities must occur through the lens of the social and economic forces driving disparate access and experiences rather than an individual-based approach. Proposed by Metzl and Hansen, structural competency requires training on 5 intersecting skills: (1) recognizing the structures (economic, physical, sociopolitical) that shape clinical interactions; (2) developing fluency in the interdisciplinary and extraclinical terminology of structures that influence health; (3) reframing "cultural" presentations in structural terms; (4) recognizing and imagining structural interventions; and (5) developing structural humility, that is, recognition of the limits of structural competency and the need for lifelong critical self-reflection and growth.[78] By incorporating this focus into medical training and clinical practice, neurologists can develop the skills necessary to identify the structural and social drivers of disease and connect their patients to necessary resources. This change in focus from the individual to the social also can build empathy and remove stigma, which in and of itself can drive health inequities[79] (Box 1).

A multidisciplinary approach to addressing SDH in clinical care is still important, regardless of how well trained neurologists are in identifying the social drivers of disease. A recent randomized trial of the use of a patient navigator for proactive case

Box 1

Example of reframing a neurologic presentation through a structural lens

Standard case presentation: 34-year-old transgender woman with epilepsy who was brought in after a witnessed seizure. The emergency room consults Neurology stating she is a "frequent flyer" and asking for recommendations on antiepileptic therapy.

Case presentation with a structural lens, patient:

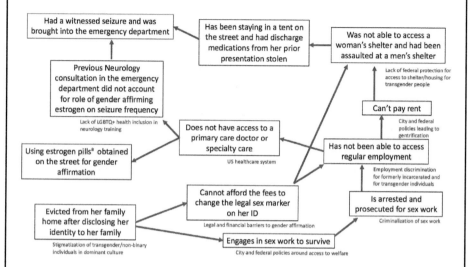

Case presentation with a structural lens, clinician:

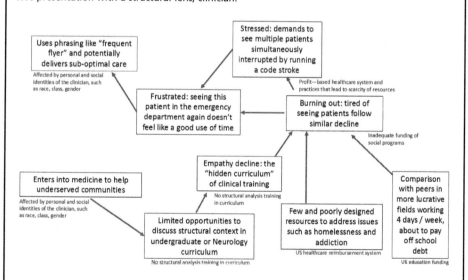

[a]Although there is a paucity of research in transfeminine people, research in cisgender women suggest estrogen has proconvulsant properties.

Adapted from Neff J, Holmes SM, Knight KR, et al. Structural Competency: Curriculum for Medical Students, Residents, and Interprofessional Teams on the Structural Factors That Produce Health Disparities. MedEdPORTAL. 2020;16:10888. Published 2020 Mar 13. doi:10.15766/mep_2374-8265. 10888; with permission

management, advocacy, and service linkage in patients with comorbid substance use disorder, for example, found a significant reduction in 30-day readmission in the patient navigator group (15.5% vs 30.0%, $P < .001$) and increased likelihood of entering community substance use treatment after discharge (50.3% vs 35.3%, $P = .014$).[80] Institutions can also intervene by changing the physical environment through which a patient navigates to celebrate diversity and reduce the risk of stereotype threat being triggered, reducing the extent to which anxiety/physiologic arousal affects communication skills and engagement in the formation of care plans.[33] Institutions can also prioritize the recruitment, retention, and promotion of a diverse workforce to ensure the clinical space reflects the diversity of the local community it serves.[33]

On an interpersonal level, understanding the influence of stress on brain development and cognitive processes can lead to targeted interventions to improve care delivery and patient education. Some suggestions include the following: providing educational materials in multiple modalities, both verbal and written, with easy-to-understand language, dividing longer discussions into shorter segments with ask-teach-ask method, and relating the educational content to the individual's particular needs and perspectives.[54] Health care institutions and community organizations can also create tools and materials to enhance health literacy and patient-centered education using existing infrastructure and leveraging technology to empower an individual patient's self-advocacy.[81]

Finally, on an individual level, it is essential that clinicians engage in lifelong critical self-reflection of their practices and the potential influence of implicit bias on their clinical care. Those motivated to use their privilege as a clinician can also be powerful advocates for change at the institutional, community, and policy levels.

Through a multipronged approach, clinicians, institutions, community organizations, politicians, and patients can work together toward the common goal of equitable health access and outcomes for all individuals.

DISCLOSURE

Dr N. Rosendale receives personal compensation for her role on the Editorial board of *Neurology*.

ACKNOWLEDGMENTS

Dr Rosendale is grateful to Dr Altaf Saadi for her guidance in the organization of this article.

REFERENCES

1. Centers for Disease Control and Prevention. About Social Determinants of Health (SDOH). 2021. Available at: https://www.cdc.gov/socialdeterminants/about.html. Accessed March 30, 2021.

2. World Health Organization. A conceptual framework for action on the social determinants of health: debates, policy & practice, case studies. 2010. Available at: http://apps.who.int/iris/bitstream/10665/44489/1/9789241500852_eng.pdf. Accessed March 26, 2021.

3. McLeroy KR, Bibeau D, Steckler A, et al. An ecological perspective on health promotion programs. Health Education Q 1988;15(4):351–77.

4. Johann Peter Frank (1745-1821) public health by decree. JAMA 1967;202(3): 228–9.

5. Farmer P. Pathologies of power: health, human rights, and the new war on the poor. 1st edition. Berkeley, CA: University of California Press; 2003.

6. Irwin A, Scali E. Action on the social determinants of health: a historical perspective. Glob Public Health 2007;2(3):235–56.

7. Galea S, Tracy M, Hoggatt KJ, et al. Estimated deaths attributable to social factors in the United States. Am J Public Health 2011;101(8):1456–65.

8. Braveman P, Gottlieb L. The social determinants of health: it's time to consider the causes of the causes. Public Health Rep 2014;129(Suppl 2):19–31.

9. Yehia BR, Winegar A, Fogel R, et al. Association of race with mortality among patients hospitalized with coronavirus disease 2019 (COVID-19) at 92 US hospitals. JAMA Netw Open 2020;3(8). https://doi.org/10.1001/jamanetworkopen.2020.18039.

10. Hafeez H, Zeshan M, Tahir MA, et al. Health care disparities among lesbian, gay, bisexual, and transgender youth: a literature review. Cureus 2017;9(4). https://doi.org/10.7759/cureus.1184.

11. Office of Disease Prevention and Health Promotion. Lesbian, gay, bisexual, and transgender health | Healthy People. 2020. Available at: https://www.healthypeople.gov/2020/topics-objectives/topic/lesbian-gay-bisexual-and-transgender-health. Accessed April 24, 2021.

12. Krahn GL, Walker DK, Correa-De-Araujo R. Persons with disabilities as an unrecognized health disparity population. Am J Public Health 2015;105(Suppl 2):S198–206.

13. Crenshaw K. Demarginalizing the intersection of race and sex: a black feminist critique of antidiscrimination doctrine. Feminist Theor Antiracist Polit Univ Chicago Leg Forum 1989;1989(1):139–67.

14. English D, Carter JA, Boone CA, et al. Intersecting structural oppression and black sexual minority men's health. Am J Prev Med 2021. https://doi.org/10.1016/j.amepre.2020.12.022.

15. Guidi J, Lucente M, Sonino N, et al. Allostatic load and its impact on health: a systematic review. Psychother Psychosom 2021;90(1):11–27. https://doi.org/10.1159/000510696.

16. Duru OK, Harawa NT, Kermah D, et al. Allostatic load burden and racial disparities in mortality. J Natl Med Assoc 2012;104(1–2):89–95.

17. Berger M, Sarnyai Z. "More than skin deep": stress neurobiology and mental health consequences of racial discrimination. Stress 2015;18(1):1–10.

18. Riggan KA, Gilbert A, Allyse MA. Acknowledging and addressing allostatic load in pregnancy care. J Racial Ethnic Health Disparities 2021;8(1):69–79.

19. Flentje A, Kober KM, Carrico AW, et al. Minority stress and leukocyte gene expression in sexual minority men living with treated HIV infection. Brain Behav Immun 2018;70:335–45.

20. Rosendale N, Wong JO, Flatt JD, et al. Sexual and gender minority health in neurology: a scoping review. JAMA Neurol 2021. https://doi.org/10.1001/jamaneurol.2020.5536.

21. Hannah G, Sacco Ralph L, Tatjana R, et al. Race and ethnic disparities in stroke incidence in the Northern Manhattan Study. Stroke 2020;51(4):1064–9.

22. Burneo JG, Jette N, Theodore W, et al. Disparities in epilepsy: report of a systematic review by the North American Commission of the International League Against Epilepsy. Epilepsia 2009;50(10):2285–95.

23. Charleston L. Headache disparities in African-Americans in the United States: a narrative review. J Natl Med Assoc 2021;113(2):223–9.

24. Chin AL, Negash S, Hamilton R. Diversity and disparity in dementia: the impact of ethnoracial differences in Alzheimer disease. Alzheimer Dis Assoc Disord 2011; 25(3):187–95.

25. Qadri S, Langefeld CD, Milligan C, et al. Racial differences in intervention rates in individuals with ALS: a case-control study. Neurology 2019;92(17):e1969–74.

26. Robers MV, Soneji D, Amezcua L. Multiple sclerosis treatment in racial and ethnic minorities. Pract Neurol 2020;49–54.

27. Saadi A, Himmelstein DU, Woolhandler S, et al. Racial disparities in neurologic health care access and utilization in the United States. Neurology 2017;88(24): 2268–75.

28. Nolen L, Mejia NI. Inequities in neurology amplified by the COVID-19 pandemic. Nat Rev Neurol Published Online January 2021;7:1–2. https://doi.org/10.1038/s41582-020-00452-x.

29. Morgenstern LB, Smith MA, Lisabeth LD, et al. Excess stroke in Mexican Americans compared with non-Hispanic whites: The Brain Attack Surveillance in Corpus Christi Project. Am J Epidemiol 2004;160(4):376–83.

30. Cruz-Flores S, Rabinstein A, Biller J, et al. Racial-ethnic disparities in stroke care: the American experience. Stroke. 2011. Available at: https://www.ahajournals.org/doi/abs/10.1161/str.0b013e3182213e24. Accessed September 6, 2018.

31. U.S. Department of Health and Human Services Office of Minority Health. Stroke and Asian Americans - The Office of Minority Health. 2021. Available at: https://minorityhealth.hhs.gov/omh/browse.aspx?lvl=4&lvlid=58. Accessed April 25, 2021.

32. Song S, Liang L, Fonarow GC, et al. Comparison of clinical care and in-hospital outcomes of Asian American and white patients with acute ischemic stroke. JAMA Neurol 2019. https://doi.org/10.1001/jamaneurol.2018.4410.

33. Burgess DJ, Warren J, Phelan S, et al. Stereotype threat and health disparities: what medical educators and future physicians need to know. J Gen Intern Med 2010;25(Suppl 2):169–77.

34. Gale MM, Pieterse AL, Lee DL, et al. A meta-analysis of the relationship between internalized racial oppression and health-related outcomes. Couns Psychol 2020; 48(4):498–525. https://doi.org/10.1177/0011000020904454.

35. Dorr N, Brosschot JF, Sollers JJ, et al. Damned if you do, damned if you don't: The differential effect of expression and inhibition of anger on cardiovascular recovery in Black and White males. Int J Psychophysiol 2007;66(2):125–34.

36. Johnston SC, Fung Lawrence H, Gillum Leslie A, et al. Utilization of intravenous tissue-type plasminogen activator for ischemic stroke at academic medical centers. Stroke 2001;32(5):1061–8.

37. Mendelson SJ, Aggarwal NT, Richards C, et al. Racial disparities in refusal of stroke thrombolysis in Chicago. Neurology 2018;90(5):e359–64.

38. Cooper LA, Roter DL, Johnson RL, et al. Patient-centered communication, ratings of care, and concordance of patient and physician race. Ann Intern Med 2003; 139(11):907–15.

39. Silver B, Miller D, Jankowski M, et al. Urine toxicology screening in an urban stroke and TIA population. Neurology 2013;80(18):1702–9.

40. Brondolo E, Love EE, Pencille M, et al. Racism and hypertension: a review of the empirical evidence and implications for clinical practice. Am J Hypertens 2011; 24(5):518–29.

41. Parker LJ, Hunte H, Ohmit A, et al. The effects of discrimination are associated with cigarette smoking among black males. Subst Use Misuse 2017;52(3): 383–91.

42. Bacon KL, Stuver SO, Cozier YC, et al. Perceived racism and incident diabetes in the Black Women's Health Study. Diabetologia 2017;60(11):2221–5.

43. Slopen N, Lewis TT, Williams DR. Discrimination and sleep: a systematic review. Sleep Med 2016;18:88–95.

44. Karve SJ, Balkrishnan R, Mohammad YM, et al. Racial/ethnic disparities in emergency department waiting time for stroke patients in the United States. J Stroke Cerebrovasc Dis 2011;20(1):30–40.

45. Lacy Clifton R, Dong-Churl S, Maureen B, et al. Delay in presentation and evaluation for acute stroke. Stroke 2001;32(1):63–9.

46. Allen L, Cummings J. Emergency department use among Hispanic adults: the role of acculturation. Med Care 2016;54(5):449–56.

47. Rodriguez RM, Torres JR, Sun J, et al. Declared impact of the US president's statements and campaign statements on Latino populations' perceptions of safety and emergency care access. PLoS One 2019;14(10). https://doi.org/10.1371/journal.pone.0222837.

48. Ellis C, Egede LE. Ethnic disparities in stroke recognition in individuals with prior stroke. Public Health Rep 2008;123(4):514–22.

49. Ader J, Wu J, Fonarow GC, et al. Hospital distance, socioeconomic status, and timely treatment of ischemic stroke. Neurology 2019;93(8):e747–57.

50. Kulick ER, Wellenius GA, Boehme AK, et al. Residential proximity to major roadways and risk of incident ischemic stroke in the Northern Manhattan Study. Stroke 2018;49(4):835–41.

51. Congdon P. Obesity and urban environments. Int J Environ Res Public Health 2019;16(3). https://doi.org/10.3390/ijerph16030464.

52. Karen XY, Graham G. Where we live: the impact of neighborhoods and community factors on cardiovascular health in the United States. Clin Cardiol 2019;42(1):184–9.

53. Stulberg EL, Twardzik E, Kim S, et al. Association of neighborhood socioeconomic status with outcomes in patients surviving stroke. Neurology 2021. https://doi.org/10.1212/WNL.0000000000011988.

54. Babcock ED. Using brain science to design new pathways out of poverty. Boston, MA: Crittenton Women's Union; 2014. p. 1–37. Available at: http://s3.amazonaws.com/empath-website/pdf/Research-UsingBrainScienceDesignPathwaysPoverty-0114.pdf.

55. Grasset L, Glymour MM, Elfassy T, et al. Relation between 20-year income volatility and brain health in midlife: The CARDIA study. Neurology 2019;93(20):e1890–9.

56. Szaflarski M, Szaflarski JP, Privitera MD, et al. Racial/ethnic disparities in the treatment of epilepsy: What do we know? What do we need to know? Epilepsy Behav 2006;9(2):243–64.

57. Szaflarski M. Social determinants of health in epilepsy. Epilepsy Behav 2014;41:283–9.

58. Camfield C, Camfield P, Smith B. Poor versus rich children with epilepsy have the same clinical course and remission rates but a less favorable social outcome: a population-based study with 25 years of follow-up. Epilepsia 2016;57(11):1826–33.

59. Stangl AL, Earnshaw VA, Logie CH, et al. The Health Stigma and Discrimination Framework: a global, crosscutting framework to inform research, intervention development, and policy on health-related stigmas. BMC Med 2019;17. https://doi.org/10.1186/s12916-019-1271-3.

60. Nathan CL, Gutierrez C. FACETS of health disparities in epilepsy surgery and gaps that need to be addressed. Neurol Clin Pract 2018;8(4):340–5.

61. Nagata JM, Ganson KT, Tabler J, et al. Disparities across sexual orientation in migraine among US adults. JAMA Neurol 2020. https://doi.org/10.1001/jamaneurol.2020.3406.

62. Hammond NG, Stinchcombe A. Health behaviors and social determinants of migraine in a Canadian population-based sample of adults aged 45-85 years: findings from the CLSA. Headache 2019;59(9):1547–64.

63. Fredriksen Goldsen K, Kim H-J, Jung H, et al. The evolution of aging with pride—National Health, Aging, and Sexuality/Gender Study: illuminating the iridescent life course of LGBTQ adults aged 80 years and older in the United States. Int J Aging Hum Dev 2019;88(4):380–404.

64. James SE, Herman JL, Rankin S, et al. The Report of the 2015 U.S. Transgender Survey. The National Center for Transgender Equality. 2016. Available at: http://www.ustranssurvey.org/. Accessed November 19, 2019.

65. Befus DR, Irby MB, Coeytaux RR, et al. A critical exploration of migraine as a health disparity: the imperative of an equity-oriented, intersectional approach. Curr Pain Headache Rep 2018;22(12):79.

66. Heslin KC. Explaining disparities in severe headache and migraine among sexual minority adults in the United States, 2013–2018. J Nerv Ment Dis 2020;208(11):876–83.

67. Meyer IH. Prejudice, social stress, and mental health in lesbian, gay, and bisexual populations: conceptual issues and research evidence. Psychol Bull 2003;129(5):674–97.

68. Hunter JC, Hayden KM. The association of sleep with neighborhood physical and social environment. Public Health 2018;162:126–34.

69. Trinh M-H, Agénor M, Austin SB, et al. Health and healthcare disparities among U.S. women and men at the intersection of sexual orientation and race/ethnicity: a nationally representative cross-sectional study. BMC Public Health 2017;17(1). https://doi.org/10.1186/s12889-017-4937-9.

70. Hatef E, Searle KM, Predmore Z, et al. The impact of social determinants of health on hospitalization in the Veterans Health Administration. Am J Prev Med 2019;56(6):811–8.

71. Blalock DV, Maciejewski ML, Zulman DM, et al. Subgroups of high-risk Veterans Affairs patients based on social determinants of health predict risk of future hospitalization. Med Care 2021;59(5):410–7.

72. Bensken WP, Alberti PM, Koroukian SM. Health-related social needs and increased readmission rates: findings from the nationwide readmissions database. J Gen Intern Med 2021. https://doi.org/10.1007/s11606-021-06646-3.

73. Rosendale N, Guterman EL, Betjemann JP, et al. Hospital admission and readmission among homeless patients with neurologic disease: Retraction and replacement. Neurology 2019;92(24):e2822–31.

74. National Academies of Sciences, Engineering, and Medicine; Health and Medicine Division; Board on Health Care Services; Committee on Integrating Social Needs Care into the Delivery of Health Care to Improve the Nation's Health. Integrating social care into the delivery of health care: moving upstream to improve the nation's health. Washington, DC: National Academies Press (US); 2019. Available at: http://www.ncbi.nlm.nih.gov/books/NBK552597/. Accessed March 30, 2021.

75. Bridgwood B, Lager KE, Mistri AK, et al. Interventions for improving modifiable risk factor control in the secondary prevention of stroke. Cochrane Database Syst Rev 2018;2018(5). https://doi.org/10.1002/14651858.CD009103.pub3.

76. Gottlieb LM, Alderwick H. Integrating social and medical care: could it worsen health and increase inequity? Ann Fam Med 2019;17(1):77–81.

77. Baker MC, Alberti PM, Tsao T-Y, et al. Social determinants matter for hospital readmission policy: insights from New York City. Health Aff 2021;40(4):645–54.

78. Metzl JM, Hansen H. Structural competency: Theorizing a new medical engagement with stigma and inequality. Soc Science & Med 2014;103(2):126–33.

79. Hatzenbuehler ML, Phelan JC, Link BG. Stigma as a fundamental cause of population health inequalities. Am J Public Health 2013;103(5):813–21.

80. Gryczynski J, Nordeck CD, Welsh C, et al. Preventing hospital readmission for patients with comorbid substance use disorder. Ann Intern Med 2021. https://doi.org/10.7326/M20-5475.

81. Marulanda-Londoño ET, Bell MW, Hope OA, et al. Reducing neurodisparity: recommendations of the 2017 AAN Diversity Leadership Program. Neurology 2019; 92(6):274–80.

Moving?

Make sure your subscription moves with you!

To notify us of your new address, find your **Clinics Account Number** (located on your mailing label above your name), and contact customer service at:

Email: journalscustomerservice-usa@elsevier.com

800-654-2452 (subscribers in the U.S. & Canada)
314-447-8871 (subscribers outside of the U.S. & Canada)

Fax number: 314-447-8029

Elsevier Health Sciences Division
Subscription Customer Service
3251 Riverport Lane
Maryland Heights, MO 63043

*To ensure uninterrupted delivery of your subscription, please notify us at least 4 weeks in advance of move.

Printed and bound by CPI Group (UK) Ltd, Croydon, CR0 4YY

03/10/2024

01040400-0003